The Philosophy of Nurse Education

Edited by

John S. Drummond

and

Paul Standish

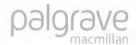
palgrave
macmillan

First published 2007 by
PALGRAVE MACMILLAN
Houndmills, Basingstoke, Hampshire RG21 6XS and
175 Fifth Avenue, New York, N.Y. 10010
Companies and representatives throughout the world

PALGRAVE MACMILLAN is the global academic imprint of the Palgrave
Macmillan division of St. Martin's Press, LLC and of Palgrave Macmillan Ltd.
Macmillan® is a registered trademark in the United States, United Kingdom
and other countries. Palgrave is a registered trademark in the European
Union and other countries.

ISBN-13: 978–1–4039–4833–5 paperback
ISBN-10: 1–4039–4833–X paperback

This book is printed on paper suitable for recycling and made from fully
managed and sustained forest sources. Logging, pulping and manufacturing
processes are expected to conform to the environmental regulations of the
country of origin.

A catalogue record for this book is available from the British Library.

A catalog record for this book is available from the Library of Congress.

10   9   8   7   6   5   4   3   2   1
16   15   14   13   12   11   10   09   08   07

Printed in China

Contents

List of figures

Foreword

Debates concerning the education of nurses have raged for decades. In particular, the change in the nature of nursing education in the UK – outlined by the *Project 2000* initiative (UKCC, 1986) – proved especially controversial.

Following countries such as Canada, the USA, Australia and New Zealand, the implementation of changes prompted by Project 2000 highlighted the importance of a university education for nurses, as nursing moved towards becoming an all-graduate profession. In the eyes of some commentators, and indeed some nurses, this was a negative step, as it changed the perspective of student nurses in a deep way. Due to their now supernumerary status, they were no longer expected simply to perform nursing work alongside their colleagues, qualified and unqualified alike, but also to *observe* practice, and indeed to adopt a more studious gaze on the nursing domain generally.

With rare exceptions, the suggestion that nurses consider undertaking academic research, publishing their own work and completing higher degrees had largely been unheard of. 'What would be the point?' was the standard response – certainly in the UK – to the idea that they should do all of this, or even be required to embark upon a degree at all. The view seemed to be that nursing was a practical business, best learned in the workplace, the ward, the clinic or the community. Time spent in the classroom, in libraries or in doing research of all things was time wasted; it was thought to have little to do with the *real* work of nursing. (It should be noted of course that the concern generated by the perceived emphasis on academic study at the expense of practice in Project 2000 led to the subsequent *Fitness for Practice* initiative that sought to bring basic competence in clinical skills into the heart of programmes of preparation (UKCC, 1999).)

Perhaps unfortunately, during that time of radical change, while there was much conflict and debate around what it was that nursing students should be taught and where they should learn, such debate, although ideologically and often politically motivated, tended to be largely instrumental in nature. There was little discussion about the fundamentals of nurse *education*. By 'fundamentals' I mean discussion of very basic philosophical questions: What is the best way to educate nurses and other health care professionals? Importantly, for what range of purposes should they be educated? What elements should the curriculum espouse and contain?

These fundamental issues raise questions about the goals of health care, because the education of nurses should help them to ensure that such goals are met, or at least are more likely to be met due to their involvement. A good education would make them good health care professionals. But what is a good health care professional? Is it one who meets managerial targets for patient 'throughput', or use of resources? Is it one who 'gets the job done', but whom patients see as lacking sensitivity? What matters most in the nurse–patient/client relationship? And what exactly is competent practice and expertise? Is it purely evidence-based?

To these questions can be added others concerning the place of university-based study for nurses. This of course brings in issues regarding the changing nature of the university, its ethos and its purpose, its seemingly endless search for certainty and quality assurance and the impact this has on educators. And what of the teachers themselves? Should the teachers of nurses be moral role models or is their character and moral integrity not of particular concern? And what of nurses when they engage in the teaching of patients and clients? Should they be guided entirely by the patients' values, or try to encourage the patient to change their value system?

These questions all prompt philosophical enquiry into the education of nurses and other health care professionals. Surprisingly, this is a largely neglected area of research within the philosophy of education, and also within the philosophy of nursing, so the present book is timely indeed. It brings together an impressive and eminent group of scholars from a range of disciplines; and, hopefully, it will prompt further work in this important area. Such work would help ensure that any future changes to the education of nurses will be prompted by well-considered arguments and conclusions, as opposed to the dictates of fashion.

STEVEN D. EDWARDS
University of Wales, Swansea

■ References

United Kingdom Central Council for Nursing, Midwifery and Health Visiting, *A New Preparation for Practice* (London: UKCC, 1986).
United Kingdom Central Council for Nursing, Midwifery and Health Visiting, *Fitness for Practice* (London: UKCC, 1999).

Acknowledgements

The editors and publisher gratefully acknowledge permission to use adapted reprints from the following:

A different version of the chapter 'Practice and its informing knowledge: An Aristotelian understanding' by Joseph Dunne was first published under the title 'An intricate fabric: Understanding the rationality of practice' in *Pedagogy, Culture and Society*, 13, 3, pp. 367–390, Triangle (2005). By permission of the Taylor & Francis Group.

A different version of the chapter 'Care of the self in a knowledge economy: Higher education, vocation and the ethics of Michel Foucault' by John S. Drummond was first published under the same title in *Educational Philosophy and Theory*, 35, 1, pp. 55–68, Blackwell Publishing (2003). By permission of Blackwell Publishing.

Notes on contributors

Peter Allmark is Principal Lecturer in the Faculty of Health and Wellbeing at Sheffield Hallam University. He has researched and published extensively in the field of health care ethics. His first degree was in philosophy; his doctorate used an Aristotelian approach to examine informed consent. He has worked on two large funded projects examining consent issues that combined philosophical and empirical questions. He has recently turned his attention to health promotion and health education and is developing a philosophical and empirical project with Angela Tod (q.v.) looking at the lay epidemiology of teenage smokers in Rotherham. He and Angela Tod are also developing a project examining the ethics of using in-depth interviews.

Tina Besley is Professor of Counseling in the Educational Psychology and Counseling Department, California State University, San Bernardino, USA. She was formerly Visiting Research Associate in Educational Policy Studies, University of Illinois, Urbana-Champaign, USA, and spent five years as Research Fellow and Lecturer in the Department of Educational Studies at the University of Glasgow, Scotland, UK. Her research interests include youth issues, in particular notions of self and identity and contemporary problems; educational policy; educational philosophy; and the work of Michel Foucault and poststructuralism. Her book *Counseling Youth: Foucault, Power, and the Ethics of Subjectivity* (2002) is now in a paperback edition (2006). With Michael A. Peters, she has written *Building Knowledge Cultures: Education and Development in the Age of Knowledge Capitalism* (2006) and is co-editor of *Why Foucault? New Directions in Educational Research* (forthcoming).

John S. Drummond is Senior Lecturer at the School of Nursing and Midwifery of the University of Dundee, UK. His teaching involves mainly postgraduate courses and modules along with the supervison of PhD students. His research interests lie in philosophy, the humanities, and social theory as applied to nursing and health care, including practice, policy, research and education. His publications include articles on Nietzsche, Lyotard, Foucault and Deleuze. He is a co-founder and current treasurer of the International Philosophy of Nursing Society (IPONS).

Joseph Dunne is Senior Lecturer in the Faculty of Education and Head of Human Development at St. Patrick's College, Dublin City University, Republic of Ireland. He is author of *Back to the Rough Ground: Practical*

Judgement and the Lure of Technique (1997), and co-editor of *Questioning Ireland: Debates in Political Philosophy and Public Policy* (2000), *Childhood and Its Discontents: The First Seamus Heaney Lectures* (2002) and *Education and Practice: Upholding the Integrity of Teaching and Learning* (2004). His *Persons in Practice: Essays in Education and Public Philosophy* is forthcoming in Spring 2008.

Keith Hammond is Lecturer in Philosophy in the Department of Adult and Continuing Education, Faculty of Education, University of Glasgow, UK, where he teaches and supervises Masters students. His research interests, along with his publications, have a focus on Gadamer and hermeneutics, modernity, and the European concept of *Bildung*. He has studied and researched in both Europe and the USA. He has also worked on various international projects that have included trips to Palestine and Sarajevo.

Gerard Lum teaches in the Department of Education and Professional Studies at King's College London and is Senior Lecturer in Philosophy at the University of Northampton. Trained originally as an electrical engineer, Dr Lum has extensive experience of vocational curriculum design. For a number of years his role was one of advising senior industrialists and trade union leaders on the educational and legal issues relating to employee competence. His research interests are centred on the nature of professional knowledge and problems in epistemology and philosophy of education.

Michael Luntley is Professor of Philosophy and Head of Department at the University of Warwick. His main teaching revolves around issues in epistemology and metaphysics, including the philosophy of Wittgenstein. His research interests focus on Wittgenstein, philosophy of mind and philosophy of education. He has published extensively in these fields. Recent books include *Reason, Truth and Self* (1995), *Contemporary Philosophy of Thought* (1999), and *Wittgenstein: Meaning and Judgement* (2003). He has also published numerous papers on issues related to the philosophy of education.

John Paley is Senior Lecturer in the Department of Nursing and Midwifery at the University of Stirling, UK. After obtaining a degree in philosophy, he pursued a career as a social researcher. He has also worked in publishing, specialising in open learning materials. In his current post, his teaching focuses on postgraduate programmes, including the Doctor of Nursing, along with the supervision of MPhil and PhD students. His research interests include clinical cognition, evidence in nursing, complexity, narrative, qualitative methodology and nursing ethics. He has published extensively in these areas. In real life, however, he plays bass guitar in an old codgers' rock band.

Michael A. Peters is Professor of Education in the Department of Educational Policy Studies at the University of Illinois at Urbana-Champaign, USA, and the University of Glasgow, UK, where he teaches and runs seminars for Masters and PhD students. His research and teaching interests centre on educational philosophy and theory, educational policy, and higher education. He is the author of some thirty books and edited collections, including most recently, *Building Knowledge Cultures: Education and Development in the Age of Knowledge Capitalism Education* (with A.C. Tina Besley) (2006); *Edutopias: Utopian Thinking in Education* (2006); *Postfoundationalist Themes in the Philosophy of Education: Festschrift for James D. Marshall* (with Paul Smeyers) (2006); *Deconstructing Derrida: Tasks for the New Humanities* (with Peter Trifonas) (2005); and *Globalization and the State in the Age of Terrorism* (2005). He is the editor of the journal of *Educational Philosophy and Theory*.

Gary Rolfe is Professor of Nursing at the University of Wales Swansea, UK, where he currently leads and teaches on the Doctorate of Nursing Science. He graduated from the University of Surrey with a degree in philosophy in 1977. He then trained as a mental health nurse before moving into nurse education in the late 1980s. He became interested in clinical supervision and reflective practice, and has taught these subjects to students at all levels for nearly 20 years. He has published extensively on reflection and evidence-based practice, and has more recently published two books on postmodernism and deconstruction: *Research, Truth and Authority: The Postmodern Turn* (ed.) (2000) and *Deconstructing Evidence-based Practice* (with Dawn Freshwater) (2004).

Rick Sawatzky is Assistant Professor at the Nursing Department of Trinity Western University, Canada, and is completing his PhD at the University of British Columbia School of Nursing. His scholarship, which is supported by the Canadian Institutes of Health Research and the Michael Smith Foundation for Health Research, focuses on philosophical and methodological issues in the measurement of health, quality of life and spirituality, and in examining the relationships between these concepts.

P. Anne Scott was appointed Deputy President of Dublin City University, Republic of Ireland, in February 2006. Prior to her present post, she was Professor of Nursing and Head of the Nursing School at Dublin City University. She continues to teach health care ethics, and supervise postgraduate research students in health care ethics, philosophy and ethics of health care, and also in the ethical dimensions of clinical judgement and decision making. Her research interests remain in these areas. She was recently appointed as a foundation member of the Irish Council for Bioethics by the Royal Irish Academy for her significant contribution to research in health care ethics, in which she has published extensively.

Paul Standish is Professor of Philosophy of Education at the Institute of Education, University of London UK. His teaching combines analytical and Continental philosophical approaches in the study of questions concerning the nature of teaching and learning, citizenship and democracy, technology, and higher education. His recent books, in various collaborations with Nigel Blake, Paul Smeyers and Richard Smith, include *Thinking Again: Education after Postmodernism* (1998), *Education in an Age of Nihilism* (2000), *The Blackwell Guide to Philosophy of Education* (2003) and *The Therapy of Education* (2006). He is Editor of the *Journal of Philosophy of Education*.

Sally Thorne is Professor and Director of the School of Nursing, University of British Columbia, Vancouver, Canada. Along with her numerous publications, she maintains an active programme of research in the field of chronic illness and cancer experience, especially as these experiences intersect with the ideological and organizational structures underpinning our evolving health service delivery systems. Privileged with the opportunity of engaging with a generation of graduate students on questions pertaining to the philosophy of nursing science and the nature of clinical evidence, she has also developed a programme of scholarship in the area of theoretical and philosophical nursing applications.

Angela Tod is Principal Research Fellow in the School of Health and Social Care Research, Sheffield Hallam University. She developed her research career following years of experience in cardiology nursing and practice development. Her area of expertise is in qualitative research. She has been involved in a range of qualitative and mixed method health services research projects. Recent areas of activity include access to health care, symptom reporting behaviour, health inequalities and social inclusion, and recovery from illness. Her recent teaching experience has focused on evidence-based practice and research.

Introduction: Philosophical enquiry into education

John S. Drummond and Paul Standish

This is one of the first books to address philosophical questions regarding the education of nurses. Over the past decade or so, philosophical issues in health care have become more evident in the academic and professional literature, particularly in the fields of ethics, philosophy of medicine and philosophy of nursing.[1] That aside, little of substance has been written on philosophical questions as these relate to nurse *education*.[2] What has been written in the field of nurse education pertains for the most part to empirical research, to learning, teaching and assessment methods, or to the sociology and psychology of education. Less attention has been given to the philosophical questions that a careful scrutiny of these practices inevitably raises. Education and preparation for professional practice are inextricably linked, and the salience of this in health care education is something that needs particularly to be taken into account. It is in the light of this that this book draws together a range of contributions that indicate how philosophical enquiry into education can contribute to educational thought and practice for nursing.

A particular feature of this book is that the contributors come from a range of academic and professional backgrounds, embracing philosophy, education and health care. Some are philosophers with an interest in education, and some are philosophers of education with an interest in nursing and health care, while others are nurse educators with a serious interest in philosophy. Many of the chapters in the book refer to nursing in particular because nursing is the largest health care profession, but the significance of the arguments cuts across the different professional sectors in multiple ways. What needs to be noticed in addition is that many of the questions that are typically raised through philosophical enquiry into education in more general terms speak powerfully to those concerned with professional education and practice across the range of nursing and health care.

In recent years, nursing has increasingly moved into the higher education sector, and it has become an almost entirely graduate profession. This, however, has not always been without controversy. For example, in the UK more than a few commentators have taken the view that nursing should settle for a predominantly technical training with no need to embrace the

1

virtues of a higher education, even to the extent that professional preparation at higher education level has been seen to attenuate or interfere with
basic clinical proficiency. As David Moore reported, in the late 1990s such a
view was brought to the attention of government ministers in the UK parlia-
ment (Moore, 2005). Views of this kind resonate with the increasing technicism of health care delivery: the technical advances that have been made
are certainly not to be denied, but 'technicism' implies the inappropriate
extension of technical ways of thinking to other aspects of practice, one
manifestation of which is the pressure to embrace a purely skills-orientated
culture. Added to this are two further factors. The first concerns the question of what it can mean to care for vulnerable people in increasingly
pressured health care environments where economic constraints drive the
demand for increased efficiency with limited resources, and where 'getting
it right' calls for an evidence-base to practice. The second involves the
recent growth in the discourse of multi-professional education and collaborative practice, which brings to the fore issues of not only commonality
and difference in professional identities but also the reconciling of forms of
knowledge and research that, while certainly not mutually exclusive, often
appear disparate. Other factors that impact on the education of nurses
include the consumerist movement in health care, permanent political
and media scrutiny and an increasingly litigious social context. A related
issue is evidenced by the dramatic and at times overwhelming increase in
information concerning health education and improvement: the incitement to adopt a healthy lifestyle has become inextricably tangled with an
idea of the good life in a political economy generated by the health care
industry. But perhaps most significant of all is the not uncommonly held
view that, in spite of quite remarkable scientific and technological advances
in certain forms of health care investigation and intervention, the ethos
of care itself, as a human undertaking, has somehow declined. Similar
trends are recognizable not only in practice but also within the academy
itself with its increasingly technicist infrastructure and its large numbers of
students. How can an ethos of care and *educere* be sustained and promoted
under such circumstances, where the Latin expression refers not only to
the drawing out of certain values, talent or latent potential, but also to the
care to be taken in such educative engagements?[3]

   Against such a background, this book examines the nature and potential
implications of these trends for the education of nurses. It does this from
a variety of philosophical perspectives, both analytical and post-analytical.
Although the issues expressed and explored have a contemporary context
to them, they are also in a sense timeless in that they keep returning in
different ways. Philosophical enquiry into education can make a contribution that, without seeking to deny the value and importance of more
instrumental texts on learning and teaching, goes beyond their range.
Indeed this book seeks to provide an enhancement of ideas of learning and
teaching through its elaboration of such central concepts as professional

care, practice, competence and responsibility, along with the virtues and development of the person that these require. In this respect the practical realities of what it means to seek to educate for health care practice lie very much at the heart of this collection. Philosophical ideas and their relevance to education are explained and explored, but we have sought to avoid unnecessary jargon or highly abstract arguments. This is not to say that the chapters ahead do not present certain challenges. They seek to remind us that, as educators, we need to think on the outside of what we do as well as on the inside of what we think we are doing. Such a reflexive invitation highlights the fact that nurse education, in all its polyvalence and diversity, incorporates many, often conflicting elements worthy of philosophical attention. This in turn alerts us to the fact that education *per se* lies at the very heart of the human condition. We do not pretend to have covered every aspect of education that philosophical enquiry might usefully attend to with regard to the professional field of nursing and health care. We have, however, sought to include a variety of perspectives and views on different issues. Health care educators seek to prepare their students to care for people in what are not only intimate and important ways, but also ways that often involve their own embodiment and personhood. This consideration is central to the concerns of this book.

Later in this introduction we shall offer an overview of the variety and intent of the chapters that comprise this book. But first, and to situate the book in its philosophical context, let us say something about the disciplinary approach that orientates the book. What is the relationship between theory and practice, and how in particular does this cast light on the ethics of the education of nurses and health care professionals? And in more general terms, what are the characteristics of philosophical enquiry into education, and how do these relate to the specific challenges of the professional field in question?

■ The place of philosophy in the study of professional education

The modern institutional development of education as an academic field of study has been inextricably bound up with the professional preparation of teachers. In consequence, it has, more than most subjects of study, been affected by changes in government policy. In a way that parallels the field of health care but that is perhaps more dramatic, a dominant factor in this development over the past two decades has been its increasing technicism: the aims of education are clear, and what must be sought is the most efficient means to their realization. A number of factors testify to this. For example, David Reynolds, the British Government Advisor on Numeracy during the 1990s, worked closely with Sam Stringfield in the US to press, in somewhat colourful terms, for an avowedly more technical approach to education. At a time of increasingly significant international comparisons, the achievements of teachers in Taiwan – teachers who were allegedly 'proud to be applied technologists, not philosophers' (Reynolds, 1997, p. 21) – were held up as something to emulate. Moreover, since a research base had been developed that showed how schools could avoid failure, the price for not implementing this was dire: 'The more recent estimates of the cost of avoidable school failure within the United States (and I know these beg serious questions)', Reynolds explained, 'estimate that cost as the equivalent of a plane crash every week, yet historically little has been done to prevent school failure by comparison with that done to prevent air traffic control failure' (Reynolds, 1997, p. 106). It was a peculiarly British parochialism, he claimed, a hostility to grubby empiricism, that gave 'more status to the pure than the applied, to the useless more than the useful and to the educational philosopher more than the educational engineer, that dirty handed and overall clothed school effectiveness researcher' (Reynolds, 1997, p. 99). Whether or not this was a British malaise, Reynolds' confidence was paralleled, in more prosaic terms, by policy statements on the broader stage of the European Union, where the blithe assertion was made that questions concerning the aims of education had now been finally settled. In the United States more recently, funding for research in education has increasingly reflected a more or less ideological commitment to a particular kind of quantitative research, the randomized controlled trial. It is no surprise then, though perhaps somewhat ironic in the present context, that health care research, in which the randomized controlled trial has a pre-eminent role, has sometimes been held up as the model for education (see, e.g., Hargreaves, 1996; Simons, 2006).

In the face of these challenges, educational research and social science more generally have not always served themselves well, especially where they have turned inwards in a sometimes narcissistic self-examination. The so-called paradigm wars of the 1980s and 1990s saw quantitative and qualitative researchers attacking one another, each side becoming preoccupied with a kind of ideological entrenchment of its position, and with a progressive inflation of claims about the rightful place of values. While such disputes have now to some extent faded from the scene, there has remained a tendency towards methodological posturing. Courses in research methods, which have proliferated in recent years, have not always been exempt from this. What is so often striking about such courses is their *empiricism*: it is not just that empirical research is taken to be the standard form of enquiry into education; it is that the gathering of empirical evidence is assumed to be the only way that research can be undertaken – this is the burden of the suffix in 'empiricism'. There is quantitative research, and there is qualitative research, and it is between these that the disputes will be played out. These, it is assumed, are the limits to the possibilities of enquiry in the field of social practice. This has the effect of rendering eccentric not only philosophical enquiry into education but also historical work, policy analysis and other forms of discursive critique. A brief examination of the range of work published in the major journals, however, will reveal the extent to which that work is *not* empirical: many articles simply do not present the results of field research enquiry but rather address an issue and argue for a particular point of view – sometimes a methodological issue and a methodological point of view, sometimes and perhaps more often matters of substantive concern. Even where the substance of a paper *is* the reporting of empirical findings, the interest will often lie in the broader examination of these that passes under the name of 'discussion' or 'conclusion'. Inevitably in such research it is questions of value that are addressed, and regretfully it is often the case that these are broached without the disciplinary background that would render their examination more robust. If we are concerned with rigour in these matters, philosophical enquiry is unavoidable. We do not doubt the value of empirical research in education, but we firmly reject empiricism of this kind.

There is a nest of problems that attend this empiricist orientation – to do with the relation between theory and practice, between facts and values, between the pure and the applied and between science and other forms of enquiry – and these need further attention. One thing that can be said at the start is that all research begins with values. This is true of qualitative and quantitative educational research, and it applies across the range of scientific research, even where this is understood in positivist terms. It is true without exception. This is so because all research begins with something that matters. Why else would it be undertaken in the first place? The crux of the matter is this: any practice depends upon a certain conception of the good, but the determination or critical assessment of that good requires the direct consideration of values. This is simply not something that can be undertaken through empirical study.

Ethics, one of the central elements in philosophy, is enquiry into the nature of value, and hence it is relevant to all research at its starting point. In empirical research it concerns the values at the beginning of enquiry (the topic, the questions asked, what is to count as data . . .), as well as those inherent in any discussion of results. In educational policy and practice also values are there at the start. Indeed, without values the idea of a practice makes no sense at all. Two initial points emerge from this. In the first place, values are definitely not just something that is 'added', and attempts to do so, however well-intentioned, have often served to support the positivist ways of thinking that they were intended to ameliorate. In the second, the concerns of courses in research ethics, typically informed by codes of practice and increasingly mindful of the law, are normally confined to methodological matters – to do with consent, confidentiality and the like. All this is important, of course, and yet an exclusive emphasis on such matters has a reductive effect: for researchers in education, as in other fields, this is what ethics has come to mean. Concentrating on the middle, empirical phase of the work, it is less than half the story. It deflects attention from the values that condition enquiry, surreptitiously implying that they are unproblematic. Gruff practicality takes over, as we saw: what is really needed is to show what works – what evidence best supports policy and grounds practice, what the best means to a given end.

A further point, more particularly related to professional health care education, should also be noted. This concerns the way that ethics is often understood in terms of headline issues, as arising in the context of major moral dilemmas rather than as being part of the fabric of everyday experience. Medical ethics as a field of study developed particularly in relation to such life-and-death dilemmas. There is no questioning the importance of these, especially with advances in technology, but this emphasis has tended to obscure rather than to reveal the pervasive ethical questions that attend health care practice. Now it may be that the remarkable technical achievements in medicine, and the *relative* lack of disagreement about what constitutes successful treatment, make this understandable. It is our view that in nursing and across the field of health care, these broader matters are less easily ignored. For the same reason it is less defensible within such practices for the professional to retreat to the role of technical expert.

The foregrounding of technical expertise may have a further pernicious effect, in respect of the ways that the relation between theory and practice are understood. How do theory and practice relate to one another? What, in any case, is meant by 'theory'? It is to these matters that we next turn.

☐   Theory and practice

A quick response to questions such as these will simply contrast theory with practice, associating the former with bookish, highly general, abstract enquiry. 'That's all very well in theory', the familiar response runs, 'but will it work in practice?' To be involved in practice is to do something; to do theory is not. In consequence, theorists seem insulated from the real world of practice, the value of their work routinely called into question. But such a theory–practice contrast does not stand up to scrutiny. A first reason is that to engage in theory is itself to be involved in a practice, the practice of theorizing; it is, after all, to *do* something. A second concerns confusion over the relationship between the ends of theory and of practice – that is, between bookish and discursive enquiry, on the one hand, and teaching at the chalk-face or empirical data-gathering, on the other. In Aristotle's terms, the *natural* sciences are theoretical in that their purpose is the advancement of understanding; ethics and politics, in contrast, are *practical* sciences, the purpose of which is better action. Where, we might ask, does this leave nursing, and where does it leave the education of nurses? It follows that to study Aristotle's *Nicomachean Ethics* in this way – bookish perhaps, but with the discursive engagement it should prompt – is itself part of this practical science. Not that the theoretical and practical sciences are tidily separated: to *act better* we need a sound *understanding* of what human nature and the socio-political conditions of our action are like. Acting well requires realism, and being realistic involves a complex blend of practical and theoretical wisdom.

To refer to such (bookish) enquiry as *theory* is, then, something of a misnomer. Educational theory, it would seem, is properly so named to the extent that it is concerned only with the understanding of practice and not with its improvement. It is true that academic research into politics or art, for example, is often dedicated not to the improvement of practice but simply to the increased understanding of salient aspects of our social world. Why should there not be educational research along similar lines? In general, however, and for a variety of reasons, the work to which researchers in education, nursing and health care departments are committed is concerned directly or indirectly with improvement in practice. The institutional reasons for this are plain enough. Students in university departments of these kinds are, for the most part, practitioners; the courses they take are usually designed to develop professional expertise. Much research, therefore, takes off from concerns with what that expertise consists in and with the conditions in which it is best exercised. Moreover, there is a strange reflexivity about the fact that, to the extent that educational researchers are employed as teachers in universities, they are directly involved in the professional activity that is otherwise their object of study. In this respect they have an exceptional position within the academy.

It follows from the above, then, that just as any ethics of research confined to methodology must be woefully inadequate, so enquiry into professional practice that does not foreground the pervasive nature of questions of value will be severely deficient. It will fail to sensitize practitioners to the practical reason they need. If we ask how this practical reason is to become more fully present in practice, then it seems reasonably clear that this will not in the main be through empirical research. Enquiry into these matters needs to be philosophical, ethics being, as we saw, one of the central elements in philosophy. And given that all research begins with questions of value, other branches of philosophy will also be conditioned in this way – not least in their commitment to truth. Epistemology, so obviously relevant to education generally, and so pertinent also to questions concerning the kinds of knowledge that matter most in health care, is simply incoherent without assumptions and judgements about the value of knowledge. Ethics, we see again, is pervasive.

This is not to make a case exclusively for philosophy: in recent decades other forms of enquiry also have been sidelined in favour of supposedly more practical study and research – one thinks of history and sociology, as well as aspects of comparative education. Nor is it to advocate philosophical approaches of a narrow disciplinary kind. It is to accept the breadth of the ways in which enquiry can fruitfully take place, albeit that any systematic study of ethics is bound in some degree to be philosophical.

The mantle of 'theory' can be accepted to the extent that the addressing of questions of value that is advocated here will necessarily be directed towards greater *understanding*. Teachers, nurses and other health care professionals are not technical operatives who do not need to understand the tasks they are carrying out. The understanding they need is internally related to practice. The teacher or nurse with practical wisdom is someone whose knowledge is manifest in the doing. Her activity is in-formed by this better understanding, whether or not this is articulated. But this is not a matter of theory applied. To see things in such terms is to resuscitate a picture of the theory–practice relation that has sometimes dogged the philosophy of education, as we shall shortly see, amongst both advocates and detractors. The point is not to pass on, *de haut en bas*, an understanding of the ethics of education that the humble practitioner can put into operation. It is to enable the practitioner to think better about what she is doing, and in this to improve her practice. This may indeed involve thinking about ideas in books such as Aristotle's *Nicomachean Ethics*. We can call this theory if we so choose. We prefer to see it as a form of investigation by engaging in the work of thought that is inextricably related to the value of any practice.

While it should be clear then that the technicist drift sketched above presents a major barrier to the enquiry that is needed if greater understanding and improved practice are to be achieved, a further complicating factor is the placing of the study of education within the social sciences. What are the consequences of this, and how, more specifically, is *philosophy's* relation to the social sciences to be understood?

□   Philosophy and social science

Undoubtedly, administrative convenience must play its part in such institutional arrangements, and to some, of course, the appropriateness of seeing the study of education – including the philosophy of education – as social science will seem obvious. But four consequences of this need to be borne in mind and two supplementary points developed in its light.

First, to the extent that philosophy is acknowledged, this conceptualization reinforces a role for the discipline that is familiar and nicely contained. Philosophy, on this view, is the 'underlabourer' to the sciences of psychology, sociology, nursing research, and so on: it clarifies the central concepts of these disciplines and the distinctive modes of reasoning that sustain them. We do not question the legitimacy of such work of clarification, as far as it goes, but the understanding of philosophy in this way surely harbours a danger. This is that the consideration of ethics tends to be limited or, at least, sidelined. The underlabourer conception has the effect of ignoring the central importance of ethics in philosophy, which we have been at pains to emphasize above. By this we do not simply mean Ethics as a 'branch' of philosophy, but rather that an ethical dimension, the question of values, is omnipresent in all modes of enquiry, whether it be in nursing or other health care fields.

Second, there is the fact that education, as social science, becomes contrasted with the humanities or the arts. The separation from the humanities means that, for example, the way that history studies the life of a culture will not be seen as appropriate to education; the separation from the arts means *inter alia* that the type of creativity and imagination found in literature or the practical arts will be thought inappropriate to the more technical problems that education is to address, where the need is for efficient means towards pre-determined ends.

Third, there is the burden of expectation that is carried by the term 'science'. The term itself has a recent history that separates it from its German equivalent, *Wissenschaft*. 'Social science', in Anglophone contexts, is a clear borrowing from the natural sciences, where procedures and standards have been established that the human sciences attempt to emulate. It may be that nothing very much turns on this, but, on the other hand, there are circumstances that make the question of terminology one of key importance – say, for example, where prestige attaches to anything called 'science' in such a way as to justify the funding of research. Related to this is the fact that popular expectations of science dovetail neatly with the prevalent (scientistic) concern with accountability. An educational science might, for example, promote the use of statements of outcomes of a behavioural and measurable kind. The positivism that prevailed in philosophy nearly one hundred years ago has clearly been superseded, but it has retained its hold over many aspects of contemporary life. With this comes a revering of what is imagined to be scientific method, and the technical expertise that goes with it, as the embodiment of certain intellectual virtues: science epitomizes rigour and disinterestedness, a proper concern for explanation and evidence, and a securing of foundations for thought. This false picture stands in the way of the true rigour that is needed.

Fourth, the understanding of education as a social science covers over its hybrid and multidisciplinary nature as a field of study. If someone is said to have expertise in education *tout court*, it is not clear what they are expert in. In contrast, the person who approaches the study of education from a specific discipline draws on a tradition of enquiry. This is not, however, to advocate a disciplinary purism. This amalgam of contributing subjects, the disciplines, could never be said to exhaust the nature of education, where time and attention are given to a plethora of matters concerning teaching, learning and professional practice. Nor does it convincingly encompass those narratives and visionary tracts – from Plato's *The Republic* to Ivan Illich's *Deschooling Society*, say – that can illuminate the consideration and development of educational practice. There is, nevertheless, a danger that research in education, when not secured in disciplinary ways of thought, becomes open to the influence of instant experts and passing fads. The political prominence of matters of educational policy and the fact that education is something of which everyone has experience (and about which everyone has an opinion) make the study of education particularly vulnerable in this respect. This is something that affects professional education too.

The first supplementary point concerns the curious asymmetry between Education as a subject and other disciplines (or fields of study). For any academic discipline one can speak of being educated in it. Although a potential source of confusion, this perhaps says something deep about the pervasiveness of education: in other disciplines one is never outside the practice of education; where educational studies involves a questioning of the practice and concept of education, this is quintessentially part of educational practice! This is the reflexivity we saw above. Education *qua* subject must be a part of education *qua* practice. A further point emerges if we consider more specifically the place of philosophy of education in relation to philosophy in general. Unlike the situation with other philosophies-of, there is no major branch of philosophy that is not relevant to education. This is obviously so with regard to central elements of philosophy such as ethics and epistemology, but other branches such as aesthetics or the philosophy of science will also be relevant to aspects of education; this is true in the minimal sense of their significance for the teaching of art or science, but a moment's reflection should show the ways in which these forms of enquiry have a bearing on educational practice more broadly – say, concerning the aesthetic aspects of classroom or health care environments or concerning evidence and argument in (social) scientific aspects of research. In some respects then 'philosophy *of* education' might be held to be a misnomer. This further affirms the importance, indeed the unavoidability, of philosophy if questions regarding professional education are pursued where they lead.

The second supplementary point, which we expand on through the remaining paragraphs in this section, involves the distinction between, on the one hand, the philosophy *of* social science and, on the other, philosophy as a form of enquiry into the nature of the good that should characterize social (and other) institutions themselves. The former casts philosophy in something of the underlabourer role we considered above, but the latter suggests a far more prominent, indeed a leading role.

Sometimes philosophy has proved to be sharply critical of social science. For example, in the closing pages of the *Philosophical Investigations*, Wittgenstein remarks that the inadequacies of psychology are not to be explained in terms of its being a 'young' science but because it combines 'experimental methods and conceptual confusion' (Wittgenstein, 1958, p. 232). His writings are, however, richly suggestive for what a more coherent approach to the study of social phenomena and the improvement of practice might be like. The key role played in this by the exploration of language – the extensive, piecemeal, grammatical exploration of psychological concepts in his later work – is exemplary for any study in the human sciences, where the phenomena are intrinsically linguistic. The force of these lines of thought is strongly present in Peter Winch's influential book, *The Idea of a Social Science*, in which the difference between social and physical sciences is elaborated. The natural scientist, according to Winch, proceeds by observing regularities in the natural world. But the idea of regularity depends upon criteria, for without these how can two occurrences be judged the same? What generates the criteria is the practice of science, the shared language of the research community, in which the individual researcher participates. As Winch puts it, 'to understand the activities of the scientific investigator we must take account of two sets of relations: first, his relation to the phenomena which he investigates; second, his relation to his fellow scientists' (Winch, 1958, p. 84). The social scientist's practice, however, cannot be like this. Winch gives the example of the parable of the Pharisee and the Publican (Luke 18: 9). The Pharisee says, 'God, I thank Thee that I am not as other men are'; the Publican, 'God be merciful unto me a sinner'. Are these men doing the *same* thing? *Are* they both praying? To answer this it will be necessary to consider the concept of prayer, and this is not a scientific but a religious or, indeed, a *philosophical* question. Questions of this kind are internal to the phenomena being observed in a way that questions concerning natural objects are not. In other words, they cannot be addressed without reference to the way that the people in question themselves understand what they are doing.[4]

That philosophy might include forms of enquiry into the nature of the good that should characterize social (and other) institutions themselves, including the goods towards which health care and education are directed, helps to show the limitations of regarding it as something to be *applied*. Apart from the fact that this reinforces an unwarranted distinction between theory and practice, the assumption fails to recognize the extent to which central aspects of philosophical enquiry necessarily incorporate questions about learning and teaching: such enquiry includes questions not only about the nature of the good (for the individual and for society) but about how we become virtuous, and not only about the nature of knowledge but about how it is acquired. These essentially educational questions of teaching and learning are not external matters to which the philosophy is applied but are internal to philosophy itself. What is characteristic of the philosophy of education, as indicative of what is at stake here, is that it typically relates to the particularities of educational practice in such a manner that a complex mix of philosophical problems needs to be addressed. Against the background of the now often over-specialized work of mainstream philosophers, it is not surprising that this work can seem insufficiently focused, even somewhat amateur. That is the price of a true and practical engagement with the problems. The breadth of this engagement becomes its virtue.

It is salutary to keep in mind the variety of ways in which the study of education can meaningfully take place, and that variety can easily be illustrated in relation to the professional education that is the concern of this book. For example, a researcher in education may be concerned with the disinterested observation of current practice. Observation cannot occur in a vacuum, however; it must begin with some sense of what matters. What presents itself as a focus for research will arise, say, out of an interest in a possible improvement of existing practice, perhaps by gaining a better understanding of what is currently happening. Then again, research may be more narrowly instrumental in kind, where teaching techniques (directed towards agreed, imposed, or tacitly assumed ends) are developed. Research may pursue a questioning of the practice of professional education in tandem with an enquiry into the nature of good nursing. This may perhaps include the consideration of what constitutes good health or what is appropriate palliative care. Questions of education, in this third case, shade into matters addressed more or less directly in other subjects – most directly perhaps in philosophy, extensively but obliquely in the humanities and tangentially in science – concerning the nature of the good life. These matters, as we saw above, are far from being of purely theoretical significance: they impinge on the very nature of practice itself, and on the personhood of patients and practitioners alike.

In a book such as this it seems inevitable that some of what is being said here will be tantamount to preaching to the converted. Many educators of nurses and other health care practitioners draw extensively on work in the philosophical traditions that interest us – one thinks of Aristotelian conceptions of practical reason, for example, or of the more contemporary work of Hubert Dreyfus on practical competence and professional expertise, which was introduced into the nursing literature by Patricia Benner (1984); but one thinks also of work that is more obviously located within the philosophy of education, as is the case, for example, with Nel Nodding's writings on the ethics of care (Noddings, 1984). But the philosophy of education, like any discipline, is in some respects a contested field, and in the light of this, it is desirable, we believe, to say something about different conceptions of this subject, not least because of the particular conception of the theory–practice relationship that at times has adversely affected its influence. Let us do this, in order to clarify what is at issue here, by speaking of rival traditions.

□ Rival traditions in the philosophy of education

In the paragraphs that follow, we comment particularly on developments in Anglophone contexts. The justification for this is twofold. In the first place, if one wishes to identify prevailing trends and dominant traditions, it is impossible to write about everything at once. Hence, we concentrate on the context that is likely to be most salient for readers of this book and for the professional settings that are the focus of the chapters that follow. In the second, the hegemony of the English language, in circumstances of globalization, creates cultural imbalances that both raise the profile of work in English and also lead to patterns of activity – through conferences and publications in books and academic journals – that encourage others to work in that idiom and hence to draw from its traditions. It was in this context, and especially with the relative prosperity of the UK in the 1960s, that British philosophy of education became widely influential, reciprocating in various ways with activity in the subject in North America, but in certain respects carving out a distinctive body of work of its own. Things have moved on since then. While that tradition and approach has developed in various ways, there has also been a broadening of the field, and it has been further internationalized.

We shall begin by saying something about the policy and institutional context of the subject, tracing in the process some arguments concerning what the philosophy of education is taken to be. The contrasting conceptions of the subject that have developed in the UK are then identified – though these differences of viewpoint, it should be stressed, are by no means confined to the UK. One virtue of focusing on the British scene is that it reveals in greater relief the contours of disagreement that characterize the field internationally, especially as it becomes more globalized. Finally, some brief remarks are made about the ways in which the philosophy of education bears upon policy and practice, especially in relation to matters of pressing concern.

In the decades after the Second World War the academic study of education in the UK and in much of the English-speaking world developed along disciplinary lines. That is to say, the study of educational policy and practice was understood to involve approaches from the disciplines of history, philosophy, psychology and sociology, which many current teachers of nursing will be familiar with. This was based on the view that Education as an academic study cannot be a discipline in its own right because it does not have its own characteristic modes of enquiry or its own ways of reasoning; its reasoning necessarily draws upon one or another of these four disciplines. Over the past twenty years, however, the primacy of these disciplines in educational enquiry has been weakened – at least, their position in universities has changed: there have been fewer jobs in these disciplines (within education departments) and fewer courses directly based on them; they have been pushed out by new areas of emphasis – relating, for example, to school effectiveness and improvement, to specific and sometimes topical matters of curriculum (such as mathematics education, personal, social and health education, or citizenship education, or innovations in teaching and assessment), and to specialisms in particular stages of education (e.g., early years or perhaps vocational education and training). We do realize that we are speaking at this point of education in the most general terms rather than in terms of the education of nurses in particular, but we would emphasize the importance of this for the theorization of educational practice in any department, and not just in departments of education. Indeed it is not often sufficiently recognized or considered that trends in educational policy and practice tend to come from outside the departments that are obliged to embrace them.

Our own view of these changes, and of the weakening of the disciplinary approach, is that they constitute a serious threat, as we have begun to indicate above, to the academic credibility and cogency of education as a form of study. This is true in terms both of educational research and of the initial preparation and continuing professional development of teachers. Earlier in this introduction we drew attention to problems with attempts to address matters of policy and practice *without the resources of traditions of enquiry*, and this is what one finds in both the research and the courses themselves. By 'tradition of enquiry' we do not mean any established set of views or orthodoxy but rather a sustained practice of asking questions of a particular kind, about a particular set of problems, with progressively refined modes of approach, with a developing line of familiar texts, and with, as Michael Oakeshott might put this, a characteristic kind of conversation (Oakeshott, 1972). In order to take part in such a conversation, one needs gradually to be initiated into it: one cannot just jump in from the outside, for more or less the same reason that one cannot simply jump into a conversation about respiratory care nursing – that is, do respiratory care nursing – without prior study of the subject.

Crucial to the vitality of a tradition in this sense, moreover, is the way that it is *not* unified – because of its rivalries and disputes, its paradigm shifts, its *avant-garde*. Indeed, any tradition worth the name must embody its own forms of criticism.[5] The educational research that we are criticizing tends to start from the recent past, with the assumption that the 'latest research findings' must be the best. It is a characteristic of the epistemological, ethical and metaphysical questions that we have been at pains to foreground – questions in professional education that are ultimately unavoidable – that they are not amenable to definitive resolution. In approaching them we may well find that Plato or Confucius have important things to say to us, and hence research should be ready to engage with traditions of thought that began long ago.

This is not to say that all was well with the former (disciplinary) approach. Very often, and especially in initial teacher education, the disciplines were taught in a dry, abstract and overly theoretical way and without due regard for the motivation and the stage of academic development of the students. With some justification, students found aspects of the work that they were required to do irrelevant to their real concerns about how to cope in the classroom or areas of practice; they did not always feel that this was preparing them well for their lives as teachers. But the reasonable dissatis-faction with this approach expressed by students and others was exploited by those who sought to make educational provision and the behaviour of teachers more amenable to the requirements of the state. In the UK Margaret Thatcher was the major influence behind this change, and as one consequence of what seemed to be her systematic attack on a range of professions, the autonomy and intellectual scope of teaching has been reduced. This is to say especially that the scope for judgement on the part of the teacher has been limited: more commonly now teachers follow more or less clearly specified syllabi, or construct syllabi in the light of pervasive standards of proficiency and assessment regimes, and less commonly are they encouraged to reflect on deeper questions concerning the nature of their role and the point of the education they are providing. It is worth adding that, as in the case of nursing and health care, their personhood and embodiment tend not to be acknowledged. While this is especially true in the UK, it has also been the broad trend generally in the Western world. As we hope we have made clear, this is a trend that should be resisted.

Those concerned to address philosophical questions need to engage practitioners, both in initial training and in continuing professional devel-opment, to think better and more philosophically about the real questions that confront them. This will involve, amongst other things, greater sens-itivity to context and the wider use of examples in the presentation of complex ideas. In doing so, the philosophy of education has the potential to extend and develop practitioners as people, and so perhaps to make them better at what they do in their professional lives. There are clear signs in the vitality of current philosophy of education that it has moved away from the abstract, dry forms it once took, and so that it is well-fitted for this task. The attention of policy-makers needs recurrently to be drawn to the benefit to professional practice that it can provide.

But how are we to describe this vitality? Having provided an initial characterization of what we take philosophy of education to be, let us now consider certain aspects of the development of the subject in recent years. From an Anglophone point of view, and especially a British point of view, a contrast can be drawn between two accounts of the philosophy of education.

According to one account, philosophy of education developed as a systematic form of study during the second half of the twentieth century. A key development in the early stages of this was the appointment of R.S. Peters to a chair in the philosophy of education at the London Institute of Education. Peters had previously worked in a Philosophy department but he quickly established his reputation in this new field. This was a time of economic growth in the UK, and teacher education was expanding. Peters and his colleagues – most notably Paul Hirst and Robert Dearden – worked together to develop an approach to the study of education that was both distinctive and highly influential, at home and overseas. Their approach was distinctive especially because it applied the assumptions, methods and approaches of *analytical* philosophy to the study of education. Analytical philosophy, which was the dominant form of the subject in Philosophy departments at the time, understands philosophy to involve a process of conceptual analysis in order to arrive at clear and distinct ideas; it takes the point of enquiry to be the uncovering of the underlying logic of the matter at hand, specifically of the concepts that are involved. Hence, in education the assumption is that it is the concepts of teaching, learning, authority, knowledge, understanding, creativity, imagination and so on that need to be addressed. Through the analysis of these and similar concepts, the logic of education will be revealed and a sound basis for policy and practice will be established. To some extent, on this view, the role of philosophy of education will also involve looking at the concepts that are operative in *other* modes of enquiry into education; thus, for example, the concept of intelligence in psychology is clarified so that the psychologist's empirical work can be based on sound conceptual foundations.

Possibly, the philosopher whose work epitomizes this approach in its purest form is John Wilson. He identifies the task of philosophy in characteristically formal or procedural terms: 'all that philosophy can do (if indeed it can) is to explain to me the criteria of reason which apply to value judgements, so that I then know how to evaluate them' (Wilson, 2003, p. 284) Thus, one might suppose, 'the logic of value-judgements' might lead us to understand, say, that moral judgements are universalisable or that they are concealed imperatives. There is a neatness to this approach that seems safely to distance itself from the substance of particular moral beliefs in their socio-historical contexts in order better to understand their underlying logic. Moreover, this position predisposes Wilson to the view that where philosophers have engaged more substantively with questions of education, as opposed to confining themselves to formal problems concerning the logic inherent in such questions, they have tended to treat it lightly: Plato, Rousseau and Locke, for example, write 'as if education were not really a respectable *philosophical* topic at all, but just a stamping ground for utopian theory or personal prejudice' (p. 280). It is evident then that 'serious thought about education must first and foremost be a strict and circumspect *logical* discipline, informed by a facility for reasoned argument' (ibid.).[6]

There is no doubt, however, that the work of analytical philosophers of education has gone beyond this, and in some respects it seems that some of their most notable achievements have departed from the conceptual analysis that they have typically claimed to be their method. Perhaps the richest part of the work of Peters and his colleagues was their advancing of a substantive conception of good education in their restatement of the idea of a liberal education, a restatement that drew its greatest strengths from the inspiration of the British political philosopher, Michael Oakeshott. (There is, incidentally, a mild irony in the fact that Oakeshott was not exactly the archetypal analytical philosopher. In the 1920s he had studied in Germany, and he was plainly influenced by Continental thought.) While the story that is being told here tends to locate the origins of this work in the UK, it is important to recognize the development in the United States at this time of ideas and approaches that were parallel. Israel Scheffler was the most dominant figure there, and his influence spread across North America and beyond in a comparable way. This then is the first account of the development of philosophy of education as a discipline.

According to the second account, the picture sketched here is too tidy and too limited by far. It is true that R.S. Peters and the London School were highly influential, and that the body of work that has arisen within this tradition of enquiry is impressive and of great value and importance. But to see the development of philosophy of education just in these terms cannot be right. In a sense philosophy of education is at least as old as Plato or Confucius, for the reasons indicated earlier. And philosophers throughout the ages have sometimes indirectly and sometimes directly given extensive thought to matters of education. One thinks especially of Locke and Rousseau, of course, but in fact the picture is much broader than this. Both Kant and Hegel were required to teach courses about education, and in the German-speaking world since their time there has been a robust tradition of enquiry into education that deserves to be recognized more fully in the English-speaking world, just as the work of the Frankfurt School and its subsequent influence is a further factor that warrants careful attention. Moreover, it is surely the case that if one looks at the development of American philosophy one finds not only a method of enquiry – pragmatism – for which education has a special importance but also a mainstream, major philosopher who has had immense influence on education during the past century, and whose work has undergone a kind of revival, especially through the efforts of Richard Rorty: this is, of course, John Dewey. More recently, the writings of a range of philosophers in the so-called Continental tradition – from Marxism to poststructuralism – have been found to have immense educational resonance. So too, in this broader account, a thinker such as Alasdair MacIntyre, who was at one time dismissed by the London School as non-philosophical, has come to have immense influence, being at the heart of the neo-Aristotelianism that has become an important element in contemporary thinking on ethics and so much else. As this last example indicates, the philosophers included in this second account have tended to be marginalized or condemned by those adopting a more exclusively analytical approach because of the alleged lack of clarity or precision in their arguments. Sometimes – as, e. g., in the case of Heidegger – they have been regarded simply as incoherent and as not worthy of study.

In sum, the first account favours a kind of exclusiveness: it is based on faith in a particular kind of approach. The second account recognizes the variety of ways in which philosophical enquiry into education has taken place, and it acknowledges the long history of this; furthermore, because of its less demanding or less narrow conception of what counts as philosophical, it is inclined to understand the boundaries between disciplines – for example, between philosophy and politics or sociology or theology or literature – as less firmly fixed. Being inclusive and pluralistic in its understanding of philosophy, it can recognize the role and the merits of work in the analytical philosophy of education tradition. As perhaps has become clear, it is this second account that accords with our own views. But it is important to recognize that to say this is not to subscribe to any faction or school of thought: it is very much the point of this second account to acknowledge the variety of ways in which philosophy of education can proceed and to recognize value in many of them, the analytical approach included.[7]

What might be the reasons for the claim that working across this broader range is likely to be more beneficial in terms of practice in education and in relation to the health care professions? Much as we value analytical approaches to philosophy, we have been struck by various ways in which they can reinforce a set of metaphysical assumptions that have had a prevailing influence in the modern world. What needs especially to be challenged within these assumptions is – to put this briefly and in exaggerated terms – the idea of human beings as individual and perhaps isolated subjects, standing in a relation of observation and cognition to the objects of experience, and having relations to other human beings of a quasi-contractual kind. In our view, such assumptions are both false to experience and ethically objectionable.

Practical problems in education have sometimes been addressed by the analytical philosophy of education that has prevailed in ways that have, in our view, failed to engage sufficiently with the urgency and implications of these problems. We offer three examples.

In much educational policy over the past two decades, especially in relation to vocational education, there has been a vogue for 'skills' and 'competencies' and a decline in reference to the acquisition of knowledge and understanding. We put these terms in inverted commas to emphasize the way that the words seem to have acquired a special power of their own; in educational practice it has been very difficult to look at these critically. Analytical philosophers such as Robin Barrow and Terry Hyland did a fine job at an early stage in exposing the lack of clarity and the muddles in the use of these terms – especially where everything, so it seemed, was suddenly regarded as a skill or competency. But there has been something deeper at stake here. Is not all this talk of skills in fact a symptom of a new form of behaviourism, and as such profoundly at odds with the most important parts of the educational endeavour? Does it not distort the competence that counts? The connection with behaviourism and the kind of metaphysics that this presupposes need to be exposed, and for this to be achieved what is required is something beyond clarity over concepts. The resources of the wider range of traditions to which we refer have been of immense value in answering to this need.

Our second and third examples are interlinked. During the 1980s, in various forms of post-compulsory education and training, there was a sudden growth in a new kind of approach to management, and this was evident across a range of educational and health care institutions. The new manager was typically cast in a role that was distanced from the specific practice in which the institution was engaged – its teaching and learning or its health care – and the skills, knowledge and expertise she was expected to have had more to do with the world of business than with the substantive commitments of the profession in question. Hence, the sense of involvement with a particular group of staff that had been enjoyed by predecessors in similar positions of responsibility, and the collegiality and trust that went with this, gradually disappeared; it was replaced by loyalty to the managerial 'team'. Revolving responsibilities also meant a lack of real commitment to any particular aspect of the institution, especially to any particular *educational* aspect, and hence a rather more self-centred focus on the manager's own career: indeed within such approaches it became commonly accepted that the aspiring manager should move from institution to institution in order to progress rapidly. The new managerialism was a factor in destroying important aspects of professional community. It made it more easy for extraneous considerations to displace priorities internal to the practical ethos of the institution, whether education or health care.

This rise of the new managerialism also coincided with changes in the daily life of such educational institutions brought about by information and communication technology (ICT). Of course, during this time everyone was encouraged to think about the ways in which ICT might contribute to the development of teaching and learning, or to other aspects of professional practice, but the changes that were really happening at that time had much more to do with systems of record-keeping and accounting; these laid the way for what we have now come to call the 'culture of accountability' or the 'audit society', in which relationships of trust are surreptitiously eroded, and aspects of learning that cannot be readily spelled out are gradually denied. Needless to say, then, ICT was an important factor in the development of managerialism. At the same time, it encouraged a conception of teaching and learning that tended to draw a clear distinction between the skills of learning (or of accessing information) and the content that was to be learned (which could be stored as information on a computer). This distinction has a superficial plausibility, sufficient to satisfy many of the managers we have been describing (especially those who were over-keen to make their mark through the innovations they introduced), and many teachers who had not reflected much on philosophical questions concerning education came to accept it too. To understand why this was so, it is necessary to explore deep connections between the kind of atomism of thinking that ICT encourages and the systematic (and similarly atomistic) understandings of the social world upon which managerialism thrives. Once again, the analyses that were offered by analytical philosophy failed to provide this; far more valuable in our view were Heidegger's writings on technology and Lyotard's various reflections upon the postmodern condition; far more important more generally was the sensitization to the significance of language that was offered by the later Wittgenstein and his successors, and by various aspects of poststructuralism. It was these latter sources that offered the possibility of understanding and addressing circumstances that had become part of the daily experience of teachers and health care practitioners, as well as administrators. None of this, it should be emphasized, is to condemn ICT *per se*. We do not doubt its untapped potential. But so much depends on how it is allowed to develop.[8] What does need to be understood better is the way in which technological thinking in general, and ICT in particular, can colonize other aspects of our lives and work. Once again, analytical philosophy seemed not to give much attention to these problems – still less to offer ways to see beyond them.

These same sources (Heidegger, Lyotard, etc.) were also valuable in bringing to light what is perhaps the most pressing threat to education in our time: that is, the dominance of performativity. 'Performativity' is a word coined by Lyotard to denote the way that so much of our lives is arranged according to principles of efficiency and effectiveness, where the overriding criterion is the saving of time.[9] It is pertinent here to think of the ways that educational practices have come to be dominated by an obsession with process: clearly specified aims and objectives are to be matched by efficient method, as if in a smoothly running machine. The questions of what the end result (the product) is and whether the experience for the learner is rich or valuable are subordinated to the question of whether the system is working well: it does not matter what students are taught provided that it can be demonstrated that this is clearly specified and that the fact that they have learned it can be shown; in other words what goes on in the school or the university, or the hospital or the clinic, must be made to fit in with the increasing weight of the quality infrastructure that has emerged as part of the cult of standardization and transparency. But let us be quite clear about this. We are not referring here to those entirely reasonable systematic procedures that are integrated into good practice in such a way, say, as to guard against human error in the interests of patient safety. It is the managerialist adoption of industrial practices of quality control that is at issue, for this has two serious consequences. In the first place, there are aspects of learning as well as of good clinical practice that cannot easily be assessed or recorded by the kinds of tests that the system requires. This is not to say that they cannot be assessed at all, but that to do so cannot be a merely routine or systematic procedure: it will require a sensitive and experienced teacher who is *on the inside of the practice* with which the student is engaged; indeed a good teacher, responding to the responses of students, is constantly assessing as teaching goes on. Hence, one of the worst effects of performativity is its denial that anything is learned unless it can be demonstrated in clearly measurable learning outcomes. In the second place, it restricts what happens in the lesson to what is clearly specified in advance as the means of realizing the learning outcomes or competences. This is objectionable because it is a part of good teaching and good professional guidance that learning should be allowed to develop in new and unforeseen directions – in the light of the responses and developing understanding of the students, their interaction with the teacher and the dynamism of the particular occasion. Good curricula require exactly this.

In short there is an overwhelming reductivism in performativity, inter-linked as it is with managerialism and the impoverished understanding of ICT, and this now presents us with a situation where many cannot think outside its terms. Of course, this involves an erosion of trust, and a weakening of the communities of practice that are so important for education. It is perhaps a response to the general weakening of communities that has come with globalization, but also, perhaps paradoxically, an accelerator of the change that globalization brings.

These then are three examples of ways in which the philosophy of education, though still important, is likely to be diminished in its relevance to practice if it restricts itself to the more limited self-conception that we have sketched above. We said at the start that we would end by drawing attention to what we believe to be pressing matters of concern. Thus, the three examples we have given here are intended as salient examples of what is at stake in everyday educational practice. It follows from what we have said also that, if these problems are to be understood and addressed by those involved in educational policy and practice, whether as teachers or administrators, improved provision in initial training and continuing professional development is needed. It also follows that these problems will not be solved by technical means alone – that is, by the passing on of new skills or new techniques. Above all they require the clearer understanding, the more wide-ranging reflection and the development of practical reason (*phronesis*) that philosophy especially can encourage. Hence, there is an overwhelming case for reaffirming the role of philosophy in these forms of professional training and education. If in the past some students were alienated by what they saw as philosophy's tendency towards dry abstraction, there are many contemporary examples of more lively and more imaginative approaches. We have provided a qualified defence for the 'disciplines' approach described above, but our real concern is definitely not sectarian or exclusive. The essence of the argument here is for the importance of philosophy in the study and practice of education – academic, professional and practical – as a whole.

But before concluding this section, let us anticipate a possible response. We recognize that it might be thought by some that philosophical enquiry into education can, in the exploration of these questions, lead only into a reflexive hopelessness and indecision, if only in the sense that there appears to be no 'right way'. We accept that there is sometimes no obvious 'right way', but we strongly resist the assumption that goes with this as negative and self-defeating. Indeed we see it as a failure to acknowledge the responsibility that a mature consideration of these matters properly exposes. It is only in the raising and exploring of such questions that reflexive and creative thought can remain enlivened in the face of institutional conventions – conventions that aspire to be self-legitimating by claiming to be born out of their own necessity, with subsequent constraints that appear to set limits on the possible. But there is also a sense in which the core of convention (whether it be moral, epistemological, political, organizational, or aesthetic) is in constant interaction with its own limits. One of the purposes of philosophy of education, in the second sense outlined above, is to keep this interaction alive. It is only by coming up against the limit, questioning the limit, that the core of convention begins to loosen, to shift and change, or that what is good in convention is reaffirmed when it may be in danger. This is all part of the dialogue, the purpose of which is not to establish once and for all some higher truth, or ultimately objective standpoint, or essence of things, on the strength of which all will become transparent. Rather, and as we have reaffirmed, it is to keep enlivened the interaction between the cores of convention and the limits of the possible, where indeed one may be seen to be contingent upon the other. These shifting conventions and limits apply to all areas of education, including pedagogy, curriculum, assessment, research, quality, political economy, support, evaluation, profession and practice – as noted at the beginning of this introduction, the list is potentially endless. This is the rationale we have adopted in this book, aimed primarily at educators of nurses but also relevant to educators of all health care professionals. It is the substance of this that we now go on to explain.

■ Overview of chapters

In the collection that follows, we have obviously not aspired to cover the whole range of issues that it would be possible to cover, although many of them are threaded through the various contributions. Neither have we gone for an 'ism' or 'ology' approach. By this we mean that we have not structured the book into different perspectives on philosophical enquiry such as positivism, phenomenology, feminism, hermeneutics, structuralism or poststructuralism. We have adopted a more eclectic approach in which some strands of these perspectives may be ascertained, although this is not the book's purpose. We have sought rather to adopt an approach that reflects the importance of the human condition in educating for health care, whether it be the student, the educator, or the patient. The last of these is obviously the most important because patients are the most vulnerable, but the first two are also important, as indeed is the interaction between them, and ultimately between the three. It is in accordance with this that the chapters we introduce below have been assembled under four main parts, in which what we shall from time to time refer to as 'the lens of enquiry' shifts its focus as the book progresses. We have arranged the chapters into broad themes that, while they do not capture all aspects of philosophical enquiry into education, do provide a certain thematic structure pertaining to what are ever-pertinent issues in the education of nurses and health care professionals in more general terms.

☐   Ethics of education and practice

The chapter by Anne Scott begins the collection with what may be broadly described as an ethics of education and practice. It does this by examining the notion of virtue as a regulative ideal into which students of nursing should be encultured as a central part of their educational preparation. Drawing on the work of Aristotle, it reinforces the importance of realizing that ethics or moral theory is not simply a subject to be taught in health care programmes, but is rather *a way of practising* that is eminently sensitive to the vulnerability of those being cared for. It is thus a training and enculturation of character, the aim of which is the subsequent manifestation of these virtues in day-to-day practice. This echoes the point about the inextricable relation between theory and practice in terms of practical reason.

The next chapter by Peter Allmark and Angela Tod remains on an ethical theme, but in a different way, and from a different philosophical direction. Here we are invited to consider that the educational preparation of nurses to undertake a health education role has, in itself, an ethical dimension that is not immediately obvious. This concerns the argument that health education, following the standard view of behaviour change by which its efficacy is judged, can actually lead to unintended and harmful consequences, which they refer to as 'the prevention paradox'. Through the use of an example, Allmark and Tod offer three criticisms of this standard view, one of which is empirical and two of which are philosophical. The kernel of their argument is based on the premise that health education is judged as if it were a treatment or intervention in behaviour change, rather than as an educational exercise, the consequence of which should be cognitive rather than behavioural. Through a contrast between libertarianism and paternalism, respectively, the tensions between a non-consequentialist and a consequentialist ethic are drawn out. This presents us with a dilemma in which the evidence for health maintenance or improvement in the large comes up against the values of a good life for a given individual. This needs to be acknowledged and taken into account in preparing nurses for a health education role.

Here again, we have a perpetual interaction, or reciprocal dialectic, between the shifting core of convention and the limits of the possible. This is not to minimize the importance of preparing nurses for a health education and promotion role. Rather, and as the authors say, 'it is to enrich it by promoting a philosophical dimension that calls us to the work of thought in that curious space where the individual stands face-to-face with the collective'.

The final chapter in this opening part, by Tina Besley, argues the case for the relevance of *narrative therapy* as a model for nurse counsellors. First, the chapter introduces the growth and significance of nurse counselling. Second, it explores the impact of the work of Michel Foucault on narrative therapy and the challenge this mode of counselling presents to psychological discourse and humanist counselling. Third, the chapter outlines and discusses narrative therapy as a mode of counselling suited to the demands of nursing. The discussion explores ways in which nurse educators and other health care professionals can be encouraged to see the relevance and importance of these issues and considers how they can be helped to develop an understanding of the practices in question. Besley's point here is that the narrative of a human life, whether it be that of a patient/client, student or educator, can be opened up for hermeneutic consideration at the horizons of what events might mean. Through narrative therapy, the experience of events for an individual can be reconstructed in a variety of ways that take one beyond the limits of normative convention while also returning to them in a more ethically positive way, a way in which the normative horizon has shifted.

☐ Profession, knowledge and practice

The next three chapters continue with a set of issues that, while still containing an ethical dimension, focus more on the relationship between profession, knowledge and practice. Michael Luntley opens with a close examination of the role of judgement in giving an account of professional practice that, although contextually situated, can nevertheless be conceptually articulated. It is in this respect that practice-experience is important for health care professional education. This is because it is only in practice that judgement is learned and executed. Moreover, practice is the only ground that provides the non-conceptual elements of experience that ultimately make judgements possible. The link from the last three chapters comes in the argument that the caring nurse is not just someone who practises techniques and interventions (with a happy smile), but someone with the sensibility to experience aspects of a patient's needs that makes certain sorts of contextualized judgement possible. Such sensibility in practice is often manifested in the nurse's non-conceptual experience, which may be difficult for the nurse to articulate, particularly when normal procedures are breached but where it still turns out to be the best thing to do. In terms of judgements based on learning from practice, how is such a phenomenon to be explained? Luntley, in exploring this important question, argues that to refer to such instances of judgement as 'intuitive' is not an answer, for to appeal to intuition is merely a different way of asking the question, how is it that the 'inarticulate expert' can make judgements that result in good practice, even when the conventional limits of good practice have been breached or transgressed?

The chapter by Joseph Dunne stays on the general theme of profession, knowledge and practice in a manner that takes us back to Aristotle's philosophy of practice, but also forward to Alasdair MacIntyre's seminal work in *After Virtue*. With regard to practices such as medicine and nursing, along with other examples, Dunne focuses on the distinction between their internal and external goods. Internal goods refer to the quality of a practice that is well executed as an end in itself, and where the end result is itself part of the internal goods. External goods refer to the potential consequences of a practice that are not intrinsic to the practice itself, but which can still influence it in various ways. External goods (such as reputation, remuneration, research funding etc.) are not necessarily bad. But intricately related to this, there are other external goods such as efficiency, protocols, league tables, competition and rationalizing economies of scale that can violate the fabric of the internal goods towards which a practice aspires. Moreover when such techno-rational pursuits become dominant in what then becomes the core of convention, this can distort the very idea of internal goods without our necessarily realizing it. This obviously sets a serious challenge for health care educators and practitioners, and it breaks open once again the limits of the possible in terms of practice, experience, character and judgement.

Paul Standish examines the concepts of profession and practice in higher education in a way that, while it connects with issues raised in the previous two chapters, refocuses the lens of enquiry. Here we are taken through Herbert Dreyfus's celebrated account of the development of practical competence, which draws extensively on the work of Martin Heidegger and Samuel Todes. Echoing the essay by Michael Luntley, the chapter deals with ideas that most nurse educators will be familiar with, through the work of Patricia Benner's (1984) *Novice to Expert*. But here the direction shifts, and it moves beyond what Paul Standish argues to be the limits of Dreyfus's pragmatist reading of Heidegger. Extending the line of argument, Standish pursues a second approach to the topic. This takes seriously the idea of professing suppressed in the term 'profession' with its suggestions of the profession of faith and of broader perfectionist commitments that open onto a larger picture. The importance of recognizing this larger picture is explicated, and the threats to it not only from technicism but also from economies of satisfaction are exposed.

☐ Curriculum and expertise

While there is an obvious sense in which all of the chapters hitherto have implications for nursing curricula and expertise, the next three take this topic as their particular area of enquiry. Although they do this in very diverse ways, they all challenge once again the limits of convention. Gerard Lum opens with the familiar theme of the ever-present tension between, on the one hand, theory, and, on the other, practice or work-based learning and performance. Advocates from each camp often differ in their conception of what it is that health care practitioners need to know. As Lum goes on to argue, attempts to reconcile these two positions characteristically take the form of conceding a place for both theory and practice, thus reinforcing the idea that professional capability consists of two fundamentally different kinds of knowledge. Curriculum designers are thus typically incited to achieve an appropriate balance between what are ostensibly different components of knowledge. Lum argues that this dualistic notion of professional capability is mistaken and, on the strength of this, that attempts to reach some kind of ideal epistemological equilibrium are in fact illusory. Lum does not disagree with the convention that professional preparation should include both academic and practice-based provision in the development of expertise, but he seeks rather to present a view of curriculum design that transcends the dualistic conception of 'theory' and 'practice'. Thus, and running counter to official policy, the argument is put forward that curriculum design should be less about trying to specify professional knowledge than about identifying the kind of educational strategies that best promote such knowledge and expertise.

This is followed by the chapter from John Paley in which the dualism implicit in conventional views of expertise, with its implications for curriculum or training programmes, is again challenged, but this time from a perhaps surprisingly different perspective. A common view of how expertise is gained is that of putting knowledge into people's brains or heads, which they then exercise through an accumulative interaction with practical 'hands-on' experience. The equally taken-for-granted view, therefore, is that expertise is a property of individuals. It would appear to follow from this that if some aspect of nursing or health care practice requires amending, improving, or solving, the obvious route is to educate people to improve, amend, or upgrade what is inside their heads. Paley refers to this conventional reaction as 'the education reflex': in the context of specific in-house training or continuing professional development programmes, this can be costly and time-consuming, and it often makes little difference. With the use of examples, he goes on to consider a theoretical, a philosophical and a practical alternative. The argument here is that expertise is not just about what does or does not go on inside people's heads, and so that delivering expertise to health care environments is not just about amending or adding new knowledge to that already possessed by individuals. It is rather the case that expertise is *distributed* – and in a very non-Cartesian way. It is a property of cognitive systems, extending well beyond the brains (and bodies) of individuals. If this is accepted, then it follows that the 'we-need-to-educate-them' solution is often misconceived: it would be better replaced by the 'we-can-fix-something-else-in-the-system' solution. Paley seeks to show that it is often the case that such 'system-solutions' are not just more persuasive from a philosophical point of view, but are also usually quicker, cheaper and more effective.

The third chapter in this broad thematic of curriculum and expertise shifts the focus yet again. Indeed the contribution by Sally Thorne and Rick Sawatzky, although concerned with issues of curriculum and programme content, broadens the lens of enquiry in a manner that opens the field of vision for the next set of chapters on the politics of education, knowledge and society. It does this by noting that current demands for public account-ability in health care and the proliferation of advances in health research have created pressure upon the profession of nursing to ensure that its practice is evidence-based. Nurse educators, therefore, are increasingly responding to this pressure with curricula and pedagogical strategies aimed at emphasizing that for which there is empirical evidence throughout the training of the next generation of practitioners. Echoing back to previous chapters, it is within this context that nursing's traditional focus upon the uniqueness of the particular individual can be easily displaced in favour of knowledge pertaining to general populations. This leads to a consider-ation of how neophyte nurses are taught the systematic thinking processes of professional practice and to an examination of some of the competing agendas that have complicated our understanding of the relevant models and frameworks generated for this purpose. Through an exploration of the philosophical underpinnings of science as it pertains to rendering general knowledge into particular practice applications, options for teaching the praxis of nursing are considered in that tensive domain of the universal and the particular.

☐ Politics of education, knowledge and society

Extending the focus in the chapter by Sally Thorne and Rick Sawatzky to the chapter by Gary Rolfe, we find the lens of enquiry broadened out quite considerably as his chapter opens the theme of the final set of chapters: this is what may be described in general terms as the politics of education, knowledge and society. Rolfe takes us on a journey that examines the nature of the university in a fibrillation between the grand narratives of modernity and what is arguably a postmodern culture. There are many 'narratives', some grand and some little, asserting what it is best to do in terms of curriculum, both undergraduate and postgraduate. In the face of this clamour for attention, Rolfe draws on aspects of the work of the poststructuralist philosopher Jean-François Lyotard and of Bill Readings in order to make a distinction between, on the one hand, the liberal capitalist university with its idea of universal standards of quality – or at least of how such ideas of quality, or indeed acceptability, might be judged – and on the other hand, the idea of a postmodern university with *no such idea* – or at least no grand idea or narrative universally applicable to all cases of judgement. Through Lyotard's notion of the 'differend', we are invited to bear witness to cases where judgement on issues of acceptable knowledge, educational practices and enquiry must be kept open, where unity comes through an acceptance of diversity or difference rather than a contrived and imposed universality.

The chapter by John S. Drummond traverses the same domain of education, knowledge and society with specific regard to changes in the treatment of knowledge in what is now commonly referred to as a 'knowledge economy'. Drummond begins with an overview of important elements of a knowledge economy and their concomitant emergence in education in the United Kingdom. He argues that education and the practice of teaching and research is now permeated with various strands of this discourse. To inform the analysis from a philosophical perspective, we are introduced to Michel Foucault's concept of ethics as a relationship that one has with one's self (*rapport à soi*). In filtering the implications of a knowledge economy through Foucault's notion of *rapport à soi*, the idea is developed that educators are now being asked to carry out a work on themselves that is presented as a prescriptive moral code. Two questions are asked. First, in the changing context of a knowledge economy, what might it mean to carry out a work on one's self? Second, what are the potential relations between such a work and what it means to engage in what now appears to be the ever-changing business of education? It is at this point, in the final part of the chapter, that we are introduced to the ancient Greek concept of 'care of the self' (*epimeleia heautou*) as a counterpoint to the impact of a knowledge economy on education policy and practice.

This brings us to the final chapter by Michael Peters, Keith Hammond and John S. Drummond. While continuing the same theme of this final set of chapters, the focus shifts to a consideration of the very concept of health in the discourse of the health care professions in a manner that relates back to the chapter by Peter Allmark and Angela Tod in this book, but in a different way that considers the political economy of health. Peters, Hammond and Drummond use the work of the German hermeneutic philosopher Hans-Georg Gadamer, one of the very few contemporary 'mainstream' philosophers to write extensively on health as a concept, especially in his book *The Enigma of Health*. It is somewhat surprising that this important book has been largely ignored, or perhaps has remained 'undiscovered', in the critical literature on health and health education. In *The Enigma of Health* Gadamer presents us with a series of essays that were written as meditations on health over the period 1963–1991 but that, as we shall see, remain particularly relevant today. As Peters, Hammond and Drummond point out, what emerges from Gadamer's analysis is that health is not something that can be made or produced. Moreover, it manifests itself by virtue of its escaping our attention: the aim of healing is to regain one's health in order to forget that one is healthy. This is, therefore, a central antinomy or perplexity that stands at the heart of the discourse and practice of health care, including health education. Along with a brief journey through some of the arguments of Ivan Illich, this chapter examines Gadamer's 'enigma' and uses it to explore dimensions of the 'political economy' and 'institutionalization' of health. In particular, a distinction is made between, on the one hand, the current image of the 'healthy lifestyle' and, on the other, the more philosophical idea of 'the good life', where it is argued that the former has begun to colonize the latter in ways that are open to question. The implications of this tension for educators of health care practitioners are considered.

While there is a clear rationale for the grouping of chapters under the above broad headings, there remains in each of them a certain openness to thought that encourages manifold connections. Hence, they could have been arranged differently. But this in turn serves to reinforce the point that philosophical enquiry into education transcends easy categorizations and stipulations.

■ Notes

1 In the case of nursing, see Edwards (1997, 1998, 2001); Benner (1984, 1994, 2000); Kikuchi and Simmons (1992); Parse (1981); Reed and Ground (1997); Rolfe (2000); Freshwater and Rolfe (2004). The year 2003 also saw the launch of the International Philosophy of Nursing Society (IPONS); see http://www.ipons.dundee.ac.uk

2 There are of course exceptions. See, for example, Horrocks (1998); Holt (1998).

3 For a critique of these issues in nursing, see Drummond (2000, 2002).

4 For an extended discussion of the idea of an educational science, see Standish (1995, 2003).

5 For an exploration of the concept of the *avant-garde* in nursing and nurse education, see Drummond (2004).

6 For a critique of Wilson's views in this paper, see Standish (2006).

7 For an attempt to present a state-of-the-art collection of work brought together in the light of an inclusive conception of philosophy of education, see Blake *et al.* (2003). For an indication of some aspects of the differences between these two accounts, see the symposium with John White, Wilfred Carr, Richard Smith, Terence H. McLaughlin, and Paul Standish in the *Journal of Philosophy of Education* (White *et al.*, 2003).

8 See, for example, Standish (1997, 2001, 2002). See also Hubert Dreyfus, whose extensive writings regarding computing technology are related especially to education in his book *On The Internet* (Dreyfus, 2001). For criticisms of this text with a response by Dreyfus, see the suite of articles published with Dreyfus (Standish, 2002). For imaginative but critical discussion of the possibilities of the Internet in education, see Andrew Feenberg's website at http://www.sfu.ca/~andrewf/ (Accessed 24th April, 2006).

9 For examples of attempts to examine the broader educational significance of Lyotard's work, see Dhillon and Standish (2000). For a controversial example related to health care, see Drummond (2001).

Part 1

Ethics of Education and Practice

Chapter 1

Nursing and the notion of virtue as a 'regulative ideal'

P. Anne Scott

■ Introduction

> In our view, the best way to conceive of a virtue ethics criterion of right action is in terms of a "regulative ideal". To say that an agent has a regulative ideal is to say that they have internalized a certain conception of correctness or excellence, in such a way that they are able to adjust their motivation and conduct so that it conforms – or at least does not conflict with – that standard. So for instance, a man who has internalized a certain conception of what it is to be a good father can be guided by this conception in his practices as a father, through regulating his motivations and actions towards his children so that they are consistent with his concept of good fathering. A regulative ideal is thus an internalized normative disposition to direct one's actions and alter one's motivations in certain ways.
>
> This general regulative ideal is what Aristotle calls "practical wisdom" or *phronesis*, and this involves an understanding of the general good for humans and the capacity to deliberate well such that one realizes virtuous ends in one's response to particular situations.
>
> (Oakley and Cocking, 2001, pp. 25, 29)

How does – or would – such an idea work in nursing? To begin with it seems that we need (a) to know what it is that nurses do when they practise nursing, and (b) to have a clear image of what might count as good nursing. Oakley and Cocking suggest that this would be tantamount to a philosophy of nursing or a model of nursing.

To begin then let us consider what it is that nurses do. While there is still a great deal of empirical work to be done in order to better describe what nurses do, we are becoming clearer about the kinds of activities nurses engage in as nurses. For example, 2001 saw the publication of two studies

33

exploring the activities that nurses within the National Health Service of the United Kingdom are engaged in with respect to their daily practice (Buller and Butterworth, 2001; Jinks and Hope, 2001). The findings of Jinks and Hope in particular were mirrored in a study carried out in Scotland in the year 2000 (Dowding *et al.*, 2001). This study is currently being replicated in an Irish health service context. Preliminary findings indicate a pattern of involvement similar to that described by both Dowding *et al.* (2001) and Jinks and Hope (2001).

Early work in a programme of research examining clinical judgement and decision-making, also within the Irish context, indicates that nursing contribution across both mental health and general hospital settings can be broadly categorized into the assessment/monitoring of patient problems, indirect and direct nursing interventions, the co-ordination of care activities and the evaluation of care outcomes (Scott *et al.*, 2004, 2005; Treacy *et al.*, 2004, 2005). Though these studies are all fairly small scale in nature and diverse in kind, it is possible nonetheless to see similar themes being identified. Nursing emerges as a highly complex, multifaceted practice that places significant demands on the person of the practitioner – from an intellectual, experiential, emotional, technical and human perspective. For example, if we summarize the domains of practice identified by Buller and Butterworth (2001), they are

(a) Doing the job: assessing, being confident, informing, planning, intervening, reflecting;
(b) Relating and communicating: treating people with dignity, listening and responding, being reflective, gaining confidence, being aware of clients;
(c) Skilled nursing practice: caring intuition, ordinariness, role modelling;
(d) Being professional: being with the client, being adaptive, conveying confidence, being responsible, handling situations, being informed;
(e) Managing and facilitating: auditing, educating, providing confidence, supervising, making sure things get done, looking forward.

There is also a literature indicating the frustration of practising nurses who feel restricted or actively prevented, by resources or organizational structures, from carrying out what they see as one of their core contributions to patient care – that is, patient support. For example, Bowman (1995) describes the impact of under-staffing on staff morale and what his participants described as the fragmentation of care that resulted. There are, however, perhaps relevant questions to be raised here regarding the various perceptions of the appropriate role of the nurse – or indeed what is core to that role. As Hendel and Kidron (2000) point out, there may be discrepancies between expected and actual role behaviours related to a position. Expected role behaviours are defined as 'those responsibilities that are perceived to be important in daily work performance'. Actual role behaviours are defined as 'those responsibilities that are participated in during daily work performance' (Hendel and Kidron, 2000, p. 325). In Bowman's study, participants' perception of the nursing role suggests that the role of the nurse is to care for patients. Caring is understood here to consist in direct, 'hands-on' types of nursing activities. Bowman (1995) found that the nurses in his sample viewed their role as 'caring' and 'nursing', with the implication that 'hands-on' care was what nurses did. The Department of Health (1999) suggests that registered nurses should be able to carry out basic, routine personal care and clinical interventions, have responsibility and accountability for the assessment, planning, delivery and evaluation of that care, and also supervise others in carrying out this care. This overview of what it is believed a professional nurse does is mirrored in publications from An Bórd Altranais (2000), UKCC (2001), NMC (2002), National Council for the Professional Development of Nursing and Midwifery (2003), who also emphasize the ethical and professional issues attached to this process of care.

It is at this point that we can see that there is really something rather odd going on here. Ethical issues are seen as 'attached' to this process of care – important, it is acknowledged, but somehow supplementary to the core business of care. It is as if that core business could adequately be described in primarily technical terms, with values added as an embellishment, as it were. Yet these delineations of the role of the nurse – with their implications for nursing practice, education and research, as well as for the health service generally – cannot be sustained, I shall argue below, unless they are linked to the notion of virtue as a regulative ideal.

■ Nursing and ideas of the good

The actions of a nurse may be to the benefit or the detriment of the patient. Think, for example, of careless or incompetent care or neglect that leads to injury, pressure-sore development, lack of recognition of significant post-operative complications or malnutrition (see RTE Primetime Programme, May 2005 and BBC 1, 1999). And think, by contrast, of the kinds of cases described by Oakley (1993) where a young nurse is perceived by a patient as having a profound, beneficial impact on her care. This is perhaps the nurse who sits and listens, sensitively and intelligently, to a patient's concerns and then provides the needed information and support (Oakley, 1993). That these are indeed matters of good or harm should turn our attention readily enough to the moral dimensions of the domain of practice. I have argued elsewhere (Scott, 1993, 1996, 1997, 2000) that a virtue ethics approach, perhaps more than other ethical stances, enables us to flesh out this moral dimension of practice.

For a virtue ethics approach to work, however, we must articulate a notion of the good. A description of the virtues appropriate to a particular role is dependent on a conception of the good towards which that role is orientated and in terms of which it must be defined. Thus in this case, we need to ask, what is the good of nursing? Aristotle would approach this task by asking what the function of nursing is. It needs to be noted that this may be, but is not necessarily, the same question as asking what it is that nurses do.

It seems fairly uncontroversial to say that nursing must play a crucial role in the health service of the twenty-first century. But what kind of answer should we as educators provide in discussing the role of the nurse or the ends of nursing. Current descriptive accounts range from those of Buller and Butterworth (2001), described above, to those of Latimer (2000), who claims that nursing exists to perpetuate modern medicine. More philosophical responses regarding the proper ends of nursing also abound, including those of Henderson (1966), Levine (1977), Benner (1984), Gadow (1986), Peplau (1987) and Edwards (2001). These philosophical responses focus on the vulnerability of patients with the role of the nurse understood in terms of care and support for the patient. The common theme in all of these responses is the requirement for skilled practice across physical and psychosocial domains of human existence and experience. The nurse is there to do patients good, whether their health condition is a matter of acute, short-term illness or of more chronic illness and disability.

That the ends of nursing are understood in terms of this focus on patient support and adjustment makes it possible to begin to consider how they might be realized. What kind of person and what type of personal characteristics would help fulfill these ends? Personal characteristics that are of moral import may be called virtues of character. Hence, what virtues might need to be developed to help meet these ends? One thinks perhaps of compassion (Pellegrino, 1979), respect (Holm, 1997), honesty (Aristotle, 1953), humility (Murdoch, 1970), linked perhaps with the intellectual virtues of humour, wit and wisdom; some have suggested that clinical competence also can be seen in these terms (An Bórd Altranais, 2000; NMC, 2002). Professional education and professional socialization (Melia, 1987) should then be a concerted and orchestrated attempt to develop these virtues, among others, because the development of these virtues will lead to better nursing practice and to a greater chance of meeting the goals of nursing.

There is a measure of agreement in the literature to the effect that direct patient care activities, or activities that are directly patient-focused, such as advocating on a patient's behalf, are at least some of the important contributions that nurses make to health care delivery (de Raeve (1998, 2000), Edwards (2001), An Bórd Altranais (2000), Benner et al. (1999), Buller and Butterworth (2001), Scott et al. (2005)). I would suggest that in fact this is at the heart of nursing practice, and that indirect care activities, and activities around the co-ordination of care, provide the environment within which direct patient care activities can occur. This is true not only from a nursing care perspective, but from the perspective of the care provided by the multidisciplinary team. On this issue, and on the basis of a study exploring nurses' activities in caring for patients, Jacques makes the following comments:

> The nurses observed in this study often assumed responsibility for conveying information between one party and another, information relevant to the overall care of some patient, but not immediately neces-sary for the work at hand [. . .] despite the fact that this role was taken for granted both by those who perform it and those who benefit from it. All workers on that unit, physician, clinical nurse specialist, tech-nician, therapist, or maintenance worker, were routinely aided in the performance of their work by a network of nursing communication that
>
> - scans the environment
> - selects the information appropriate for the various workers, and
> - delivers this information to the recipients, who can concentrate on their specialized work, confident that such knowledge will just appear when needed.
>
> The existence of such networks of nursing communication is not a new discovery. They are described by Georgopoulos and Mann as far back as 1962. In this respect, nursing differs qualitatively from the other health care professions in that its domain – caring for the whole patient – involves connecting between all other expert domains. To the extent that nurses must claim recognition only through their legitimate tech-nical expertise (such as IV certification or diagnosis), the critical role of unifying the fragments of expert care delivery is hidden and under-valued. (Jacques, 1993, pp. 2–5)

People require nursing care, for example, when they are not capable of meeting all their own health care needs – when they are not able to manage basic activities of life, such as feeding, hygiene, dressing, mobil-izing; when they are in pain and distress, disabled, feeling ill and helpless; when their knowledge of how to cope with a particular situation or condi-tion is lacking. Henderson's famous definition of the nurse describes this quite well:

> The unique function of the nurse is to assist the individual sick or well, in the performance of those activities contributing to health or its recovery (or to a peaceful death) that he would perform unaided if he had the necessary strength, will or knowledge and to do this in such a way as to help him gain independence as rapidly as possible (Henderson, 1966, p. 15).

This notion of the nurse doing for the patient what the patient cannot do for himself suggests that nursing care should be a direct response to patient need. Nursing care should be undertaken with a clear view of what the patient needs and what the patient actually wants. Clearly these are not necessarily the same thing. It is at least possible to interpret Henderson's definition as requiring insights from the nurse. The nurse knows what the patient needs – otherwise she would not be able to care effectively for the unconscious patient or the patient compromised by illness, or to prepare the patient to regain independence. However, from the definition it also seems necessary that the nurse knows what the patient wants – at least where it is possible to ascertain this. If the nurse is to engage in the 'performance of those activities contributing to health or its recovery (or to a peaceful death) that he would perform unaided if he had the strength, will or knowledge [. . .]', then this suggests that the patient's views in terms of what care is desired are important. This also has clear implications regarding what drives the care patients receive from nurses, and what the focus of that care is.

Our literature is replete with claims about the centrality of care in nursing practice. We are, however, perhaps less clear on what this implies or actually requires of the individual nurse. Despite John Paley's concerns regarding the lack of wisdom in pursuing a concept analysis of care in nursing (Paley, 1996), it is important to articulate what *may* be required of the nurse and what essentially *should* be required of the nurse in the provision of nursing care. If we fail to do this, we cannot really know what to teach our students; we cannot clarify for individual members of the public what they can expect from a nurse when nursing care is accessed or forced, by circumstances, upon them.

■ A brief attempt to analyse care in the health care context

I have argued elsewhere (Scott, 1995) that students of nursing (and of medicine) should be encouraged and helped to examine and develop their understanding of care. Considering the concept under the four headings proposed by Blustein (1991) – that is *care for, care of, care about* and *care that* – may provide, at least initially, some structure and focus to the exercise. Discussion of one's role in terms not only of the kinds of duties, skills and procedures involved but also in terms of one's own investment in the role, and in one's patients, may help the nurse to consider some of the less tangible aspects of her role. The Scottish moral philosopher, Robin Downie seeks to capture this in the interrelated concepts of 'quality of role enactment' and 'moral strategy' (Downie, 1964, 1971). Downie explains role enactment as follows:

[ ] a person brings to his actions in his chosen role qualities which are not analysable in terms of the role. For example we may praise the shopkeeper for his courteous and cheerful service, but 'courteous' and 'cheerful' are terms of praise for the person's *enactment* of his chosen role; they cannot therefore be reduced to the concepts of the role itself (Downie, 1971, p. 133, emphasis added).

This is related to moral strategy. As Downie states,

[ ] the basic demands of duty can be exceeded not only by the saint or the hero but also by the 'moral strategist'. Thus it may be our duty to tell someone the truth about something, but when and how we go about this is a matter of 'moral strategy'. The importance of moral strategy is due to the fact that morality is a mater of relationship among people and no two people are quite alike in their outlook and response (Downie, 1964, p. 24).

We can see from Downie's explanations that moral strategy is a more reflective aspect of one's good role enactment. This is to say that while good role enactment refers importantly to expressive qualities of character that are not, of necessity, reducible to performative competence in the clinical sense, moral strategy, in combination with the former, marks out a higher order of sensitivity that aspires to a fuller recognition of the patient's current state as rendered by illness and associated forms of relative dependence. Thus when one focuses on the quality of one's role enactment and moral strategy it seems that almost automatically the focus of attention shifts from the practitioner to the patient. One tunes in to the particular patient in his or her particular situation, with his or her particular needs. To add to Downie's examples, if a nurse is giving information to patients, the way of approaching the matter appropriate for one patient may well not be appropriate for another. One method of approach may result, say, in making a patient very upset or in leaving a patient none the wiser, perhaps because she is unable to remember large chunks of what she has been told.

It may often appear that the 'virtues' of role enactment and moral strategy come naturally to some, while less so to others. I would argue, however, that both qualities require a certain degree of cultivation, and indeed enculturation through educative experience such that they are ultimately conceived of as an intrinsic dimension of the role itself. One important aim of teaching ethics to health care practitioners is to help them become better practitioners (for further discussion of this topic, see Scott, 1996). In this present chapter the idea of the better nurse is being understood in terms of care – care *of* and *about* the patient, and care *that* patient-directed, patient-orientated nursing is provided for patients. I have termed this approach to nursing care, which must, of course, involve competence in clinical and technical skills, *constructive care*. Constructive care, in taking account of the quality of role enactment and moral strategy, articulates the manner in which the ethical is *constitutive* of clinical practice as opposed to a subject that is simply taught in classrooms in the hope that it will somehow manifest in practice.

This mode of caring is, on occasion, profoundly demanding on the nurse in terms of energy, imagination, time and emotion. Evidently there are degrees of patient need and, therefore, degrees of demand that this type of caring places on the nurse. In order to be able to care constructively the nurse needs to be equipped accurately to assess the degree and type of need of the particular patient, and it will be this that directs the nurse's response. Patient need is very closely tied to human vulnerability. Human vulnerability is not a morally neutral state. Moreover, feelings of vulnerability, often heightened by illness, disease state, fatigue and emotional exhaustion, can be seen to demand particular kinds of responses, especially from doctors and nurses. In an empirical study exploring doctors' and nurses' ethical reasoning and decision-making, Holm (1997) expresses this moral call thus:

> When you meet the patient you meet another human being who is vulnerable, who trusts you, and whose life you can influence in a significant way. This creates a specific responsibility towards this other human being, which can be difficult to understand for outsiders, but which nevertheless plays a significant role in the deliberation of health care professionals. In their minds it is both related to the power they have, and to the respect they have to show (Holm, 1997, p. 127).

For care to be patient-based and patient-orientated means that the nurse begins from a point of respect and compassion. Respect for the personhood of the patient includes recognizing that the patient, before becoming a patient, was an individual who generally managed to maintain their life as a member of society, with all the competencies which that entails. The nurse needs to remember that illness or hospitalization does not automatically mean that a person has lost these competencies. This insight may demand advocacy activities from the nurse when other practitioners – or the organization as a whole – undermine patient respect or patient autonomy (Levine, 1977; Gadow, 1986; Jacques, 1993; Hirskyj, 2004). Sometimes this type of advocacy activity can place extreme demands on the nurse and others called upon to act in this way – Pink (1992), Hunt (1995), Bolsin (1998), Gueret (2003), Faunce and Bolsin (2004a,b).

■ Nursing and the idea of virtue as a regulative ideal

From the above discussion one begins to develop a picture of nursing, or a model of nursing (Oakley and Cocking, 2001), from which the goods of nursing can begin to be delineated. These goods of nursing include

- Clinical competence – without this the nurse cannot carry out basic elements of the job. The nurse thus cannot *have care of* her patients;
- Practical knowledge – the ability to use one's knowledge base for the benefit of *this* particular patient, in his/her *particular* circumstances;
- Respect for the personhood of the patient, which demands active attention to and accurate perception of patient vulnerability and consequent patient need;
- The courage to advocate for a patient when patient respect or patient good is being undermined (Faunce and Bolsin (2004b));
- Oakley (1993), Scott (2000) and Niven and Scott (2003) argue that an important element in being able to accurately perceive involves the ability of the nurse to feel empathy with or compassion for the patient in their particular situation;
- Such active respect in turn supports high-quality role enactment and moral strategy. High-quality role enactment and moral strategy are articulated through nurses *having care of* their patients, and also *caring about their patients* and *caring that* their patients receive appropriate, constructive nursing care.

It does, therefore, seem possible to begin to delineate the virtues that appear to be important to the realization of the goods of nursing. What then of the notion of virtue as a regulative ideal? Any model of nursing *per se* is liable to be somewhat abstract. Perhaps a better way to proceed here is to think in terms of role models as an important part of educative experience. Good role models may be very important in fleshing out the goods of nursing. Nursing has an 'oral' culture, and when nurses are together they often exchange stories – frequently educative stories about good or bad practice, and stories about our heroes and demons (Montgomery Hunter, 1996). Practitioners and students can very quickly call to mind and describe their 'ideal nurse': the practitioner who inspires them, the practitioner they would want to be like; the nurse who is skilled at her job, who cares for her patients, who listens to, respects and supports them; the nurse who in addition works well with, mentors, advises and teaches colleagues and students. This model is not so different from that described above by Buller and Butterworth. Niven and Scott (2003) have many descriptions of such performance. Consider, for example, the following concerning the performance of a breast care nurse specialist (E), taken from the diary of a woman (CN) who had been diagnosed with breast cancer:

> E's skill and respect for me as a patient were evident in a number of ways, on this occasion and on all succeeding occasions. I told her I was scared, I would have told anyone but she made it easy to say to her and her reaction, which was minimal, didn't make me feel foolish. Her behaviour made it entirely clear that she had understood my terror and was reacting accordingly. E knew I was an academic before she met me, so her conversation during the biopsy, clearly designed to distract me, utilized that knowledge. She told me about her Masters degree and the essay she stayed up all night word-processing and which had got lost. The topic was familiar enough to hold my attention and to remind me of situations in which I was a competent 'grown up' person; thus boosting my self-esteem and confidence. I nearly passed out at one point. Her skill in dealing with that was very evident – position, comfort, maintaining the circumstances which allowed the biopsy to continue; afterwards a glass of really cold water, keeping someone with me when she had to go. And everything done in a way which allowed me to maintain my dignity . . . E's behaviour during the biopsy established the basis for my total trust in her. This was vital when she became the person to communicate the confirmed diagnosis and the options for surgery (Niven and Scott, 2003, p. 205).

The skill, knowledge, understanding and humanity of this practitioner is very clear from the above description. It seems legitimate to ask if this is extraordinary practice or the practice of an extraordinary practitioner? Or, is this the practice of the virtuous nurse, conscious of the goods that nursing provides in patient care? The notion of an acceptable standard of practice is pertinent here. What comes through clearly, however, in this example is the sensitivity and humanity of the nurse. How this nurse comports herself in this role is salient; and part of this salience has to do with how she relates to her patient, in the strategies she uses to help the patient relax, to gain the patient's confidence and to support the patient's sense of autonomy – strategies that bear witness not only to the nurse's clinical skills but also to her humanity. Both her technical know-how and her personhood, in effect, are engaged to therapeutic ends. This again encapsulates Downie's concepts of the moral agent's role enactment and moral strategizing (Downie, 1964, 1971).

The issue for both the nurse and the patient is how to do the best possible for this patient. Incompetent care is clearly not acceptable. But what would competent care look like in this situation? Would skill in the clinical and pathological elements of the diagnosis and biopsy proced-ures be considered acceptable without the close attention to the person of the patient and without the provision of psychological and emotional care? Would the provision of the latter, but not the former, be deemed competent practice? CN remembers this nurse for the excellence of her care, the all-round excellence – not for mere competence in one element of nursing rather than another. So perhaps this goes some way to providing us with an answer. This practice is not reflective merely of a basic level of competence. The practitioner in this example impresses and provides a model of care that one can, as a nurse, be inspired by and that one will, as a patient, desire. From the perspective of a vulnerable, frightened patient, of someone who is potentially facing a life-threatening diagnosis, however, this quality of care is not an extra; its absence would be a life-diminishing loss.

Part of the answer to the question, 'What type of psychological or social support should nurses provide?' must surely come from consultation with our patients.

An essential element here may be to make the invisible visible. CN struggled to articulate the ways in which nurse E had provided such vital care:

> The sense of unlimited time and a depth of knowledge about a huge range of vital things – surgery, recovery, side effects and how best to manage them, the individual differences, the emotional consequences, the hands-on skills and her availability for anything – to be with you the first time you looked, when you got your prosthesis, for my husband, for my daughter, for me when I want, not according to a schedule . . . I have seen E many times now and her skills are always impressive but it's at times of shock and distress – diagnosis, admission, post-operatively – that they are most evident. It's like the matching pieces of a jigsaw – what she provides fits your needs so well that it makes something approaching a whole (Niven and Scott, 2003, pp. 206–207).

This analogy of the jigsaw reminds one of the interactional synchrony described by Schaffer (1977) in observing the attentive, bonding interaction in the early stages of the developing relationship between mother and new-born. It is also suggestive of the 'patient-led' style of assessment, one of three identified assessment styles used by district nurses (see Bryans, 1998). The patient-led approach, identified by Bryans, involves close attention on the part of the community nurse to the new patient who is being assessed, in order to develop trust and to obtain the information necessary to ensure that intervention is appropriate. In the above description of nurse E, however, what is striking is the consistency of behaviour and approach across a range of interactions. As CN indicates, she had met nurse E many times and her skills were 'always impressive'. The consistency of competence, sensitivity and responsiveness to the patient's needs seems to go beyond the operation of individual virtues. Do we not have here an exemplary image of the good nurse, one akin to Oakley and Cocking's 'good father'? The internalized conception of excellence, in this case excellence in nursing practice, helps the nurse to adjust her motivation and practice to that regulative ideal: 'A regulative ideal is thus an internalized normative disposition to direct one's actions and alter one's motivations in certain ways' (Oakley and Cocking, 2001, p. 29).

This conception of the virtues helps to explain the combined operation of many virtues that often seems to be required for the effective, competent and humane provision of nursing care. It also helps to explain the sometimes extraordinary lengths nurses will go to, despite constraining organizational structures, processes and culture, to try to 'humanize' the care environment for patients – for example, through buying small items such as birthday cakes or toiletries out of their own pockets, when unit resources are not forthcoming (Scott *et al.*, 2003); or through staying with a patient well beyond the end of their shift (Kellett, 1996); or again through going out of their way to visit or find information for a patient in need (Begley, 2004; Scott *et al.*, 2005). These instances of 'going the extra mile' are made more comprehensible by the notion of virtue as a regulative ideal.

All this can become extraordinarily demanding of the nurse. If this is the type of nurse we require, if we are to provide excellent nursing care, it is important that this is openly acknowledged. As noted above, the development of such virtue does not normally come about by accident. It must be supported and planned, according to Aristotle, from the earliest exposure of the individual to models of virtuous behaviour, through habit formation to education. Thus, certain elements must be put in place. Our organizational structures, processes and resources must support the nurse in developing the appropriate personal characteristics (virtues) and ultimately in the internalization of an image of the good nurse that regulates the nurse's conception of appropriate practice.

■ Conclusion

As we move through the early years of the twenty-first century, we are becoming much clearer about what is important in nursing practice and the nursing contribution to health care – from both a patient care and a professional perspective. We need, therefore, as this chapter has attempted to show, to ensure that the elements of this are carefully articulated, examined and supported, and that this informs the education of students, including the development of those virtues appropriate to the profession.

Oakley and Cocking's (2001) notion of virtue as a regulative ideal is helpful, as we have seen, in describing what is at work when a practitioner provides excellent patient care. The notion of virtue as a regulative ideal helps make sense of the drive in many practitioners to go beyond the call of duty, and beyond the constraints of organizational structures, processes and resources, in an attempt to provide good care for the patient. The provision of such care should not, however, depend solely on the sense of responsibility of individual nurses. Each one of us, as members of society, has a responsibility to ensure that such care is possible.

Chapter 2

Philosophy and health education: The case of lung cancer and smoking

Peter Allmark and Angela Tod

■ Introduction

At first blush it may seem odd to introduce the notion that the educational preparation of nurses to undertake a health education role has, in itself, an ethical dimension worthy of further exploration. That is what we set out to do in this chapter, in the following way. We critique the philosophical underpinnings of what we term the 'standard view' of health education: that health education is a treatment like any other treatment and should be judged as evidence-based medicine. Implicit in this view are answers to two philosophical questions. The first concerns the method for the judgement of health care treatment (of any sort); the standard view is that all treatments should be judged by whether or not they are evidence-based. The second concerns whether or not health education should be judged in the same way; the standard view is that it should.

The chapter begins by setting out the standard view of health education. We then set out a case study that illustrates how health education can have some unintended and harmful effects. This enables us to draw out three criticisms of the standard view. The first is essentially an empirical criticism: it is that health education is not actually evaluated in the same way as other treatments. This does not constitute a rebuttal of the standard view, of course; one who holds that view may reply that health education should be evaluated in the same way as other treatments even if it has not been heretofore. However, this leads us onto the next two criticisms, both of which are philosophical.

The first philosophical criticism is that the standard view ignores the role of values in our attributions of health and illness. What is termed 'education' is actually an attempt to impose a particular risk-averse view of how it is best to live, and, therefore, has an ethical dimension. This is because health education does not attempt to give a treatment for something which both patient and health care professional agree is an 'illness'; rather, it attempts to change people's values so that their view of health and its place in a good life concords with that of the health educator. This, in our view, is unacceptable. The second philosophical criticism is that health education should not be judged in the same way as other treatments, because it is education, not treatment. Education should be judged primarily in terms of its effects on the knowledge of those educated, not in terms of whether they change their behaviour to accord with the desires of the educator.

In our discussion of these criticisms we suggest that, first, the empirical criticism is probably well grounded, although it is not the primary focus of this chapter. We offer a rebuttal of the first philosophical criticism largely through a rebuttal of the libertarian view of health and health education from which the criticism generally emanates. However, we find the second philosophical criticism to be more compelling. Insofar as health education is education rather than treatment it should be judged differently. Further-more, viewing health education as treatment is compatible with practice that involves deception or lying; this is unacceptable to those who hold to a non-consequentialist ethic. Let us begin, then, with the standard view of health education.

■ The standard view of health education

Health education practice has been directed and influenced by a number of theoretical models (Tones, 1983; Ewles and Simnett, 1985). All take into account a range of issues. These relate in varying degrees to health, disease, risk factors, and social and environmental factors (Ewles and Simnett, 1985; Downie *et al.*, 1990). However, health education has been criticized for focusing too much on lifestyle and neglecting larger structuralist issues that influence health (Macdonald and Bunton, 1992). This distinguishes health education from health promotion, which has been referred to as 'health education plus' (Cribbs and Dines, 1993, p. 27). In health promotion, health education activity is seen as combined with preventative health care and health protection (Tannahill, 1985, 1990).

The working definition of health education that we adopt here is one that interprets the activity in its broadest sense. That is,

> The sum total of all influences that collectively determine knowledge, belief and behaviour related to the promotion, maintenance and restoration of health in individuals and communities (Downie *et al.*, 1990, p. 27).

Our focus here, however, is particularly on the intentional health educa-tion activity performed by health professionals as an inherent component of their practice. In the UK, a recent Government White Paper outlining

prospective health policy points to several examples of good health education practice in which nurses play a key role, for example, stop-smoking
clinics (Department of Health, 2004). The White Paper, and related documents, sets out a number of targets in six key areas including smoking,
drinking and obesity; for example, to reduce smoking prevalence to 21%
by 2010. Local bodies are also encouraged to set their own targets. The
role of nurses is central to realizing the targets inherent in this policy.

Health education is also a mainstay of nursing curricula. As such, nurse
education seems to be doubly involved with this intervention: first, it is
something for which nursing students, at both undergraduate and post-
graduate levels, need to be prepared through education, and second, such
preparation is an educational intervention in itself. At the same time, health
education is not an area that has often come under a more considered
ethical and philosophical scrutiny. There are a few notable exceptions
to this. In particular, libertarians of both the right (Skrabanek, 1990;
Le Fanu, 1999) and left (Seedhouse, 1997; Fitzpatrick, 2001) have raised
many concerns. At the heart of these is the feeling that health education is
part of a paternalist (or 'Nanny State') strategy. The White Paper dismissed
these concerns lightly, saying,

> [ ] too often work to tackle longstanding, intractable or emerging prob-
> lems was increasingly caught up in a sterile national debate [ ] that
> created a false dichotomy between those proposing a heavy handed
> Nanny State on one hand, and those supporting inactivity bordering on
> neglect in the name of individual freedom on the other (Department
> of Health, 2004, Para. 6).

The force of this dismissal lies in an emphasis on 'informed choice', references to which lie throughout the document. The idea is that the role
of health education is not to enforce change upon people for their own
good, as a 'Nanny State' would, but to give people the best opportunity to
make healthy choices should they so wish (Allmark, 2006). And in practice, few clinicians seem to have expressed the libertarian concerns. Health
education has an intuitive appeal: 'a stitch in time saves nine'; in other
words, it is better to prevent people becoming ill than to treat them once
they are. This is backed up by evidence that shows that health education
is a cost-effective intervention. The nature of this evidence ranges from,
for example, randomized trials of smoking cessation advice (Pieterse *et al.*,
2001) to cost effectiveness studies[1]: Health education appears to be good
evidence-based medicine (EBM). Given this, nurses may even feel it ironic
that the majority of their time is organized around care for people with
acute and chronic illness rather than around its prevention.

However, it is worth noting that this EBM approach takes health education to be 'medicine', a treatment or intervention just like any other. But
here two philosophical questions arise. The first is whether treatments of

any kind should be judged against the EBM standard; the second is, if so, whether health education should be judged against this standard just like any other treatment. Whilst these two questions are not generally posed explicitly, there are implicit answers that can be gleaned from current practice. These constitute, for want of a better term, the philosophy underpinning current practice. Let us examine this philosophy.

Our first philosophical question asks whether treatments should be judged against the EBM standard. It seems pretty clear that most health care professionals would answer this in the affirmative. There is some concern over precisely what constitutes 'evidence' and whether some evidence is too lightly dismissed (Barry, 2006; Buetow, 2006; Goldenberg, 2006; Paley, 2006), but the general idea that treatment should be based on evidence is widely accepted. Our second philosophical question asks whether health education should be judged in the same way as other treatments. At present, current practice seems to imply an affirmative answer here. Health education initiatives are to be judged like any other interventions, on the basis of their effect on health and illness. However, a caveat is needed. Health education is likely to produce its effects only in the very long term. Therefore, usually the only realistic way of judging it is to see whether it results in a desired change in behaviour correlated with illness or its prevention, such as smoking or taking exercise. This is generally the method of judgement chosen: health educationalists are charged with changing the behaviour of a given population, such as reducing the incidence of smoking.

We shall call the philosophy underpinning the practice of health education described in the previous paragraph, the standard view. We now begin our critique of this view with a case study.

■ Case study

A 62-year-old man (Bill) gave up smoking 25 years before presenting to his GP with left-sided chest pain. Both he and his wife had been prompted to give up smoking when they had their first child. They were motivated by the risk of passive smoking to their child, and by the desire to be fit and well and able to support and raise their children.

They were advised by health education messages at the time of stopping smoking that, if they gave up, their risk of developing lung cancer would revert to that of someone who had never smoked. This belief was reinforced by subsequent public information messages that echoed this view and linked lung cancer firmly to smoking. As a result, Bill and his wife did not consider themselves at risk of lung cancer.

Bill was previously fit and active until six months prior to presenting to his GP. He had enjoyed hill-walking as a pastime before his illness and worked with his son as a plumber. Bill and his wife had developed a cough, which they put down to a routine winter infection. His wife recovered but Bill did not. His continuing symptoms were explained by a number of factors including dust from his work. After two months Bill started to get increasingly short of breath and developed haemoptysis. He thought this was due to straining and trauma from the cough. The symptoms persisted. When he started to get discomfort at the left side of his chest he went to his GP, who prescribed antibiotics and sent him for an X-ray. By the end of May his symptoms had not improved. One night he had a large haemoptysis. His wife phoned for an ambulance and he was admitted to hospital. Following a CT scan and bronchoscopy, Bill was diagnosed with terminal lung cancer and commenced a course of palliative treatment. Had he presented his symptoms and been diagnosed earlier it is possible he would have been eligible for a curative intervention.

At no time did Bill consider himself at risk of lung cancer. It did not occur to him that his symptoms indicated such a severe problem. This was because of the information he gleaned from health education messages, his status as a long-term ex-smoker, and a lack of awareness of lung cancer symptoms and other risk factors in addition to smoking (e.g. passive smoking). He did not know that non-smokers and ex-smokers could develop lung cancer.

■ Case examined from the standard view

How does this case look under the standard view? The first question it would ask is whether the treatment or intervention has been effective in terms of illness avoided. It seems likely that the intervention has been highly effective; Bill has almost certainly had extra years of life free from smoking-related illnesses. As a bonus, his family has been protected from the effects of second-hand smoke. Furthermore, the intervention has been very cheap, particularly when set against the costs of treatment for smoking-related illnesses earlier in life; Bill may, for example, have developed angina before eventually succumbing to lung cancer. Of course, there is a caveat: at the end of Bill's life the treatment, health education, had an unfortunate side effect in that Bill did not recognize the symptoms of lung cancer as early as he may have done if it hadn't been for the intervention. However, from the standard viewpoint, this side effect seems minor when set against the many extra years he probably benefited from not smoking.

Turning to the second philosophical question, the standard view judges the health education intervention as it would any other treatment; it asks whether it is effective or not in terms of illness treated or avoided. Judged in this way, health education appears to be a cheap and effective way of avoiding premature death and illness due to lung cancer. Clearly, the behaviour of not seeking help that Bill displayed at the end of his life was unfortunate. If we could find a way of avoiding its recurrence then the treatment would be even better. Nonetheless, it is good as it stands.

■ Empirical criticism of the standard view

Some critics of health education have implicitly accepted the standard view but have raised questions about whether practice has been judged as would be other treatments. Skrabanek (1990), an early critic of health education and health promotion, suggested that its interventions were not properly evaluated in the way that other interventions are. The evidence base for health education is epidemiology; this shows the links between modifiable behaviours and health outcomes (e.g. smoking and lung cancer). These links provide the justification for health education measures (such as media campaigns) to take place. Those measures are evaluated largely in terms of whether people change their behaviour in significant numbers and whether the required impact on health is achieved. However, this is to judge health education only in terms of its positive effects; the assumption seems to be that it cannot harm and so we only need to look at whether it has good effects or not. Bill's case suggests otherwise. Taking the example of lung cancer and smoking there seem to be at least three possible harms.

The first is that lung cancer has become a 'cancer of blame'. Smokers who are harangued each time they visit their GP become reluctant to do so (Butler *et al.*, 1998). They may be embarrassed to mention certain symptoms for fear of a 'what do you expect?' response (Smith *et al.*, 2005). As a result, those symptoms may be missed.

The second is that ex-smokers (and their health professionals) may believe they are not at risk of lung cancer. This is reinforced by health education literature and by 'objective' measurements such as carbon monoxide monitoring (which shows the lungs to be 'clear' after the smoker gives up). As such they seek other explanations when symptoms of lung cancer emerge. However, those who have given up smoking for more than 30 years have a risk ratio for lung cancer of 0.1 compared to current smokers; the risk ratio for lifetime non-smokers is 0.03 (Peto *et al.*, 2000). In other words, ex-smokers still have a risk of lung cancer several times greater than lifelong non-smokers. Ironically, it is possible that ex-smokers could fare worse than smokers once initial signs of lung cancer emerge because they and the health care professionals are less likely to take heed of them.

The third is that even non-smokers sometimes get lung cancer, particularly if exposed to other risks, primarily second-hand smoke (Scientific Committee on Tobacco and Health [SCOTH], 2004). They too may respond inappropriately to symptoms if health education messages do not alert them to their risk because of their sole focus on smokers.

Thus health education can harm even when based on overwhelmingly good epidemiological evidence. Perhaps then we should simply say that health education should be scientifically evaluated and economically judged just as any other health measure. This can be done in cluster randomized trials, as in the case of the REACT study, an evaluation of a population-based intervention to reduce delay in reporting chest pain (Luepker *et al.*, 2000). This showed that a particular health education intervention was ineffective in producing a desired behaviour change. Where a health education intervention is shown to be effective through such evidence, we may say, it is right to use it.

However, unease about Bill's case does not just lie in the question of whether or not the particular health education intervention had been properly evaluated. Indeed, it seems likely that were we to evaluate such interventions they would be effective in behaviour and health terms. As we have seen, from the standard view the case could be judged a success for health education. The concern we have seems to be more ethical or philosophical than empirical. Roughly it is that Bill's lifestyle change in giving up smoking was based on untrue beliefs that were at least in part down to the health education he received. Let us turn, then, to philosophical criticism of the standard view and see how Bill's case looks from a different angle.

■ The standard view and the judgement of the effectiveness of treatment

As we have seen, the first pillar of the standard view is the idea that health care interventions should be judged by the empirical evidence in terms of whether or not they prevent illness or promote health. At first sight this seems obvious. However, a major problem lies in the role of value judgements in our attributions of health or illness to people (Allmark, 2005). Critics argue that illness is not a fact but rather a judgement of the facts. Take the example of a tumour in the brain. We take this to be an illness. But imagine that this particular tumour is always associated with an increase in intelligence and protection against neurological degeneration in old age. Would we then be seeking to develop treatments in order to get rid of it? We would not. Any condition becomes an illness or disease only when it is linked to things we disvalue, such as pain or death.

The importance of this is that health and illness cannot be viewed as objective facts about individuals. Whether or not we judge someone to be ill will be a function of our values; and given that values vary between individuals, so too will attributions of health or illness. This makes it far from straightforward to judge a treatment on the basis of how it affects health or illness. Let us illustrate this with a (partly) fictitious example. It is well known that runaway slaves in America in the 1800s were sometimes said to have a mental illness termed 'drapetomania', a pathological urge to escape (Kingwell, 2003). Imagine it is found that drapetomania is associated with lack of protein in slaves' diet. Slaves fed meat twice weekly are less likely to run away. Health educationalists concerned with a high incidence of drapetomania in a particular State put out information to slave owners recommending they adopt this diet for their slaves. The slave owners respond favourably and the incidence of drapetomania declines. Presumably we would not view this as an example of successful health education. We do not share the view that drapetomania is an illness nor that its absence is a sign of health.

It follows that the basis for judging health education against its effect on health and illness should be a shared view of health and illness based on shared values. Libertarian critics of health education suggest that this is absent. Their starting point is a view of human beings and the human good akin to that given by Mill (Mill, 1972). For Mill, the human good lies in individuals undertaking unfettered experiments in living through which they find (what Gray [1983] terms) their quiddity. This is the set of goods that match each individual's personality. This will vary between individuals. Mill thought that humans would share certain intellectual pleasures (e.g. finding that poetry is better than pushpin[2]); however, later libertarians have tended towards Bentham's hedonist view that people should pursue whatever pleases them and that for many this will not be intellectual pursuits. For libertarians, the problem with health education is that it is based on a particular view of the human good in which one avoids doing things that may risk one's health. They believe that for many individuals, life would be miserable without smoking, taking drugs, drinking too much, indulging in risky sports or sex and so on. This is not just hedonism, either. Hilary Graham's research showed the importance of smoking for single mothers in deprived areas. For these mothers, smoking may have presented a risk to their long-term health, but in the short term it relieved stress sufficiently to keep them going without, say, hitting their children (Graham, 1987). Furthermore, the prospect of a long life may seem far less attractive if one is facing the suffering of an impoverished old age in a rundown housing estate. Thus health education can be accused of trying to persuade people to adopt a view of the good that may not match either their quiddity or their circumstances. How might one respond to this criticism?

The libertarian view has at least two major problems. The first is political. Libertarianism values the autonomy of the individual above all: each person must be free to pursue her ends in order to discover her quiddity. Having found it, she must be free to live in accordance with it. The state must not interfere 'for her own good' as only she can know what her own good consists in. But note the forbidding of state interference: one such interference is protecting individuals against the consequences of their decisions. Hence, any state provision of health care is forbidden.

In effect, state provision of health care is forcibly making people pay for health insurance. A consistent libertarian must forbid this for it is imposing choices on people that they may not wish to make. If I choose to take the risk of not having health insurance then that is part of my experiment in living. Under a libertarian system, a young person who takes this risk and who develops, say, leukaemia must live and die by his decision. Thus the political problem with libertarianism leads to the following *ad hominem* argument against it: libertarianism forbids state provision of health care; if you believe in such provision you are not libertarian. And insofar as you are not libertarian, you believe that certain values have an importance that is greater than simply being able to choose to live in accordance with whatever values one happens to have. For example, to believe in a State health care system is to believe that health has a value over and above its value in terms of whether or not individuals choose, say, health insurance. This leads directly to the next point.

The second major problem with libertarianism is more directly philosophical. It is that it treats values as having three attributes: first, they are given to each individual; second, they are individually varying; and third, they are unassailable. It treats them as given in the sense that there is a given quiddity to be uncovered in each individual. Through experiments in living, the individual will uncover this quiddity. The values he ends up with will accord with this quiddity. For example, as a teenager someone may value poetry but later in life he discovers that his quiddity is such that he much prefers pushpin. It treats values as individually varying in the sense that we all have our own, differing, quiddity. It treats values as unassailable in the sense that there is no rational argument one person can put to persuade another to adopt his view of the good. I may say you should stop smoking because it risks your health but if your quiddity results in your not valuing the risks and benefits of smoking in the way I do, my suggestion will be utterly unpersuasive.

All three of these attributes can be questioned. Perhaps the best way of doing this is through analysis of the concept of health itself. If one person continues to smoke or indulge in dangerous sports and cannot be persuaded to give up he will almost always accept that his practices risk his health. What he does not accept is that his health should take overriding priority over his dangerous pleasures.[3] However, we have seen that our picture of health depends on our values. Despite this, it seems, there is a very widely shared picture of what constitutes health and illness. Across almost all individuals and cultures, pain and death are disvalued. Other things being equal, it is better not to be in pain or to die prematurely, it is better not to be limited in the use of one's limbs or to get breathless before others do. This almost universal picture of health and illness shows that we can talk about them in quasi-objective terms. The statement from the risk-taker is not, say, 'I don't think lung cancer is illness' but rather, 'I think smoking is a pleasurable risk to health that is worth taking'. Similarly, the statement from the women in Hilary Graham's study is that the immediate therapeutic effects of smoking outweigh its long-term harms, not that those harms don't exist.[4]

If there are shared values allowing us to construct a shared notion of health and illness then the idea that values are unassailable also becomes questionable. The fact that we share many core values allows us to see, for example, that a teenager bent on suicide or self-harm having been spurned in love is almost certainly making a mistake. Whilst his current value-set results in him perceiving his well-being as worth nought without his loved-one we may view this as very probably a temporary straying from shared values. As such, we would feel free to try to persuade him from his course of action and perhaps even forcefully to prevent him pursuing it.

The libertarian may concede that these are generally shared values. However, he would argue that such shared values do not allow us to construct a notion of the importance of health that would justify the view that smoking is wrong for all people. Such a libertarian, though, does not realize the extent of this concession. It amounts to saying that, other things being equal, it is better to be healthy than ill; unless there is a worthwhile pay-off, one should avoid courses of action that lead to illness. The health professional can therefore approach the public knowing that there is a value put upon health that is widely shared; other things being equal, almost all would rather maintain good health than not. This provides sufficient ground for health professionals to undertake health education. Roughly, the health professional can say, 'I know that you value health. I will provide you with information that will help you adapt your behaviour to protect it.' Individuals will then have the information with which to decide whether to change or maintain health-risking behaviour.

One could take the account further. One might say that we don't just happen to share the values that allow us to construct our notion of health; human beings share these values because of the sort of creatures they are (see more on this in Chapter 12 of this book). This would be to take a naturalist path. Pursuing it allows one to say that not only do people share these values but that, insofar as they are human, they ought to share them. It may also allow us to say that it is possible for people to be mistaken if they do not value health enough. It would give us ground to say that, for example, most smokers are mistaken in the value they place on smoking.

This naturalist and Aristotelian route has been pursued by a number of writers (Megone, 2000; Allmark, 2005). For our purposes we do not need to go down that route; enough has been said to suggest that libertarian critics of the standard view can be rebutted. It is reasonable to judge health care interventions against their effects on health and illness even though these notions are dependent upon values. Let us turn next to the question of health education in particular and whether it should be judged in the same way as other treatments.

■ The standard view and the judgement of the effectiveness of health education

In the case study presented above it seemed plausible that the health education intervention should be judged a success in that it was cheap and probably resulted in many extra years of disease-free life for Bill. However, perhaps we would not call it a success in terms of education; Bill and his wife had a false belief that, at the end of his life, caused him to misinterpret the early symptoms of lung cancer.

Here it is useful to draw on a distinction suggested by Campbell (1991) between indoctrination and education. Education takes place when one undertakes an intervention with the intention of appealing to the agent's reason, helping the agent to learn something new or see something rightly. Indoctrination takes place when one seeks to induce change in an agent in a way that bypasses her reason.

This suggests there are at least two ways in which health education interventions may be evaluated. The first is behavioural: an intervention would be deemed successful were it to lead to behavioural changes that improve the nation's health. The second is cognitive: success would be judged by the extent to which the public acquires accurate epidemiological knowledge about health matters.

The behavioural criterion seems to be predominant. For example, the White Paper *Choosing Health* and related papers set out numerous behavioural targets; it sets out no cognitive ones (Department of Health, 2004). The argument for using such targets is that in health terms what matters is what people do rather than what they think or say. The problem is that this argument is one that would support indoctrination should it be more effective than education. Faced with intransigent public behaviour, health educators may be tempted to frame information using advertising techniques; whilst the messages may, strictly speaking, be true, the impression conveyed is false. A well-known example of this is the use of the striking relative risk figures (behaviour x trebles your risk of illness y) rather than the more sober absolute risk (behaviour x causes your risk of illness y to be a certain level).

The temptation to frame information is reinforced by the prevention paradox (Rose, 1985; Hunt and Emslie, 2001; Allmark, 2006; Allmark and Tod, 2006). This arises because behaviours tend to have a normal distribution. Persuading people who are at the high-risk end of this distribution to change their behaviour will benefit their health in individual terms. However, in terms of the whole population's health one would have greater impact by persuading people who are in the middle section of the distribution. This can mean that one must persuade people who are not at particularly high risk of harm from their behaviour to change it anyway. Some have argued that this has occurred in the case of current alcohol limits (Fitzpatrick, 2001). Clearly the message, 'What you're doing isn't particularly bad for you but we'd like you to stop anyway' is unlikely to be effective. For this reason it may be tempting to exaggerate the benefits of behaviour change.

Hence the behavioural criterion for judging health education can lead to interventions that are misleading and, sometimes, harmful; to indoctrination rather than education. One outcome of this is the phenomenon of excessive advocacy whereby people come to believe that some behaviour, such as smoking, is more hazardous than it is and, conversely, that changing behaviour is more beneficial than it is (Seedhouse, 1997). By contrast, the cognitive criterion requires health educators to convey information that is clear and non-proselytizing.

■ Implications

Those engaged in health education, especially at a senior level, are increasingly judged by their success in meeting behavioural targets at a population level. Inevitably this leads to some tension in the role. We have seen that values have a central function in both (a) our attributions of health and illness and (b) our decision making in relation to behaviour that presents a risk to our health. Libertarians object to the health education role because they view values as individually given, individually varying and unassailable. We have shown that this position can be rebutted. As such, health education interventions are, in principle, defensible. More worrying, though, is the judgement of the effectiveness of health education as a treatment *simpliciter*. Judging health education in this way may tempt health care professionals to pursue the route of indoctrination rather than education. An alternative way of judging health education is as education. This would involve adopting a cognitive rather than a behavioural criterion.

We have focused on a case involving smoking and lung cancer; similar points could be made about health education in other areas. In Bill's case, on the behavioural criterion the health education should be judged a success. On the cognitive criterion its success is partial. He learned some of the risks and seemed to make a well-thought-through judgement. On the other hand, there seemed to be some excessive advocacy resulting in a false reassurance about the possibility of lung cancer in the future. In cognitive terms it would have been better had he known the truth.

In Bill's case, having the complete picture may also have been better in health terms as well. However, the problem for the cognitive approach is that this may not always be so. There may be occasions where conveying partial, carefully framed information to the public is more effective in behavioural and health terms than is conveying the complete picture; the prevention paradox suggests this may be so. In deciding whether to prefer the behavioural or cognitive criteria one may have to choose between a consequentialist and non-consequentialist ethic. In consequentialist ethics, deception and lying may be acceptable for a greater good. The behavioural criterion for judging health education leads us down this route. In non-consequentialist terms, deception and lying are generally unacceptable. If one chooses to go down this route one may have to accept that the ethically best option is not necessarily the one that is most effective in health terms.

■ Conclusion

This chapter began by identifying nurses as key players in health education. It has ended by showing that health education performed under present guidelines, in which behavioural ends predominate, risks practice which is, in non-consequentialist terms, unethical. At the very least, we hope to have shown that the answers to philosophical questions that arise through educational preparation for practice sometimes matter a great deal. Health education is one area where they do. In terms of the educational preparation of nurses to adopt a health education and promotion role, this leads to a rather odd dilemma. It is a dilemma in which both evidence and ethics appear to engage, if not in a contradiction, then certainly in a perpetual fibrillation that gives rise to the question of what is best to do. We would argue that this needs at least to be acknowledged and taken into account in educational programmes for nurses. This is not to minimize the importance of preparing nurses for a health education and promotion role. Rather it is to enrich it by promoting a philosophical dimension that calls us to the work of thought in that curious space where the individual stands face-to-face with the collective canon of accepted knowledge.

■ Notes

1   See (Cromwell *et al.*, 1997, and also Tengs *et al.*, 2001, along with Yu *et al.*, 2004). For contrary evidence, however, see Salkeld *et al.* (1997).
2   Pushpin is a simple game popular in the Victorian era. Mill was concerned to show that intellectual pursuits, such as poetry, give superior pleasure to simple ones, such as pushpin. Bentham was a more consistent utilitarian here, believing that for many people this would not be true. We refer to it once more a little later in the text. We do this to suggest the idea that most libertarians would probably take Bentham's line rather than Mill's.
3   As we wrote this, an interesting example arose. A well-known television presenter crashed a jet-powered car and was nearly killed. In the press discussion of this at least two threads of opinion were discernible. The first was that the television centre had recklessly violated standards of health and safety; the second, that the presenter's behaviour was a triumph over the Nanny State and that people should resist the attempts of health and safety officials to take risk out of our lives.
4   Although the harms may be less significant to the women because a long life may not be particularly valued, as we pointed out above.

Chapter 3

Foucault, nurse counselling and narrative therapy

Tina Besley

■ Introduction

This chapter makes the case for the relevance of narrative therapy for
those nurses involved in counselling, whether it be in practice or education, as a model for nurse counsellors. First, it introduces the growth
and significance of nurse counselling. Second, it explores the impact of
the work of Michel Foucault on narrative therapy and the challenge this
mode of counselling makes to psychological discourse and humanist counselling. Third, the chapter outlines and discusses narrative therapy as a
mode of counselling suited to the demands of nursing. The discussion
explores ways in which educators of nurses can be encouraged to see the
relevance and importance of these issues, and considers how they can be
helped to develop insights into the practices in question that may then
influence or inform their engagement with patients, students, carers and
others. The chapter draws on themes I have developed in earlier work.[1]
The purpose of this chapter is obviously not to teach people how to
become narrative therapists. Rather it is to introduce and elucidate the
ideas that underpin narrative therapy. Chief among these is an ethical
concern and engagement with the other, whether it be the patient or the
student, and in which no prior form of stereotyped identity or categorized problematic is assumed. Thus every engagement with a client, patient
or student is a new journey to the hermeneutic horizon of a personal
narrative in the making. We often forget that words and concepts, especially when spoken in presence, carry within them a certain power to
inspire, defeat, humiliate, normalize, unlock, affirm, stifle, create, damage,
enlighten, heal, deflate and degrade, anger, gratify, awaken or sedate, to
name but some. Second, the power that discourses carry also have a history
in which they contingently emerged for various purposes and ends. Unless
untangled, both ethically and politically, this historical power can appear
to 'naturalize the present' as if every would-be therapeutic engagement
was a progress to some pre-determined end, or normative state. One of
the main purposes of the ethico-political ideas behind narrative therapy

is to problematize this assumption. In doing so, my intention is not to criticize the growth in nurse counselling in various areas of practice, but rather to enrich it by introducing broader concerns that may be taken on board.

Nurse counselling is a highly generic term that does not always apply to trained counsellors; rather it is the case that educators and practitioners often find themselves in what amount to counselling situations, including the assessment of students in clinical practice. This in turn necessitates a certain awareness of what may be 'going on' when these events occur. My main purpose in this chapter therefore is to provide a different, and indeed poststructuralist perspective on this, in which individual lives may be re-authored rather than 'authorized' by the expert, whether educator or practitioner. But first, I begin by overviewing the growth and significance of nurse counselling.

■ The growth and significance of nurse counselling

Caring for patients, nursing's *raison d'etre*, requires a high level of expertise in interpersonal skills (Leininger and Watson, 1990; Tschudin, 1995; Morrison and Burnard, 1997; Watson, 1999). Not surprisingly, once counselling became established as a profession, the idea of using counselling in nursing emerged strongly from the 1980s and is now well established in theory and to a lesser extent in practice (Tschudin, 1995). Yet in many parts of the world, in a context of neoliberal financial constraints, nurses have been forced to cut back patient contact times, so time for counselling is often simply not available and may not even be tolerated except in certain situations. With the current dominance of concerns about meeting performance targets and budgetary constraints, as part of applying medical procedures, except for some areas of patient care, supporting patients and their families as they face emotional stress and upset in relation to their health issues can sometimes take a lower priority.

While a core element of most nursing is the clinical-medical aspect, arguably nursing has always been located in a dialogical situation where practitioners have been more concerned with and closer to the patient's subjective world than most other health care professionals. Herein lies a structural tension for nurses. Patient dialogue historically has been largely an informed one based on listening skills and notions of care for the other, as exemplified in the first chapter in this book. There are, therefore, some pre-existing elements and tendencies that tend to favour the use, development and application of counselling in the broadest sense as a general aspect of nursing, but more recently as a professional post-qualifying and post-graduate specialization.

Several research studies attest to the value of nurse counselling. As comment on an article in the *British Journal of General Practice* (Holloway *et al.*,

2003), an article in August, 2003, issue of *Practice Nurse* posed the question, 'Nurse counselling key to fewer smear tests?' The study in 29 practices in Wales aimed to find out if high-quality information about risk could help reduce women's fears about cervical cancer and found that when practice nurses provided a brief (10-minute) counselling session women felt more reassured, less anxious and more comfortable with the recommended 3-year interval between tests (Holloway *et al.*, 2003). A Danish study 'Nurse Counselling of patients with an overconsumption of alcohol' concluded that frequent counselling and positive attitudes towards prevention reduced alcohol consumption. Not surprisingly, since they are the professionals most likely to be dealing with patients with alcohol problems, psychiatric nurses were most active, followed by medical nurses then surgical nurses as the least active in counselling. Nevertheless, the study concluded that

> To promote nurse involvement in alcohol prevention, increasing the capacity for intervention via skill-based training on assessment of alcohol problems and intervention techniques is necessary: all nurses, but especially surgical nurses, needed updates on alcohol-related counselling (Willaing and Ladelund, 2005, p. 36).

Based on a UK study of 894 women, an article, 'Study links nurse counselling with lower hysterectomy rate' in *RN* in 2003, summarizes a study published in the *Journal of the American Medical Association*, vol. 288, no. 21, 2003, p. 2701 (Schiff, 2003). It stated that 'women with menorrhagia were less likely to have a hysterectomy if they received nurse counselling about their treatment options'. Furthermore, women who received 30 minutes of counselling prior to their specialist consultation reported being more satisfied with their treatment and with their role in treatment decisions than those in the control group who received neither counselling nor an information pack.

A report on a conference paper presented by David Katz, University of Wisconsin, Madison, at the annual meeting of the American Society of Preventive Oncology, stated that 'smoking cessation rates rose "dramatically" in primary care practices where nurses and medical assistants used a brief counselling intervention with patients who smoked' (Moon, 2002, p. 16). The study of adult smokers (642 in the intervention group and 499 in the control group) who presented to practices for routine non-emergency care were counselled by non-physician practice staff (mainly registered nurses and licensed practitioners). The practice staff were trained to do a very brief initial smoking assessment and counselling intervention of 2–3 minutes and to put a modified 'vital signs' stamp on each patient chart so that the patient's smoking status was recorded on subsequent visits. Patients were questioned about their desire to quit or not within the next 6 months. Those opting not to quit were given a patient education pamphlet on the benefits of quitting. In addition, those opting to quit were 'given a voucher for free nicotine replacement therapy [. . .] provided with brief counselling in support of quitting, and given the business card of a trained smoking cessation counsellor' (Moon, 2002, p. 16). Katz argued that since 70% of smokers in the United States visit their primary care physicians at least once every year, approaching patients with a brief nurse counselling intervention prior to counselling from trained smoking cessation counsellors would mean that 'potentially two million more smokers would quit annually if approached this way in their doctors' offices' (Moon, 2002, p. 16).

Studies such as these seem to confirm beliefs about the efficacy of nurse counselling and yet none of these interventions comprise anything like what a professional counsellor would consider to be 'counselling'. These interventions are all too brief and stand more in the domain of 'advice' rather than traditionally non-directive forms of counselling. Furthermore, they do not require anything like the level of post-graduate training that is required to become a professional counsellor in most parts of the world. Though they are studies of worthy interventions, they are somewhat misleading in being termed 'nurse counselling'.

So, what is counselling and what is nurse counselling? National counselling associations tend to not supply a definition and counselling texts can be quite convoluted in attempting definitions. Rather than a definition, the British Association for Counselling and Psychotherapy (BACP) has an 'ethical framework for good practice in counselling and psychotherapy' which includes a statement of values that goes a long way towards a definition:

> The fundamental values of counselling and psychotherapy include a commitment to
>
> - Respecting human rights and dignity
> - Ensuring the integrity of practitioner–client relationships
> - Enhancing the quality of professional knowledge and its application
> - Alleviating personal distress and suffering
> - Fostering a sense of self that is meaningful to the person(s) concerned
> - Increasing personal effectiveness
> - Enhancing the quality of relationships between people
> - Appreciating the variety of human experience and culture
> - Striving for the fair and adequate provision of counselling and psychotherapy services
>
> Values inform principles. They represent an important way of expressing a general ethical commitment that becomes more precisely defined and action-orientated when expressed as a principle (http://www.bacp.co.uk/ethical_framework/).

The BACP then lists and explains the following six principles:

Fidelity: honouring the trust placed in the practitioner.
Autonomy: respect for the client's right to be self-governing.
Beneficence: a commitment to promoting the client's well-being.
Non-maleficence: a commitment to avoiding harm to the client.
Justice: the fair and impartial treatment of all clients and the provision of adequate services.
Self-respect: fostering the practitioner's self-knowledge and care for self.
(http://www.bacp.co.uk/ethical_framework/).

As a component of its code of ethics, The New Zealand Association of Counsellors' (NZAC) website statement on the 'nature of counselling' reads,

Counselling involves the formation of professional relationships based on ethical values and principles. Counsellors seek to assist clients to increase their understanding of themselves and their relationships with others, to develop more resourceful ways of living, and to bring about change in their lives.

Counselling includes relationships formed with individuals, couples, families, groups, communities and organizations (http://www.nzac. org.nz/).

Notions of what constitutes counselling, as indicated above, imply a philosophy of being and knowledge about who/what we are, and how we think and relate to our world. Philosophy has influenced how we think of knowledge, what can be known, the relationship between the enquirer and the known (epistemology); of ourselves and of others, of being and reality, so understanding some of the key ideas associated with these becomes an important means for contextualizing nursing education. Dossey notes that neither 'being' nor ontology is generally discussed in nursing or medical education, and that 'health care to be complete, must focus on more than doing – it must also address matters of being' (Watson, 1999, p. viii).

Nursing tends to find itself between an engagement with the physically oriented bio-medical sciences and the social sciences. Critical social science draws attention to the existence of power relations between the patient/client and the professional. Often these notions are taken-for-granted, viewed as natural or seen as being uncontested and therefore not open to question. When competing views exist of what counts as science, it is easy to see that questions of epistemology, ontology and ethics are inextricably bound up with the whole enterprise. Yet the question of the aims of science and research can only be answered if we first investigate what view of science or research the discipline embraces, and the implications of this for education and subsequent practice. Hence the case exists for including introductory courses on philosophy of medicine and nursing that encompass epistemology, ontology and ethics, on care of the self and of others.

The introduction of nurse counsellors goes some way to addressing this and of contributing to a legitimate and funded place for a return of interpersonal caring into nursing. It extends traditional scientific, physically based medicine. The concept of nurse counsellor tends to generally be separate from the form of counselling or psychotherapy that is available within the mental health arena, so this chapter excludes discussion of that speciality. Nurse counselling that generally focuses on sexual issues and dying is currently available in some countries. Nurse counselling tends to be available for people with life-threatening and degenerative diseases (e.g. multiple sclerosis, motor neuron disease and cancer, etc.) and for those in hospices. It also tends to be available for people undergoing fertility and gynaecological treatments (e.g. pregnancy screening tests for genetic disorders and prenatal invasive procedures) and for those being treated for sexually transmitted diseases including HIV/AIDS.

An integral aspect of the medical model has long been the emphasis on the physical body and the application of medico-scientific techniques in order to effect a cure or an improvement that at least does no harm, while largely ignoring the emotional has often meant a tendency towards both pathologizing and totalizing people – of seeing them, and even calling them by their illness or condition rather than as whole individuals. Narrative therapy is not anti-medication, and in fact the Dulwich Centre website acknowledges the value that some people may gain from medication (including anti-psychotic medication) but notes that 'in other circumstances, it can be used in ways that are primarily for the purposes of social control' (http://www.dulwichcentre.com.au/). Narrative therapy does, however, question and challenge the sort of pathologizing practices that are common within health professions, including medicine and nursing (White, 1995). Rather than the person being the problem, it views the problem within the wider socio-cultural context such that where medication is involved, narrative therapists are interested in exploring with people a range of questions to assist in clarifying what is and what is not helpful in relation to the medication. While the word 'therapy' tends to focus on the treatment of disease or disorder, in narrative therapy problems are not constructed in terms of disease, nor as effecting a cure per se (White and Epston, 1990). Using narrative therapy in nurse counselling rather than traditional forms such as behavioural or humanistic would start to address some of the obvious problems of power relations that the medical model engenders and would acknowledge a more holistic, socio-political, relational and emotional context that people negotiate in their lives.

■ The challenges of Michel Foucault and narrative therapy to psychological discourse and humanist counselling

The work of the philosopher-historian Michel Foucault (1926–1984) looks closely at the social archaeology of practices of the self in Western culture. Foucault provides us with 'creative, controversial, and original thinking on philosophical–historical–social ideas. Yet he did not propose any grand, global, utopian, or systematic solution to societal ills' (Besley, 2002a, p. 2). He was neither a counsellor nor a psychotherapist, but obtained his *licence de psychologie* in 1951 and a diploma in psychopathology in 1952 and subsequently worked in a psychiatric hospital in the 1950s. Foucault's early work was oriented towards psychology, psychopathology, madness and psychiatry. However, regardless of the subject matter, it is the force of his critique that opens up possibilities for how we might see, understand and, in turn, negotiate our subjectivity and the power relations in our world, and so Foucauldian philosophical notions of care for the self, confession and technologies of the self are relevant to all aspects and specialities of counselling, including nurse counselling.

The work of both Friedrich Nietzsche and Martin Heidegger helped Foucault to develop his ideas on how human beings become subjects and to move from his earlier work that emphasized the disciplinary aspect of power relations, normalization, domination and political subjugation of 'docile bodies' to an understanding of humans as self-determining beings continually in the process of constituting themselves as ethical subjects (Foucault, 1977, 1986). His earlier work discussed the relationship between the subject and 'games of truth' in the human sciences (such as economics, biology, psychiatry, medicine and penology) that have developed knowledge and techniques for people to understand themselves in terms of either coercive practices (psychiatry or prison) or theoretical-scientific discourses, for example the analysis of wealth, language and living beings (Foucault, 1970, 1988, 1997).

Nietzsche inspired Foucault to analyse the modes by which human beings become subjects without privileging either power (as in Marxism) or desire (as in Freud). For Foucault, power is not simply something negative used by one person or group to oppress others, but can also be productive, positive, and a set of complex strategies where there is also resistance (Besley, 2002b) For Foucault, power is *power-knowledge* since

> power produces knowledge and [ ] power and knowledge directly imply one another: that there is no power relation without the correlative constitution of a field of knowledge, nor any knowledge that does not presuppose and constitute at the same time power relations (Foucault, 1977, p. 27).

In Foucault's *Discipline and Punish*, the body becomes both an object of knowledge and a site where power is exercised (Foucault, 1977). The critically reflective counsellor not only asks how power in the counselling relationship constructs the knowledge of the self for both parties, but also how the relationship might be developed. Counselling might be developed in line with Foucault's ethics as a practice of caring for the self, as a form of self-mastery rather than one of self-denial (see Besley, 2005).

Foucault's analytical method of genealogy (inspired in part by Nietz-sche's *On The Genealogy of Morals*, 1956) conducted by moving backwards in a process of descent and forwards in a contingent process of emergence, rather than through evolution or an internal process of development, forms a critical ontology of our selves (Foucault, 1984a). Thus Foucault challenges the humanist idea that the self is unified and fully transparent to itself and that consciousness is linear, storing memories in the same way as a novel progresses a plot. It also challenges the progressivist agendas of the Enlightenment by emphasizing dispersion, disparity and difference, taken-for-granted universal 'truths' about life. This is not to say that Foucault was anti-Enlightenment. He just invites to look at it in a different way (see Foucault, 1984a).

Late in his life, as his understanding of the self shifted under the influence of Heidegger's work (see Besley, 2003b), Foucault sets out a typology of four interrelated 'technologies' – namely, technologies of production, technologies of sign systems, technologies of power and technologies of the self (Foucault, 1988). Each is a set of practical reasoning that is permeated by a form of domination that implies some type of training and changing or shaping of individuals. Technologies of power 'determine the conduct of individuals and submit them to certain ends or domination, an object-ivizing of the subject' (Foucault, 1988, p. 18). Technologies of the self are ways the various 'operations on their own bodies and souls, thoughts, conduct, and way of being' that people make either by themselves or with the help of others, in order to transform themselves to reach a 'state of happiness, purity, wisdom, perfection, or immortality' (Foucault, 1988, p. 18). He clarified 'that, while the human subject is placed in relations of production and of signification, he is equally placed in power relations that are very complex' (Foucault, 2001, pp. 326–327). Furthermore, he admits that he may have concentrated 'too much on the technology of domination and power' (Foucault, 1988, p. 19). For Foucault both technologies of domination and technologies of the self produce effects that constitute the self (Foucault, 1988). They define the individual and seek to govern their conduct as they make the individual a significant element for the state through the exercise of a form of power, which Foucault coined as governmentality in becoming useful, practical citizens (Foucault, 1991). By this time, Foucault not only provides quite a shift from earlier discourses on the self, but also brings in notions of disciplinarity, governmentality, freedom and ethics as well as notions of corporeality, politics and power and its historico-social context into understandings of the self.

Foucault points out two forms of 'subjugated knowledges' that are lowly ranked and considered inadequate for the accepted standards of knowledge and science:

> One constitutes previously established, erudite knowledges that have been buried, hidden, disguised, masked, removed, or written out by revisionist histories; another involves local, popular, or indigenous knowledges that are marginalized or denied space to perform (Besley, 2002a, p. 17).

In recovering these knowledges, we can rediscover the history of struggle and conflict and challenge the power-knowledge institutions and scientific discourses (Foucault, 1980c). It is these subjugated knowledges that narrative therapy seeks to harness in developing alternative narratives that challenge the dominant stories in peoples' lives (Besley, 2002a,b).

Narrative therapy was initially developed in 1989 by Michael White (Adelaide, Australia) and David Epston (Auckland, New Zealand) as a form of family therapy (White and Epston, 1990). Narrative therapy is part of the turn to 'narrative', located within broad movement within philosophy, the humanities and the social sciences known as the linguistic turn (Rorty, 1967). Detailed descriptions of the main features, arguments and practice-related examples of narrative therapy are available elsewhere (see, e.g., White and Epston, 1990; Parry and Doan, 1994; Smith and Nylund, 1997; Monk *et al.*, 1997; Winslade and Monk, 1999, 2003; Payne, 2000; Speedy, 2000). Rather than being developed from psychological discourse, narrative therapy is a synthesis of the work of several social theorists including Michel Foucault and is philosophically grounded in what is now referred to as poststructuralism (see Peters, 1996, 2001; Peters and Burbules, 2004; Williams, 2005).

Poststructuralism, which initially developed in France in the 1960s from the work of Derrida, Lyotard, Foucault, Deleuze and Baudrillard, draws from a variety of sources to provide a specific philosophical position strongly informed by the work of Nietzsche and Heidegger (Peters, 1996). Poststructuralism is not only difficult to define, but is also often confused or conflated with 'postmodernism' with which there are philosophical and historical overlaps, although it needs to be emphasized that their relation is not one of identity. Its specific philosophical position challenges the overly optimistic and social scientific pretensions of structuralism and reappraises the Enlightenment notions of universality and rationality (Peters, 1996). Peters (1999) argues that the theoretical development of French structuralism during the late 1950s and 1960s led to an institutionalization of a transdisciplinary 'mega-paradigm' where the semiotic and linguistic analysis of society, economy and culture became central to the scientific analysis of socio-cultural life in diverse disciplines such as anthropology, literary criticism, psychoanalysis, Marxism, history, aesthetic theory and studies of popular culture. Structuralism helped to integrate the humanities and the social sciences but did so in an overly optimistic and scientistic (science as an ideology) conception. Poststructuralism offers a challenge to the scientism of structuralism in the human sciences, an anti-foundationalism in epistemology and a new emphasis upon 'perspectivism' in interpretation (that there is no one textual 'truth' but that texts are open to multiple interpretation). Poststructuralism challenges the rationalism and realism that underlies structuralism's faith in scientific method, in progress. It challenges the way structuralism's totalizing assumptions had been elevated to the status of a universally valid theory for understanding language, thought, society, culture, and economy, and indeed, *all* aspects of the human enterprise (Peters, 1999). In other words, it is suspicious of metanarratives, transcendental arguments and final vocabularies (Lyotard, 1984). These views involve the rediscovery of Nietzsche's critique of truth and his emphasis upon interpretation and differential relations of power, and also Heidegger's influential interpretation of Nietzsche.

Poststructuralism can be defined in terms of both its affinities and continuities on the one hand and its theoretical innovations and differences with structuralism on the other (Peters, 1999). Poststructuralism shares structuralism's radical questioning of the problematic of the humanist (Cartesian–Kantian) subject as rational, autonomous and self-transparent. It also shares with structuralism a theoretical understanding of language and culture as linguistic and symbolic systems. The two related movements share a belief in unconscious processes and in hidden structures or socio-historical forces that constrain and govern our behaviour. Finally, they share a common intellectual inheritance and tradition based upon Saussure, Jacobson, the Russian formalists, Freud, Marx and others. Poststructuralism's innovations involve the reintroduction and renewed interest in history, especially the 'becoming' of the subject, where genealogical narratives replace questions of ontology or essence.

More recently, poststructuralism has developed a political critique of the way modern liberal democracies construct political identity on the basis of a series of binary oppositions (e.g. we/them, citizen/non-citizen, responsible/irresponsible, legitimate/illegitimate) that exclude 'others' or some groups of people. In this sense, poststructuralism can be seen as a deepening of democracy and Enlightenment values. Perhaps, most importantly, poststructuralism explores the notion of 'difference' (from Nietzsche and Saussure, and developed in their different ways by Derrida, Deleuze and Lyotard), which serves as a motif for recognizing not only the dynamics of 'self' and 'other', but also contemporary applications in multiculturalism and immigration. Poststructuralism invokes new analyses of power, particularly Foucault's 'analytics of power' and the notion of 'power/knowledge', both of which differ from accounts in liberal and Marxist theory, where power is seen as only repressive (see Peters, 1996, 1999, 2001; Peters and Burbules, 2004).[2]

On a poststructuralist account, it is held that language not only affects how we frame our notions of the self and identity, but also how counsellors deal with people and the meaning they make of the world they live in. A poststructuralist and Foucauldian stance allows for an examination of self, cultural contexts, power-knowledge, the way power relations shape, legitimize and constitute personal narratives and the assumed neutrality of institutions that often seem unaware of their power-knowledge relationships. Hence narrative therapy offers new ways of thinking about people and about therapy and counselling.

Notions of power have been 'much overlooked in the therapy literature generally, and in the benign view that we frequently take of our own practices' (White and Epston, 1990, p. 18). In therapy discourse, power has usually been considered 'in individual terms, such as a biological phenomenon that affects the individual psyche or as individual pathology that is the inevitable outcome of early traumatic personal experiences, or in Marxist terms as a class phenomenon' (White and Epston, 1990, pp. 18–19). Subsequently, feminist discourse alerted many therapists to issues of abuse, exploitation and oppression in a gender-specific and repressive analysis of power. But therapy has not considered the more general problematics of power – both its obligatory and constitutive aspects and the operation of power-knowledge (Foucault, 1980c).

■ Relevance of narrative therapy to nurse counselling

The Dulwich Centre, Adelaide, Australia, founded by Michael White, describes narrative thus:

> It centres people as the experts in their own lives and views problems as separate from people. Narrative therapy assumes that people have many skills, competencies, beliefs, values, commitments and abilities that will assist them to reduce the influence of problems in their lives. The word 'narrative' refers to the emphasis that is placed upon the stories of people's lives and the differences that can be made through particular tellings and retellings of these stories. Narrative therapy involves ways of understanding the stories of people's lives, and ways of re-authoring these stories in collaboration between the therapist/community worker and the people's whose lives are being discussed. It is a way of working that is interested in history, the broader context that is affecting people's lives and the ethics or politics of therapy (http://www.dulwichcentre.com.au/).

Like all forms of knowledge, narrative therapy has developed its own specific 'language' or terms that describe its therapeutic processes. For narrative therapy, both the words and how they used are important, so the language is deliberately non-sexist, and ethnic-neutral. Moreover, it avoids medical model terms that many mental health professionals use and which unthinkingly objectify and pathologize people, therefore, White never uses 'cases' or 'case histories' and has replaced the term 'client' with 'person' (Payne, 2000). 'Speaking' and 'voice' are used as metaphors for the agency of the client (Drewery and Winslade, 1997, p. 43). Language can blur, alter or distort experience as we tell our stories; it can condition how we think, feel, and act, and can be used purposefully as a therapeutic tool (White, 1995). These include problem-saturated descriptions; dominant stories; externalizing conversations and naming the problem using metaphorical language (e.g.,'sneaky poo', 'voice of doubt' and 'black thoughts'); using relative influence questions to map the influences of the problem; externalizing internalizing discourses; deconstructing the problem to find alternative stories and unique outcomes, experiences or 'sparkling moments'; inviting the person to take a position; client and counsellor uniting against the problem; using therapeutic documents; constructing a history of the preferred story; re-authoring the story by telling and re-telling to enrich the self-narrative; creating an audience of sympathetic outsider witnesses to revised stories; re-membering; reflecting teams; preparing for the future through possibility questions; and an ending ceremony (White and Epston, 1990; White, 1995; Monk *et al.*, 1997; Winslade and Monk, 1999; Bird, 2000; Morgan, 2000; Payne, 2000). Details of what these features are and how they operate are widely available in what has, in the last fifteen years, become a burgeoning literature. It is also interesting that there is now a growing interest and literature in what is called 'narrative-based medicine' (see, e.g., Greenhalgh and Hurwitz, 1998, 1999; Launer, 2002, 2003).

Externalizing language is used throughout narrative therapy because the problem is seen as outside the person, not embodied within as part of their psyche, personality or being and the aim is to stop people being disabled by the problem. This becomes a very powerful understanding for people because it challenges the operation of deficit theory that not only blames and/or shames people for what appears to be their chosen lifestyle, but also encourages them to think that they have to change, grow, develop or improve, thus inadvertently reinforcing the power of experts and institutions that aim to help people achieve this. However, it is important to note that abuse or violence is not addressed in this manner but is named directly (see Jenkins, 1990). Narrative therapy uses a deconstructive conversation to find ways of subverting dominating patterns of relating that the person finds problematic and to open spaces for possible change. In a move that decenters the therapist, a narrative conversation uses shared contributions. This seeks to respect that it is the person who is expert in their own life and who has personal/local knowledge, skills and ability, which they can tap into to help solve their problems. Naming the problem is something that therapists invite the person to do and negotiate with them, but the actual decision on the name or even to use naming is up to the person who may then challenge how it has been taking over things in their life. Unlike other therapies, especially the Rogerian Person Centred Therapy, that see questions as intrusive and threatening and so avoid them, the narrative therapist asks creative, curious, persistent questions, yet this is nothing like an interrogation but is part of a dialogue. The questions aim to explore the meanings of the person's world, to examine socio-politico-cultural assumptions in that world and to find subplots that are richer and closer to actual experience and to facilitate co-authoring the person's unique story. They are also used as a means of checking how the person is finding the direction of the conversation, their comfort with what and how things are proceeding, to ask their permission about taking notes and about using therapeutic documents.

One of the distinguishing features of narrative therapy is the use of therapeutic documents, especially in the later stages of counselling – the addition of a literate means rather than only a verbal means of therapy (White and Epston, 1990). The form such documents might take includes letters of invitation to engage people who are reluctant to attend therapy; 'redundancy' letters that refer to roles people have assumed over some time that have now become redundant, such as, 'parent-watcher, parents' marriage counsellor, brother's father' (White and Epston, 1990, p. 90); letters of prediction as a form of follow-up; counter-referral letters; letters of reference; letters for special occasions and brief letters (see White and Epston, 1990, Chapters 3 and 4). The literate mode enables the recording of linear time and maps experience onto the temporal. It assists short-term memory and enables people to be 'more active in determining the arrangement of information and experience, and in the production of different accounts of events and experience' as they produce meaning in their lives (White and Epston, 1990, p. 37). More recently, Martin Payne suggests therapeutic documents might include visual elements, 'letters, statements, certificates and creative writing' to 'encapsulate new knowledges, perspectives and preferred changes which have become part of the person's enriched but still perhaps slightly fragile view of her remembered experience' (Payne, 2000, p. 127). Engaging an audience that is significant to the person and harnessing the power that is so often assigned to the written word becomes an effective way of validating the person's alternative story by briefly documenting the changes that he/she has made in their life.

The professional stance taken by narrative therapists differs from that of many medical and 'psy' professionals. It aims to avoid the unintentional objectifying professional gaze that can occur when the therapist is unaware of their role as professional expert in constructing a therapeutic dialogue.

Narrative therapists do not present themselves as distant, objectively neutral experts who diagnose problems and prescribe solutions and treatments. Instead, the stance is a curious, interested and partial participant in the person's story. Narrative therapists adopt an optimistic, respectful but a 'not-knowing', tentative or curious stance using listening, language and therapeutic skills to assist people to find inconsistencies, hidden assumptions and contradictions in their stories. Alternative and enabling narratives are not just consistent stories, but are stories that are richer and closer to experience and make meaning for people. People regularly work to make sense and meaning of their lives, so to respect their knowledge and stories and to empower them, narrative therapy considers that it is not the counsellor's task to apply 'expertise' to make sense of other people's lives. Empowerment is seen in a general sense of 'teaching' people ways to understand the discursive conditions and power relations of their lives, and how they might *re-author* their lives and to find and use their own voice and to work on the problem to find their own solutions (Drewery and Winslade, 1997).

Although client-centred to the extent that the person is the focus, paradoxically, narrative therapy is directive in its use of questioning, but encourages people to find their own voice (Drewery and Winslade, 1997; Winslade and Monk, 1999; Speedy, 2000). Unlike traditional counselling practices, it does not privilege the client's voice or the binaries of the dominant versus the marginalized, hidden voices, or local versus expert knowledges. While accepting the equal validity of each voice, it acknowledges that 'some voices have more meaning-making power than others', thus it impacts on power relations for the client as well as the counsellor and his/her practices (Speedy, 2000, p. 365).

As noted above, the turn to narrative was thoroughly endorsed as a practice for GPs recently in the *British Journal of General Practice*, as a means to 'balance evidence-based medicine with the other attributes of good doctoring including attentiveness, imagination, humanity and literacy' (Launer, 2003, p. 91). He points out that in primary care, patients 'bring their "broken stories", inviting professionals to help fix them' (Launer, 2003, p. 92). Although many will want GPs to,

contribute elements of the scientific "grand narrative" that we have brought from our medical training and professional knowledge, and that they may need some practical and technical solution, such as a prescription, injection or hospital referral. However, they are unlikely to want a new narrative that is wholly constructed around a hierarchical doctor-patient relationship or a reductionist scientific understanding, now will they be willing to accept anything we say or do unless it makes sense as part of a story that they can construct and own themselves (Launer, 2003, p. 92).

Launer concludes that narrative-based medicine is a giant philosophical leap because in many ways it 'turns the conventional biomedical approach – and even the patient-centred one – on its head. Instead of listening to the "the patient's history" to determine what to do, it judges our actions by whether they contribute to an improvement in the patient's narrative' (Launer, 2003, p. 92). As an extension of this philosophical and practical change, the use within nurse counselling of narrative therapy would be a further move in helping patients make meaning of their lives, since narrative therapy 'represents an alternative to the pragmatic, empiricist, instrumental therapies and health care systems that have come to dominate the global psychotherapy scene in recent years' (McLeod, 2000, p. 333). Narrative therapy challenges and forces a re-evaluation of the dominant and to a large extent unquestioned/unquestionable truths of traditional psychological and humanist counselling discourses and ways of thinking about the self, and is an important new modality of counselling for health care educators to be aware of, and for nurses to use with their patients.

■ Conclusion

As stated in the introduction to this chapter, not every health care practitioner or educator will train to become a narrative therapist, but it is the principles and ideas behind the practice that I have sought to emphasize, for these can be incorporated into both educative and clinical practice. It is clear that the principles of narrative therapy seek to promote a hermeneutic dimension in which horizons of meaning or understanding are not fixed, but rather are always in a state of continuous becoming. In a poststructuralist sense, this is done by coming up against the limits of the structures of convention, where even identity itself can be loosened from the sedimented constructions of its own history. Thus the politico-ethical dimension of narrative therapy is not a code by which one abides; it is a practice that one undertakes.

■ Notes

1 In particular I have discussed poststructuralism and the critique posed by the work of Michel Foucault to traditional humanist notions of the self (Besley, 2002a,b; Besley and Edwards, 2005). Narrative therapy is a further theme (Besley, 2002a,b). I have examined Foucault's notions of technologies of the self, confession and notions of self-denial and self-mastery (Besley, 2003a, 2005). A further theme is an examination of the Cartesian duality of mind/body (Besley, 2003b).
2 For an analysis of the intricate relationship between structuralism and poststructuralism, see Williams (2005) in which he also gives an excellent account of five major poststructuralist philosophers, along with an excellent guide and bibliography.

Part 2

Profession, Knowledge and Practice

Chapter 4

Care, sensibility and judgement

Michael Luntley

◼ Introduction

In this chapter I want to use the following scenario as the basis for investigating the concept of experiential knowledge:

> A nurse in an intensive care unit (ICU) has charge of the care of a patient who is recovering after major surgery. The patient has a feeding tube and is unable to communicate verbally with the nurse. In addition, given the level of sedation, the patient has limited opportunity for communicating their needs in any other way. The protocol in the ICU is for feeding tubes in cases like these to be removed six days after surgery. By the third day, the nurse has a growing concern that the patient is uncomfortable with the tube. By the fourth day, the nurse's concern is so strong that she takes the decision to remove the tube. She has no articulate account of why she thought this was the right action. The most she can say is that she had a 'feeling', an 'intuitive sense', that this would greatly enhance the patient's comfort. After removal of the tube the nurse is proven right, and as the patient recovers the nurse is thanked for removing the feeding tube at that time.

I will now explore the above scenario through four main stages that relate to care, sensibility and judgement.

◼ I

We can contrast the action of the nurse in the above situation with that of a less experienced nurse who in a similar situation follows the ICU protocol and has no sense that in so doing they might not be giving the best care for the patient. I shall disregard issues about the status of the unit's protocols and whether or not the nurse at issue has infringed any regulatory requirements of her hospital.[1] What I want to focus on is the following simple thought: it is tempting to say that the experienced nurse makes her decision on the basis of experiential knowledge. This is something that, by definition, the less experienced nurse lacks. But the question is what does it mean to speak of experiential knowledge and how can we acknowledge a role for it in situations, like the above, where the nurse has limited or negligible ability to articulate why they acted as they did?

I shall assume that the above nurse acted professionally and made use of something that is commonly available to professional nurses in the management of their performance. That is to say, I think there is such a thing as experiential knowledge that can, as in the situation above, be outwith the scope of the subject's capacity to articulate what they know. As such, this is to allow that part of what we should accommodate within the notion of experiential knowledge is out of the reach of judgement.[2] In the above scenario, the nurse can offer no judgement about why she did what she did. All she has is an inarticulate sense that what she did was called for or was appropriate in that situation. But why that situation was different to others in which she had obeyed the unit's protocol is something on which she has no conceptual grip. Plenty of theorists have labelled this phenomenon but, thus far, there is no detailed account of what is really going on in such situations.

Benner (1984), following Dreyfus and Dreyfus (1986), would account for the above as a case of 'intuitive knowledge'. Dreyfus and Dreyfus's developmental trajectory from novice to expert is one that starts with explicit rule-formulated propositional knowledge and leads to perceptual knowledge that operates in an intuitive way. This is fine as a first description of what we think is going on, but it offers no real purchase on exactly what it is that the experienced nurse possesses and the novice lacks. To say that the difference is one of 'intuition' is simply to label the difference. It is not to provide an account of it. This matters, for it seems to me that it is a plausible constraint on an adequate account of experiential knowledge that the theory has some consequences for how this knowledge can be taught. Simply saying that it is intuitive gives no guidance on what sorts of experiences one needs to provide to the novice in order that they may acquire the experiential knowledge of the experienced nurse. It seems implausible to think that merely by observation alone one would pick up this knowledge. Furthermore, to treat the experienced nurse as an expert is to miss out a further stage available in the trajectory from explicitly propositional knowledge to experiential knowledge.

I shall say that the nurse in the opening scenario is an 'inarticulate expert', for she has *ex hypothesi* limited or negligible capacity for artic-ulating why she did what she did. She has experiential knowledge that differentiates her performance from the novice who rigidly follows the protocol, but she has limited capacity for articulating this knowledge. That leaves room for a further stage in the trajectory of expertise, a stage marked by noting the differentiation between the inarticulate expert and the artic-ulate expert, where the latter is the nurse able to articulate their decision and bring their understanding within the realm of judgement. Not only then should a theory of experiential knowledge have consequences for how one can educate a nurse so that they move along the trajectory from novice to inarticulate expert, it should also offer the resources to show how that trajectory can be continued to that of the articulate expert. Note, in requiring this, I am not assuming an evaluative preference for the role of the articulate expert over that of the inarticulate. Indeed, I take it an advantage of the account of the trajectory from novice to inarticulate expert that I offer that it provides sufficient resources to capture the nature of learning involved that there is no need, purely from the point of being able to offer instruction in such matters, that the expert be an articulate expert. That is to say, my model of experiential knowledge provides sufficient detail to make sense of a form of instruction and learning that is deeply practical and detached from the capacity of the learner and instructor to articulate what the latter is passing on to the former. I suspect that the majority of experienced nurses combine some mix of inarticulate and articulate expertise and that instruction of novices by experts involves both types of expertise.

■ II

One of the first things to say about our inarticulate expert is that she is engaged in pattern recognition. She has a skill for discriminating regularities governing the comfort and need of patients. This capacity to discriminate and keep track of such regularities plays a role in guiding her own action. That is, I shall assume, uncontentious. The point at issue concerns what it means to recognize regularities and to act on their detection when the agent has no conceptual grip on the regularities that would enable her to talk of them and use her knowledge of them to justify her behaviour. Simply to talk about 'skills' without giving an account of what sorts of skills are at issue gives no purchase on what experiential knowledge is.

I shall assume then that our inarticulate expert nurse has a capacity for discriminating features of the patient's condition that are causally relevant to managing care. Furthermore, her discrimination of these causally relevant features is deployed in controlling her behaviour. What we need is an account of what this capacity for discriminating the relevant causal features consists in and how it contributes to the control of expert behaviour. Given that I am assuming that the concept of the inarticulate expert makes sense, these capacities must involve a level of awareness prior to conceptual awareness.

Following Dreyfus and Dreyfus, Benner's model allows for a preconceptual level of awareness. The account is influenced by Heidegger's discussion of capacities for handling tools. Although it is descriptively suggestive and, *prima facie*, phenomenologically accurate to speak of the way the skilled craftsman finds tools that embody a 'readiness to hand' and feels that their agency flows through the tools, such ideas make little or no headway in providing a model of the discriminative capacities at issue. Simply to posit a content to experience that is beyond the reach of conceptually organized judgement gives no account of how this level of awareness is related to conceptual awareness, nor of how it figures in the control of behaviour.

Furthermore, the phenomenological appeal to our sense of involvement in handling tools is too gross a description, for it does not adequately distinguish the preconceptual from the conceptual. Often enough, our sense of involvement with tools is conceptually structured. Consider the skilled craftsman who sees the apprentice handling a tool incorrectly. The craftsman may not have a description for the appropriate way of handling the tool, but their discrimination of the appropriate handling can still be articulated demonstratively. They might say to the apprentice, 'Don't handle it like that. Do it like this.' The articulation of their discrimination might deploy contextually sensitive language, but that does not make it nonconceptual. It simply shows up the availability of contextually sensitive conceptualizations for understanding the nature of our capacities for discriminating the salient features. Simply appealing to a notion of a sense of our bearing in the world is too crude to begin to distinguish the variety of forms such a sense might take, from the nonconceptual to the conceptual.[3]

We need then a much more nuanced account of the capacities for discrimination that we need to ascribe to the inarticulate expert nurse. We need an account of these capacities that leaves them clearly preconceptual. One obvious way of ensuring that such capacities are preconceptual is to treat them as capacities for discrimination that operate at the sub-personal level in terms of the processes of the subject's cognitive systems. Such a move ensures that the content of such discriminations is not available to be picked up conceptually in a short-lived contextual demonstrative concept, for they fall below the level of conscious awareness altogether.

However, to treat the capacity for discriminating the relevant causal features of the patient's condition at the sub-personal level is in danger of missing the central thrust of the whole idea of experiential knowledge. Information carried by sub-personal systems within cognition is, by definition, information that is not available to the subject. Information exploited by sub-personal systems is to do with information that such systems exploit in order to enable certain actions to be performed, but it is not information that is exploited by the subject. It is not information that the subject, in any sense, knows. For example, most of us know how to catch a ball in flight by moving to intersect with its trajectory and positioning ourselves to intercept it just before it hits the ground. We have a sense of chasing after the ball, but at a personal level the most we know about what is going on is that we want that ball. There is, plausibly, a good deal of information that is processed sub-personally that makes it possible for us to achieve this simple feat. Our cognitive systems need to calculate the direction and speed of movement that keeps our angle of gaze on the ball constant. We have no sense of doing this, but it is what our cognitive systems are doing that brings it about that we intercept the ball and catch it.

I have no doubt that successful experienced nursing involves acquiring all sorts of sub-personal routines that prompt action without the nurse knowing how it is achieved or having any awareness of the information being exploited. For example, fine detailed detection of subtle changes in palour of skin might be discriminated by the cognitive systems of experienced nurses in ways that most people fail to detect. But this hardly addresses the notion of experiential knowledge. The acquisition of routines in sub-personal systems that exploit information unavailable to the subject is a matter of acquiring automated routines for behaviour. It is akin to learning how to balance when, as a toddler, you take your first step or, as a young child, you ride your first bike. Some of this might be relevant in understanding the nuanced poise and bearing of the experienced nurse who seems to anticipate her patient's needs effortlessly and without, seemingly, knowing what she does. But there is a danger of this model reducing the experienced nurse to an automaton with a battery of slick tricks for responding to circumstances. Furthermore, if this were the only model for handling nonconceptual content, we would get no purchase on the issue of how to educate the novice. If experiential knowledge is just a matter of acquiring a range of sub-personal systems for handling information that is inaccessible to consciousness, then how are we to inculcate such knowledge? Treating the preconceptual as content dealt with sub-personally does not provide an account of experiential knowledge as something the subject knows.

I suggest that we need an account that mediates the sub-personal and personal-level systems. What is it that we do at personal-level attention that kicks in the sub-personal routine? What provides the focus to the personal-level attention? It is here, at the level of personal consciousness, that we need a sense of what matters, even if the subject cannot capture that sense conceptually, not even with a short-lived concept such as a demonstrative concept. If this is right, what we need is a notion of personal-level awareness, something that the experienced nurse can have an awareness of though not necessarily be able to articulate conceptually. Nevertheless, it must be something that figures in her experience and not just something that figures in the computations of her sub-personal routines.

■ III

Let me put this point about the relationship between the personal and sub-personal levels in terms of training. I said an account of how to train a nurse with respect to sub-personal systems would be to say that training a nurse is like training someone in how to ride a bike. But why is this so? With the trainee bike-rider, you do not train the sub-personal system directly. You train the rider by directing their attention to the action of bike riding. By doing this, you end up laying down the sub-personal routines that provide the sense of balance. You get the trainee to concentrate on riding a bike. For sure, in doing this, they concentrate on the phenomenon of balancing, on their feeling that they are about to fall off, and so on, but they do not concentrate on the specifics of balancing their body weight. Indeed, often enough, the strategy that works is to get the subject to concentrate on the route ahead, the direction in which they are aiming to ride rather than the specifics of adjusting body position first to one side and then to the other. Once they have learned how to ride the bike, then they just decide to ride a bike. At that stage, you do not do anything about balance, the sub-personal system takes over and handles that for you. The activity becomes automated.

This is not an adequate model for thinking about the training of the sensibility of experienced nurses for two reasons. First, the automation of the process is not true to the phenomenology that sees an appropriateness to speaking of the intuitive sense of the experienced nurse. The experienced nurse is not just performing on autopilot. In the scenario with which I began, the experienced inarticulate nurse has a sense of doing the right thing, of responding to a need, even if she is not able to articulate what that need is. The hypothesis that I am exploring is that there is something at the personal level, above the automated responses of the sub-personal, that needs analysing. Second, for the sub-personal to take over, there needs to be a sense of direction from the personal level and the notion of the inarticulate expert is precisely someone with a sense of direction that is more fine-tuned than the novice. So, training in the sense of building up the appropriate sub-personal routines requires a training with respect to focussing at the personal level. It is not enough just to say that both expert and novice direct their attention to 'caring for the patient', but that the experienced nurse has more sub-personal routines that kick in than the novice. To make sense of the situation requires a sense to the thought that at the personal level there is a finer discrimination of opportunities for direction even if not all are capturable conceptually. It is in personal-level experience that the experienced nurse has different capacities to the novice, not in her sub-personal routines. The richer capacities at the personal level no doubt kick in a richer range of routines at the sub-personal, but what we are looking for is an account of the capacities within personal-level experience that distinguish the expert from the novice. If this was not the case, then training would be passive, for the only direction would be, 'Let's go care for the patient' and it would then be a matter of practice, like bike riding. If that were the case, training would amount to no more than the general injunction and a hope that the novice catches on.

■ IV

The discussion so far accommodates three possible models for accounting for the experiential knowledge of the inarticulate expert nurse in the opening scenario. The first model treats the nurse's knowledge as the content of a preconceptual personal-level intuition. This is the model found in Benner and Dreyfus and Dreyfus. The suggestion is not intrinsically problematic, but it amounts to no more than a label for the phenomenon to be accounted for. The second model treats the nurse's knowledge as the content of sub-personal routines. These routines might be brought about by personal-level attention to the patient, but such attention does no more than kick in the sub-personal routines that operate automatically and outwith the scope of the nurse's awareness. The problem with the second model is that it fails to say anything to the nurse's personal experience, it leaves it unclear that there is anything that is inarticulate experiential knowledge. The third model would be one in which a notion of personal-level awareness is characterized in terms of a pre-reflective awareness, that is, an awareness that is prior to and independent of conceptually structured awareness. In the abstract, it is easy to state what a model of this third variety has to provide. The difficultly lies in providing the details.

A model of the third variety has to give an account of the sort of experience by which our nurse discriminates the needs of the patient such that the way she experiences the patient's needs is not conceptually organized. In general, then, there is a feature of the patient (their needs) which we can represent as some property or set of properties of the patient F. The experienced inarticulate expert nurse has the capacity to discriminate F. In order to ensure that her discrimination of F is a personal-level discrimination and not just a discrimination performed by sub-personal routines, there must be a way she experiences F. So, the expert nurse discriminates F and there is a way she picks it out in experience. What makes her an inarticulate expert is that she has no way of reflecting on her way of discriminating F and talking about it in the rationalization of her actions given her current conceptual capacities. The qualification that the inability to reflect is conditional on her current conceptual capacities is important. Of course, the nurse can come to acquire the capacity to reflect on the discrimination of F and employ that in rational reflection on action, but that would then amount to conceptual enhancement. She would then be an articulate expert with respect to F. It is important that we have a theoretical account of this transition from inarticulate to articulate expert and that the existence of the transition is not just assumed. I return to this point below.

Let me clarify the notion of the inarticulate expert and what makes her inarticulate. Clearly, she has no name for the way she discriminates feature F, but neither can she conceptualize the way she experiences F with contextual language, for example as 'that way'. If the experienced nurse can employ even that limited contextual language, then she is able to make use of the way she experiences F and consider what it would be for other patients to be F. She would therefore be able to generalize her discrimination of F and treat it as something that could apply to other things and that, of course, makes her discrimination a conceptual ability. But if she could do that, she could articulate her discrimination of F and thus be an articulate expert, not an inarticulate one. In that case, experiential knowledge would be no different in kind to ordinary reflective conceptual knowledge. At times, it might be short-lived and timely knowledge, but there would be nothing in principle against the idea that it could all be rendered explicit in contextual language and treated as ordinary reflective propositional knowledge. The propositions concerned would be contextual ones, but nevertheless, the nurse could not be an inarticulate expert. At the most, she would be an expert who, for whatever reasons, chooses not to articulate what she knows. She would not be someone who could not articulate what she knows.[4]

The condition for an account of experiential knowledge that makes sense of the idea of an inarticulate expert is then threefold:

(i)   The subject discriminates F
(ii) There is a way the subject discriminates F
(iii) The subject is not able, without conceptual enhancement, to reflect on the way she discriminates F

The qualification in the formulation of (iii) is to allow that although our inarticulate expert cannot, by hypothesis, reflect on her discrimination of the patient's needs, she can of course come to do so. But doing so would be to come to acquire new conceptual resources. The point of the hypothesis that the discrimination is pre-reflective is that she is not able, with her current understanding, to reflect on her discrimination and exploit that in the rational organization of her behaviour.

If we can give an account of experience for which these three conditions obtain, we will have provided some purchase on the notion of experiential knowledge that captures the case of the nurse in our opening scenario. The challenge here is meeting condition (ii) in a way that does not automatically mean we cannot meet (iii). Many philosophers assume that the notion of *the way a subject discriminates something* introduces the idea of content into the account of experience. The idea of the way a subject discriminates something is the idea of the representational content of the subject's experience. If there is a way you experience F, that is the way your experience represents it to be. But the notion of representational content is the notion of content that can be correct or incorrect (true/false). There is no account of a content being true or false independently of how its being true or false makes it bear upon other contents. But that means that if you have an experience with representational content, the idea of the way you discriminate F must be generalizable to other things. But that means that the notion of the way the subject discriminates F will, after all, be conceptual. If that is right, there is no such thing as experiential knowledge beyond that which is conceptualizable and thereby available to be articulated by the knowing subject. But that would mean that we could not make sense of the notion of experiential knowledge hypothesized in the opening scenario.

The challenge is to understand (ii) and to allow that if the idea of the way the subject discriminates something introduces a notion of content, it does not introduce conceptual content. Once again, it is simple to define in the abstract what a notion of nonconceptual content is. It is content that can be correct/incorrect (this is necessary for the notion of representation), but it is content whose being correct, if it is correct, does not bear rationally on the content of other experiences. Similarly, if an experience with nonconceptual content is incorrect, its incorrectness does not bear rationally on other experiences. So, what is required is to make sense of the idea of a subject having an experience that either gets things right, or gets things wrong, but where their sense of getting it right/wrong cannot be integrated into their sense of other things. This means that the notion of correct/incorrect conditions for such contents is not the full-blown notion of truth conditions, for it is difficult to see how it would be possible to account for content being true/false independent of its integration with other contents. I shall assume, therefore, that representational content that has truth conditions is conceptual. What is required for nonconceptual content is a notion of representation that is not rationally integratable without conceptual enhancement.

The simplest case to understand is the case in which there is a sense of getting things wrong – the negative case. It is the idea of an experience in which the subject has a sense (personal-level experience) of things not being as they expected, but not being able to reflect on that sense and integrate it in the rational control of their behaviour. If they could reflect on the experience and rationally integrate it in behavioural control, the content of the experience would be conceptual. In the abstract, the requirement for what I have called the simplest case sounds plausible. Indeed, it sounds a good first formulation for what is going on with our nurse in the opening scenario.

The case, one might think, is something like this: the experienced nurse has a sense of the patient's needs. This is something she experiences. She experiences it as a sense of things not quite running their proper course. That is to say, the way she experiences F gives her a sense of expectations being thwarted – something is not quite right. She has, however, no ability in her current conceptual repertoire to reflect on this sense of things not being quite right. What that amounts to is that not only does she perform no reasoning from this experience to her producing the action to remove the feeding tube, but that there is no account available with the concepts in her grasp to display the rationalization of her action given the experience.

The key concept in understanding this idea of nonconceptual content is the concept of expectations.[5] Condition (ii), that there be a way the subject experiences F, is met by saying that the content of the subject's experience is given by their expectations. The trouble with this suggestion is that it is easier to make sense of there being a way the subject experiences something when their expectations are thwarted than when they are satisfied. Consider all the sorts of cases in which your experience gets things right. As you walk around the room you experience the support of the floor, the resistance of the walls, the slight breeze of the air from the open window and so on. Surely you can experience all these things without consciously having expectations that are satisfied? It seems superfluous to posit satisfied expectations in all these cases, for there is a real danger of an overload of experiential content. It makes it sound as if there are too many candidates for the notion of the way one experiences things.

I want to take seriously the challenge that to introduce personal-level nonconceptual content in experience is to run the risk of overloading the account of what's in experience to a ridiculous degree. Here, then, is what seems to be the alternative – it is the relational account of experience. On the relational account of experience, experience has no content. Content is concerned with states that are responses to experience, but not part of experience itself.

On the relational account of experience the way one experiences an object is characterized simply in terms of the object and its properties, especially its causal properties. On a relational account of experience there is no content picked out by the notion of the way one experiences an object, for one simply and directly experiences it. The relational account is attractive for it provides a direct realism to the account of experience. Experience is a direct openness to and conscious awareness of objects and their properties. The very object itself and its properties are the object of experience.[6] The relational account offers to clear away the very idea of content from the notion of 'the way we experience such-and-such'. On the relational account, the notion of 'the way we experience such-and-such' is exhausted by our direct awareness of objects and their properties, content only comes about in our responses to experience. Experience as such is characterized relationally without content. Content comes later in how we respond to experience.

This is not an easy idea to get into view, for the history of philosophy is a history of theories that find experience containing content. The idea that 'the way we experience such-and-such' can be understood without a content notion can, therefore, seem very odd. The simplest way of expressing that oddity is to ask: how, without the notion of content, can there be anything of any substance to the notion of 'the way one experiences such-and-such'? Surely, one might think, the very notion of there being a way in which you experience something introduces the idea that you experience it from a perspective. To experience something from a perspective is to experience it from a point of view, a restricted view that does not, as it were, take in the whole object, but that gives you a 'take' on the object. This notion of a restricted view cannot then amount to a direct relation to the object, for the partiality of the relation shows that there is more to the way you experience such-and-such than simply being related to it. There is the way you are related to it, and that must be the case or else there is no point to the notion of the perspective or point of view from which one's experience of the object is had. The next thought is then that without introducing a content notion there is no other way of filling out this notion of perspective or point of view. It is this last thought that is mistaken. The notion of the way one experiences an object is susceptible to a quite different account without introducing content notions.

The way one experiences something is, at its most basic, in terms of the object's impingements upon one's agency. The way something looks as having a certain shape is the way it fills out impediments to my action visually. The way something feels as having a certain shape and texture is the way it fills out impediments to my action through my handling of it. And similarly for other cases. That is to say, the notion of 'the way we experience such-and-such' can be explicated without introducing the notion of content, if one understands the idea in terms of the object's impacts upon agency. This means that the experiencing subject has to be conceived as essentially an agent, for the perspective of their experience is shaped by the way objects and their properties impose upon their agency. That is what gives them a point of view upon things; it is provided by the character of their agency. The way I experience the room as I walk around it – the support of the floor, the slight feel of the breeze through the open window and so on – is in terms of how my activity goes in relation to these things.

If this is right it provides a satisfying account of the notion of nonconceptual content in terms of expectations, but this is now a content that figures in the subject's response to experience rather than a content that is a component of experience. Rather than have a plethora of expectational contents that are satisfied as I walk around the room my experience is simply my direct conscious awareness of the room as I move around it and as I see it as a site for my agency. When things are going right I have no particular responses to the firmness of the floor precisely because when things go right I have no impediments to my agency. I have a direct conscious awareness of things and their powers to impinge on me and in getting these right there is no response that is called for. And when things keep going right, as they do most of the time, I build up expectations about how they will go next. Having such expectations just is a matter of coordinating my action with the causal structures and powers of things around me. I coordinate my actions precisely in order to avoid being surprised. When things go wrong, matters are different. Suppose there is a loose floorboard.

I feel the sponginess of the floor at that point. This is something that is particularly salient in my awareness. It is salient precisely because having coordinated my action to the causal powers of things I have come to expect solidity in floors. This expectation is not part of the experience. When things are going right, it might remain at the sub-personal level. When things go wrong, when the expectation is thwarted, this is salient at the level of personal awareness. That is when I get a nonconceptual content. It is a content in my response *to* experience rather than a content *in* experience, but it is nevertheless a candidate for a nonconceptual content. What makes it nonconceptual concerns whether or not I can, with my current conceptual resources, reflect on the sense of things not being right and make use of this sense in the rational control of further action. If I can, the content is conceptual; if I cannot, it is not.

If the above account is right, we have a model of content that satisfies both conditions (ii) and (iii) above. It is not a model of the content of experience, for I have sketched the account on the basis of a relational theory of experience. But that does not matter, for the account is still an account of content and of content that arises in response to experience. The account provides a model in which the subject experiences the properties of things in terms of the dispositions of objects to enable and thwart action. The notion of the way the subject experiences an object or situation lies in the way they coordinate their action with respect to the properties of the situation. In general, if a subject discriminates F, then they coordinate their action by acting towards the situation as if it is F. But acting towards a situation as if it is F does not require the subject to have the concept F. It is by habituating action to such situations as if they are F that the subject comes to have expectations. If all goes well, this might all occur at the sub-personal level. When an expectation is thwarted this typically produces a response, a nonconceptual content, at the personal level. This response amounts to a personal-level sense that acting with respect to the situation as if it is F is no longer possible, for doing so provides a sense of things not being quite right.

Here is a simple example of this kind of situation. Suppose a young infant has acquired the expectation that strongly coloured spherical objects are soft. They habituate their actions with respect to such objects as if they are soft. They then pick up a prickly pear. Their expectation is thwarted. At a personal level they have a sense of things not going right, of not going as expected. And this holds true regardless of whether they have concepts for representing any of this in judgement. Their sense of being thwarted consists in their personal-level sense of not being able to act with respect to the prickly pear as if it is soft.

The model transfers easily to our nursing example. The inarticulate expert nurse has a sense of things not being quite right and, although she cannot articulate quite in what respect this is so and she cannot generalize this sense to other cases, she has a feeling that her action is appropriate given this sense. On the account I have sketched, she will have this inarticulate expertise just in case she is, first and foremost, an agent. Her experience of the patient's needs, the way in which she discriminates F, is due to the way she acts with respect to the patient's needs. Her ability to discriminate F arises because she is actively engaged with F. You do not get to be a nurse with the ability to discriminate the sorts of features of patients' care and needs required for expertise without a considerable apprenticeship in acting with respect to these things. And you train the novice by getting them to join in the action, not by getting them to watch. But that training might, in the first instance, amount to training to act with respect to F, a fine-tuning of actions and interventions that does not require that the nurse have a conceptual representation of F. Such training could occur without the nurse acquiring a capacity to reflect on F and generalize their response to F in the manner of conceptually articulated judgement.

But consider the nurse whose expectations in acting towards F are thwarted. They find that their actions do not deliver the usual consequences (like the infant picking up the prickly pear). They find that they are not able to act in their normal way with respect to F. At that point, they try a different response. There are two ways a different response can be generated. One way would be by random variation or action. Another way is by directing and organizing activity with respect to F. The latter way is, I suggest, in broadest outline, what is going on for the inarticulate nurse in my opening scenario. Furthermore, it is an account of what is going on that leaves it open for the inarticulate nurse to bring their thwarted expectation into conceptual focus. By attending to their thwarted expectation they might very well be able to render it conceptual. Indeed, it seems plausible to suppose that the key step to rendering a thwarted expectation into something that can be generalized and considered with respect to how it bears upon other experiences is precisely the subject's ability to attend to the thwarting as itself an item of awareness. That, of course, is to make the capacity for conceptual thought and an articulate level of expertise dependent on the ability for a self-conscious capacity to organize and direct activity with respect to saliences. That dependence might be right, but it would go too far beyond the scope of this chapter to begin to treat that matter here.

■ Notes

1 Of course, one of the issues about regulatory requirements is precisely whether or not the imperative to observe written protocols and other output targets for care diverts the attention of the nurse away from those aspects of the situation that are central to providing the best care. The account of experiential knowledge that I sketch below shows how the rigid application of protocols can be a

diversion from the professional's best sense of optimum care where the latter, not the former, tracks the truth of the matter.

2   I think much of what the expert knows is within the reach of judgement and properly theorized in terms of the exercise of short-lived conceptual capacities that enable one to think and reason in highly contextual ways. My present concern is to explore the case for a further level of experiential knowledge that is outwith our conceptual capacities.

3   The availability of short-lived contextualized conceptually structured capacities is exploited in a series of articles in which I have developed an account of professional expertise that is both perceptually driven and yet conceptually organized, cf. Luntley (2002, 2003b, 2004, 2005). The present chapter is an extension of the theory of conceptually structured perceptual engagements that shows how such capacities are related to and arise out of a more basic set of nonconceptual forms of engagement. The account of nonconceptual engagement that I provide below is of a piece with that proposed in Luntley (2003a).

4   This would leave experiential knowledge as fully capturable with the contextual conceptual capacities that I have emphasized in earlier work. I am not dissenting from the view that such conceptual capacities are very significant in understanding the nature of expertise, I continue to think them very important. The present point is whether or not there is any more to the notion of experiential knowledge that falls outside the capture of conceptualization.

5   See my account of nonconceptual content in Luntley (2003a).

6   See Campbell (2003) for detailed argument for the relational account. I am enormously indebted to my colleague Bill Brewer for my understanding of the relational account. Although Bill and I differ on how we read the relational account, the differences are, I think, slight. And if they are not slight, it remains the case that I have learnt a very great deal from his work on experience.

Chapter 5

Practice and its informing knowledge: An Aristotelian understanding

Joseph Dunne

■ Introduction: 'Internal goods' of practices

If one says that nursing is a practice, does much hang on this claim?
A great deal, I would argue. Much of the argument consists of bringing
forward a rich conception of practice capable of stoutly resisting threats
to the integrity of nursing that stem from the institutional conditions and
epistemological presuppositions by which it, like other comparable professions, is now increasingly constrained. In presenting the argument here,
I shall refer to nursing itself only by way of recurrent advertences to how
it illustrates or instantiates points introduced in the course of elaborating
'practice' and the kind of knowledge that I see as integral to it. This
conception of practice and of practical knowledge might be called 'neo-
Aristotelian'. In this opening section, I shall locate it briefly by reference to
a well-known analysis of the contemporary Aristotelian, Alasdair MacIntyre,
in *After Virtue*; and in subsequent sections my elucidation of the nature
of practical knowledge is strongly influenced by (though it seldom refers
explicitly to) Aristotle's own analysis of the kind of knowledge – what he
called *phronesis* – that is brought into play by and in *praxis*.

A practice, for MacIntyre (and I will not reproduce here his famous,
much quoted and very long sentence of definition; see MacIntyre, 1985,
p. 175), is a coherent, complex set of activities that has evolved cooperat-
ively and cumulatively over time, that is alive in the community who are its
practitioners, and that remains alive only so long as they remain committed
to sustaining – and creatively developing and extending – its internal goods
and its proper standards of excellence (this commitment constituting them
as a community). 'Internal goods' here includes the desirable outcomes
characteristically intended through a practice, for example good health
in the case of nursing or good building in the case of architecture.[1] But
it also includes qualities acquired and exercised by practitioners through
their apprenticeship into the practice, their answerability to its standards

91

of excellence and their submission to the demands of achieving its characteristic ends. These qualities are both competences proper to each practice and (as illustrated in this volume in the chapter by Anne Scott) virtues of character that transcend any particular practice, though they may receive a unique modulation in the context of some particular practice. The former are technical proficiencies in, for example, nursing and medical assessment and interventions. But one may not be able to exercise these proficiencies in striving to realize the internal goods of the practice – rather than treating it as a means for achieving external goods (e.g., money or status, which are external in that they could be achieved by some other means) – unless one has also acquired virtues such as patience, temperance, courage or honesty. Together, these qualities direct one's energy and attention as well as disciplining one's desires. In fixing one's efforts on the requirements of the practice they bring one into partnership with others who are similarly focused. Since in itself this partnership is not based on an economy of scarcity it does not encourage rivalry or conflict between partners: one person does not excel at the expense of others – rather, every achievement of excellence potentially enriches all who participate in or care about a practice. The same is not the case, however, with respect to the *external* goods that can accrue from accomplishment in a practice, leading to a different kind of competitiveness. Pursuit of these goods can bring one into conflict with others *and* jeopardize one's achievement of the internal goods. It is not only that the practice can become a means to acquiring external goods (which in itself is not a bad thing). Rather, the practice can be made *purely* instrumental so that no violation of its internal fabric is disallowed if it can be made to maximize the external goods. With reference to health care generally, obvious examples of things easily implicated in such violation are published league tables, reduction of waiting lists and efficiency of 'throughput'.

For both MacIntyre and Aristotle the extension of 'practice' is notably broad, though in rather different respects. In MacIntyre's case, the breadth stems from the variety of specific domains that can count as practices – for example, performance arts (dancing, flute-playing), productive professions and crafts (architecture and weaving), areas of theoretical endeavour (physics, history), and games (soccer, chess). For Aristotle, by contrast, the denotation of *praxis* is not domain-specific and so its breadth stems rather from its designating the open set of engagements through which one strives, primarily as a citizen of the polis, to live a worthwhile life in the light of some conception of the overall human good in all its vernacular range. My own concern in this chapter is with a subset of practices that converge with both MacIntyre's and Aristotle's foci of interest: on the one hand these practices are enclaves of specialized, one might say professionalized, competency and concern; but on the other hand, since their ends lie in significant changes to the human beings who form one party to the interaction that constitutes them, they are deeply and pervasively implicated in very basic issues concerning the human good. Examples here are the caring and educative professions and so, conspicuously, nursing and nurse education.[2]

In practical domains of this kind, we can distinguish the core practice itself and at least three other closely related factors with a significantly determinative effect on it. First is the institutionalization of the practice, or how structures are established to frame it and to protect its essential priorities (and to ensure its adequate funding) in its mediation with wider economic, political and ideological realities; policy issues are involved here that are seen increasingly to fall within the remit of managers and administrators. Second is the reproduction of the practice through the initiation of aspiring or apprentice practitioners; this is the issue of what might broadly be called professional education. And third is the articulation of the practice, the kinds of analyses and arguments, with their own proper concepts and language, in terms of which it is conceptualized and legitimated, to itself and to the wider society that it purports to serve; this is the issue of what might be called theory or discourse. While all of these bear reciprocally on one another, my chief concern here will be with what I have just called the 'core' of the practice; and in dealing with it, I shall clearly be engaged in the third attendant activity, that of discursive articulation. A practice can indeed be seriously subverted or derailed by weakness or failure in its institutional or educational arrangements. However, such weaknesses or failures can be understood or even acknowledged – let alone effectively addressed – only if there is clarity about the practice itself; and providing this kind of clarity is one of the tasks of the form of discourse that I am engaged in here.

While nursing is the focus of interest here, I shall be concerned not singly with any one of these practices but with all of them as sharing, so I shall claim, an internal feature, essential to their integrity as practices; this feature has to do with the kind of knowledge that they embody, a kind that I shall characterize as 'practical'. My argument will be historical in interpreting a central thrust of the whole process of modernization as posing a fundamental threat to these practices by attempting to discount and displace this kind of knowledge. It will be historical too in its indebtedness to ancient philosophy and specifically to the philosophy of Aristotle *both* for what may be regarded as a prefiguration of this thrust and for an analysis that can still help us to understand and defend the kind of practical knowledge that it threatens.

■ Distinguishing technical and practical rationality

It is easy to see that the relationship between knowledge and action looms large in any understanding of these practices. Already in Plato's day we find pretensions to professional expertise by practitioners in any field being checked against the status of the knowledge they could claim to possess; and Plato himself is committed to establishing the well-groundedness of *techne* as a superior form of knowledge. Likewise, over the centuries, guilds and clerisies have justified their prerogatives by reference to their privileged knowledges. Beyond lay comprehension or mere common sense, these have been asserted to be variously recondite or esoteric, acquirable only through specialized training or elaborate rituals of initiation. And in our own time, in respect of attempts by different domains to establish themselves in the pecking order of professions, things are little different. The claims of any 'profession' or would-be profession, in terms of its authority with clients, the wider social esteem it enjoys, the exclusivity of its members' mandate to practice – and not least the level of remuneration it commands – still are, or are claimed to be, tied to the kind of knowledge it embodies.

In our modern societies what most powerfully underwrites the status of any knowledge is its claim to *rationality*. And one mode of rationality has established a hegemony, so that only knowledge assembled and activity conducted within its frame are recognized as respectable – claims for the efficacy of the activity being grounded in prior claims for the rigour of the knowledge. This mode, which is closely related to modern science – though it has roots in Western philosophy traceable back to the Socratic valorization of *techne* – may be called 'technical rationality'. It puts a premium on 'objectivity' and detachment, suppressing the context-dependence of first-person experience in favour of a third-person perspective that yields generalized findings in accordance with clearly formulated, publicly agreed procedures. These procedures give an indispensable role to operations of observation and measurement, modes of testing that specify precisely what can count as counter-evidence, replicability of findings and the adoption of a language maximally freed from possibilities of misinterpretation by its being maximally purged of the need for interpretation itself. And through these procedures, knowledge is established that is both explanatory and predictive.

In characterizing technical rationality here, I have emphasized factors that are normally associated with scientific method. But technical rationality may not be as securely tied to the scientific enterprise, inaugurated in the seventeenth century with novel modes of experimentation and of exploiting the explanatory power of mathematics, as we sometimes tend to assume. Rather, it may more properly be associated with a basic attitude that welcomed the new sciences, helped to give them impetus and shaped an understanding – or perhaps misunderstanding – of them that made them so powerfully exemplary in the new modernity. This attitude was espoused in early modern epistemology, both empiricist and rationalist: it is as evident in Francis Bacon's assurance that 'fruits and works are as it were sponsors and sureties for the truth' (*Novum Organon*, 1, 73) as in Descartes' assertion that 'it is possible to attain knowledge which is very useful in life [. . . .] by means of which [. . . .] knowing the force and actions of [. . . .] bodies that environ us, as distinctly as we know the different crafts of our artisans, we can in the same way employ them in all those uses to which they are adapted, and thus render ourselves the masters and possessors of nature' (*Discourse on Method*, 2001, p. 6). The *ars dominandi* so strikingly presaged by these two thinkers is distinct from the scientific project – though, to be sure, the latter could serve it very well because the predictive power of its knowledge could so easily translate into enormous technical mastery over matter, a mastery abundantly manifest in modern technology. I shall claim later that in an important respect the drive for mastery is not essential to the scientific project – or, as we might make the point here, is not internal to the sciences *qua* practices of inquiry. This drive is better understood as part of the ideal of disengagement by a subject who could take an objectifying and instrumental stance towards the reality from which it had disengaged. Inscribed in pure instrumentality is the goal of mastery and maximization: everything becomes a means over which one aspires to exercise total control – a control defined in terms of optimal effectiveness in achieving ends and optimal efficiency in realizing most benefit with least cost.

It is in control over *matter* that technical rationality has most successfully demonstrated its power. But the story in which I am mainly interested here is that whereby attempts are increasingly made to organize and regulate *human action and interaction*, especially in specialized domains of practice, according to its dictates. As its prestige has grown – to the point where it is no longer seen as *a* form of rationality, with its own limited sphere of validity, but as coincident with *rationality as such* – modes of knowledge which do not accord with it are deemed to be non-rational and hence to be without proper credentials for delivering progress in an area. Any area of practice, then, that does not rationalize itself according to its standards – that persists in giving a strong function to other modes of knowledge – is likely to be regarded as backward and to be under pressure to adopt its procedures and accommodate to its norms. The pressure will come from outside the practice or profession and, increasingly, from 'modernizers' within it. This is a dynamic that has been very evident in nursing, medicine, education, law, business and politics, as well as in a range of other occupations keen to assert their 'professional' status.

To technicize a practice is to make it over in such a way that control over its key operations is maximally assured by a method whose successful implementation can be monitored systematically and unambiguously. Such making over might entail the construction of an entirely new set of operations that simply replaces an older, now superseded set (as has happened, for example, in some aspects of dentistry). In genuinely interactive practices, however, it would seem to proceed more inductively by a process of *re*construction. In other words, rather than simply sweeping aside all the old procedures, it seeks to extract from them a rational core that can be made transparent and replicable. Typically, this entails disembedding the knowledge implicit in the skilful performance of the characteristic tasks of the practice from the immediacy and idiosyncrasy of the particular situations in which it is deployed, and from the background of experience and character in the practitioners in whom it resides. Through this disembedding it is supposed that what is essential in the knowledge and skill can be abstracted for encapsulation in explicit, generalizable formulae, procedures or rules – which can in turn be applied to the various situations and circumstances that arise in the practice so as to meet the problems that they present. These problems are supposed to have nothing significant in them that has not been anticipated in the analysis that yielded the general formulae, and hence to be soluble by a straightforward application of the latter without need for any new insight or discernment in the actual situation itself. Control and efficiency – and proper 'accountability' – seem to be made possible here by the fact that the system is minimally dependent on the discretion or judgement of individual practitioners, with all the hazard and lack of standardization that this might entail. The ideal to which technical rationality aspires, one might say, is a practitioner-proof mode of practice.

My articulation of the nature of technical rationality has just brought out its inherent opposition to practitioners' knowledge, or its drive to refashion and supplant what might be called an alternative mode of *practical* rationality. How then is this alternative mode of rationality to be characterized? In the Aristotelian tradition, the answer here will rely heavily on the notion of *phronesis* elaborated (somewhat sketchily) in book six of the *Nicomachean Ethics*. Like the notion of *techne*, to which it is there counterposed – and which already anticipates much of the spirit of what I have been calling technical rationality – *phronesis* is characterized as a rational orientation (a *hexis meta logou*): in its case a rational orientation to action (*praxis*) rather than, as in the case of *techne*, to production (*poiesis*).[3] Later I shall return to this distinction between action and production, which seems to underlie the distinction between *phronesis* and *techne*. Here I want to outline a few key, interrelated features of *phronesis*, features that have to do with its role as an action-orientating form of knowledge, its irreducibly experiential nature, its non-confinement to generalized propositional knowledge, its entanglement (beyond mere knowledge) with character, its need to embrace the particulars of relevant action-situations within its grasp of universals and its ability to engage in the kind of deliberative process that can yield concrete, context-sensitive judgements. If one wants an English equivalent of *phronesis*, perhaps 'judgement' is the best candidate – a word we use not only (as I have now just done) for particular judgement 'calls' but more generally for the cultivated capacity to make such calls resourcefully and reliably in all the complex situations that they address.

Such situations may of course be perfectly standard and typical – that is to say of a type that has often been met previously and for which there is an already established and well-rehearsed procedure. But they may *not* be exactly to type, deviating in an indefinite number of respects from what is standard or conventional. Judgement, then, is an ability to recognize situations, cases or problems of this kind (which are perhaps of *no* clearly specifiable kind) and to deal with them adequately and appropriately. A person of judgement respects the particularity of the case – and thus does not impose on it a procrustean application of the general rule (Procrustes was the character in Greek mythology who stretched or shortened people to make them fit the bed predesigned for their captivity). At the same time, she will try to find a way of bringing this particularity into *some* relationship, albeit one yet to be determined, with the body of general knowledge codified in rules and formulae. This general knowledge is available to her, one might say, like the measuring rule of Lesbian builders whose pliable material allowed it to be stretched over the irregular surfaces of individual stones.[4] Her adeptness, then, as a person of judgement, lies neither in a knowledge of the general as such nor in an entirely unprincipled dealing with particulars. Rather, it lies precisely in the mediation between general and particular, in the ability to bring both into illuminating connection with each other. This requires perceptiveness in her reading of particular situations as much as flexibility in her mode of 'possessing' and 'applying' the general knowledge.

Judgement is more than the possession of general knowledge just because it is the ability to actuate this knowledge with relevance, appropriateness, or sensitivity to context. In each fresh actuation, there is an element of creative insight through which it makes itself equal to the demands of a new situation. Because of this element of 'excess', beyond what has already been formulated, which it proves itself recurrently capable of generating, judgement lies partly in 'the tacit dimension'[5] – a fact closely related to its experiential character. The primary sense of 'experience' here is that whereby we refer to people as 'experienced', thinking of the way in which their accumulated past experience, so far from being a dead capital, is at their disposal, informing in intimate detail their way of meeting and interpreting what is *now* appearing within their experience *here*. It is through recurrently rising to the challenge of new situations that are not comfortably encompassed by her previous experience that she allows this experience to be reconstructed; and this reconstruction (a central motif of Dewey's whole philosophy)[6] *is* what we refer to as significant learning. It is of course possible to have experiences from which we do not learn: it is a commonplace observation, for example, that the 30 years 'experience' of some practitioners reduces to one year's experience, repeated stalely thereafter.

The kind of openness that allows one's experience to be quickened by new learning – so that one develops the fine discrimination of judgement – can be characterized as 'cognitive'; but it also brings into play some of those virtues of character mentioned earlier. There is patience in sticking with a problem, or courage in entertaining an unwelcome or unfashionable viewpoint, or a kind of temperateness that keeps one from being too easily swayed by impulse or first impression, enabling one to sustain attention to what is salient, irrespective of personal preference and bias, or compulsion to have one's present opinion confirmed, or disinclination to jettison a plausible but insufficiently supported conjecture. In all of this there is a kind of 'unselfing' (finely articulated by Simone Weil in her discussions of 'attention' [Weil, 1978]). Receptivity to the problem is called for rather than keenness to master it with a solution; and while this receptivity may call for great imaginative and emotional engagement, it does not gratify the 'fat relentless ego' (Murdoch, 1998). One might speak of it as 'impersonal', were it not that the springs of judgement, deeply recessed in one's mind and being, are expressive of the kind of person – as well as, or rather in and through, the kind of practitioner – that one has become.[7]

■ The priority of 'material' to 'method'

As between the two kinds of knowledge-orientation that I have just outlined, the technical and the practical, the former has an interrelated set of attractions. The kind of objectivity that it adheres to seems to make it proof against intrusions of the merely subjective. The transparency of its procedures frees it from reliance on personal gifts or inarticulate intuitions. The replicability of its operations and the generalizability of its findings ensure a universal reach beyond the local and customary. The prediction that it enables and the control that it guarantees provide unambiguous criteria for establishing accountability and assessing success – thus averting interminable disputes and ultimately inadjudicable contests of interpretation. Against these advantages, knowledge with an irreducible core of judgement can appear makeshift, unreliable, elitist and unaccountable. Still, a large question remains as to the competence of technical rationality to deal with the actual material of many practical domains. Can it supersede judgement or abrogate the need for it, without thereby distorting or violating the integrity of this material? And even if the answer is 'no', a more ominous question looms: might it nonetheless have the power to impose its distortions, thereby altering the very nature of a practice – indeed liquidating it precisely *as* a practice? Or, beyond this possibility, is there something irrepressible in the very nature of these domains that will find ways of reasserting itself, exposing the futile pretensions of technical rationality?

These questions are ultimately about the relationship between the *material* of a domain of reality – in the present case, a wide range of practical spheres – and the *methods or models* that we use to get a purchase on this material. It is the hallmark of an Aristotelian approach, formulated very clearly in the *Nicomachean Ethics*, to grant priority to the material and to argue that the method should be congruent with it.[8] In certain respects technical rationality seems to accord with the fabric of the material universe, in its physical, chemical and even biological aspects. However, does the attempt to impose it on the very different reality of human practices spring from a considered understanding of this reality itself – or from an *a priori* enthusiasm (even obsession) to have in these areas the same kind of standardization and control that, partly through technical rationality, we have in our dealings with some aspects of the material universe? That some kind of rigour and accountability are necessary in practical domains is hardly in dispute; otherwise we should be exposed to all manner of mystification and chicanery. And so the argument is not about *whether* but rather about *what kind of* rigour is available in these areas. Similarly there is no good reason to deny a need for effectiveness in all these areas. And since, in certain circumscribed arenas of operation, technical rationality has its own proper competence, one can grant the validity and indeed desirability of technicizing – even in practical domains – everything that can without loss be technicized. Insofar as there are routine or systematically categorizable tasks that can, for example, be computerized then clearly there is advantage (by economizing on time and other probably scarce resources) in doing so. Advantage is gained, however, only if we can reliably recognize those tasks that can and those that can *not* be so programmed – and only within an overall approach of maximally freeing the most precious resource (which, on the present analysis, is precisely good practical judgement) to do what only it can do well, and not one of attempting to supplant it or render it obsolete.

We return, then, to the issue of just what kind of material we deal with in practical domains: the material will determine the kind of activity we are engaged in and, in turn, the kind of knowledge that is required or the type of rationality that is appropriate. Technical rationality is most at home with the activity of production or fabrication, where there are materials (in the most literal sense) on which an already designed form can be imposed, so that the activity issues in a substantial, durable product that – like the materials themselves – is quite separate from the producer and even from the activity of production. This type of activity held a powerful fascination for those classical Greek thinkers who first shaped our notion of rationality. Both Plato and Aristotle were so impressed by this kind of activity, working on this kind of material, that when they developed a conception of expert knowledge in their notion of *techne* (the original and continuing inspiration, as well as the etymological root, of what I have been calling technical rationality) they privileged it at the expense of other types of activity, whose corresponding knowledges remained unarticulated, without official philosophical sanction.

The notion of *techne* was itself articulated through a cluster of conceptual dualities that, still part of our linguistic stock-in-trade, remain at the core of the technicist paradigm: matter and form, means and end, planning and execution. Matter here (e.g. wood, stone, cloth or leather) is at the behest of the producer (the carpenter, mason, weaver or cobbler as *homo faber*), who can masterfully construct a design or blueprint (the 'form') which is then to be impressed on the matter to yield the finished product. This formed product is the end that his productive activity is set to achieve; and the activity, together with the materials and whatever tools he may need, are the means that are used for its achievement. There is a clear distinction here both between form and matter and between end and means; and this is reflected in a further attempt to differentiate within the productive process itself between a planning phase (which involves a determination of the form – which in turn specifies the end – and a calculation of the sequence of actions that will be necessary to achieve it) and an implementation phase (which is the execution in the materials, usually in reverse order, of the steps laid out in the prior plan). Rationality here resides in the planning: it is just to the extent that this planning can be abstracted from the nitty-gritty of the actual productive activity and preformulated in a set of prescriptions governing the latter that the whole process qualifies as 'rational'.

It was in reflection on the figure of the master craftsman, then, that the dominant orientation of Western reason was first articulated. Exposed as they were to the awesome forces of nature, not to speak of the awful capriciousness of the gods, classical Greeks found in the notion of *techne* a source of control that was all the more to be prized insofar as it resided in their own – newly self-conscious, one might say newly discovered – rational powers. And, far from forcing a recasting of *techne*, the great achievements of modern science allow it all the more to come into its own. For the philosophical conception of *techne* did not accurately reflect the reality of what actually went on in some of the crafts of fabrication – think, for example, of a surgeon and a theatre nurse and of the amount of know-how in their hands that is irrecoverable in any explicit propositions. And by contrast, with the increasing marginalization of genuine craft skill, modern science gives us just that kind of general, nomological knowledge that was anticipated in the concept of *techne* – even if it was not instantiated in all the actual arenas of production to which it was ascribed. Moreover, the *instrumental* structure of *techne* is not only retained but reinforced in our scientific age: deep-structure knowledge of the materials opens a huge field of possibilities within which we can contrive new ends – while at the same time it provides just the kind of predictive control that enables us reliably to mobilize means towards their achievement.

What, then, of those other activities that are *not* captured by this technicist paradigm? Examples in the Greek world were rhetoric, military strategy and politics or statecraft.[9] Far from being stable or passive, awaiting the impress of a previously devised form, the materials here include volatile constellations of human passions and motivations; and far from having the clearly defined boundaries of the clinic or laboratory, sites of engagement are shifting and protean. Rather than imposing a design on materials to bring about a product, the adept here intervenes in a field of forces or immerses herself in a medium, in which she seeks to bring about a propitious result. And insofar as the play of chance ('*Fortuna*, bitch goddess of unpredictability') and the vagaries of timing are ineliminable, she needs a kind of opportunism, or talent for improvization, that responds to the dynamism in the materials themselves, teaching by seminar and tutorial being obvious examples here. It is a curious fact that although activities with this kind of fabric were important for classical Greeks (what indeed was more important to them than theatres of speech, politics and war?) – and although the concepts of chance (*tuche*) and good timing (*kairos*) occur frequently enough in Arisotle's writings – there is a clear mismatch between these activities and the master conception of rationality, *techne*, that was one of their trademark philosophical constructs. But it is just here that the significance of Aristotle's analysis of *phronesis* emerges. For it is in this analysis that we find an alternative notion of rationality, more fitted to these activities and to the texture of their 'material'.

One cannot say that Aristotle himself gives us any very developed treatment of this texture or just how and why it calls for a quite different kind of knowledge orientation. But a few points may briefly be filled in here with help from some recent thinkers of a broadly Aristotelian stripe. While the action of any agent may indeed be a real initiative, setting off something new, it is still inserted in a web of interaction, with its own power and limits conditioned by its capacity to mesh with – without manipulating – the actions of *other* agents that transpire in the same space of plurality, a space-between-agents. This is a space of possibility insofar as it can elicit initiatives that have an event-like quality, finding their intelligibility not in a predictable chain of causality but rather in the plot of a story that can be narrated only retrospectively. This possibility opens up only because it is also a space densely marked, though not fully saturated, by the effects of many other previous actions, that is to say, by a tradition and the particular language and concepts through which it is expressed. To acknowledge these points is to recognize the frailty and intricacy of human affairs – or, what amounts to much the same thing, the non-sovereignty of the single agent.[10] And it is, I believe, a feature of the practices whose nature I have been exploring here that they do not escape this frailty, intricacy and non-sovereignty – all their concern with successful accomplishment and proper standards of excellence notwithstanding.

It follows from the features of these practices that I have just adverted to that they often present us with a problematic situation where there is no discrete problem already clearly labelled as such – so that we might better speak of a difficulty or predicament rather than a problem. For the classic 'problem', however hard, is made tractable by the stable background of a clearly defined type to which the solution must belong. Thus, in the case of a problem in fabrication, an already formulated blueprint or design, by specifiying an end, lays down clear-cut criteria for determining the most efficient assemblage of means (or similarly in the case of a cross-word puzzle the number of blank letters clearly circumscribes the field in which the solution lies). A problematic situation, by contrast, may be a point of intersection for several lines of consideration and priority that, while running in different directions, are interwoven tightly in a complex web. Attempts to unravel any one of these strands (the classic task of analysis) may only introduce greater tangles in the others. In education, for example, a practitioner or policy-maker may face a situation where academic standards, considerations of safety, psychological needs and the demands of social equity, in relation to a diverse set of students, pull in contrary directions – but where *some* decision has to be made (take the sublime example of dispute at an exam board as to whether a 'borderline' student should be accorded a pass or fail).

In attempting to resolve problematic situations of this kind, one is not calculating the efficiency of different possible means towards an already determined end. Rather, one is often deliberating about the end itself – about what would count as a satisfactory, or at least not entirely unaccept-able, outcome to a particular 'case'. This will entail a kind of pondering – though imponderables may not be entirely eliminable from the reckoning (should the borderline student be given the chance to make good?). It may only be by action – and not, in the end, by any purely deliberative process – that this reckoning can eventually be carried through. While strategically directed action will provide new feedback, it may also set off its own chain of unintended *or* unexpected consequences (the borderline student goes on to become a renowned expert in her field). And so, one is involved in an experimental process. But there is a great difference between the kind of experimentation that may occur in a practical field and that which goes on in a laboratory. For whereas in the latter case, a 'negative' or discon-firming result may be celebrated by the sceptical spirit of the scientist as a step in the onward march of knowledge, in a practical field it may have to be regarded as an error that was simply too costly (the borderline student keeps making mistakes in patient-care and is held to be unsafe). And yet the situation may be such that to hazard *no* experimental probe is itself an error, if not an outright impossibility. It is such situations that call for judgement.

▪ Some concluding clarifications

Though my analysis in this chapter treats of a very general issue, closely related to the whole historical phenomenon of modernization, its aim has been modest. I have tried to say enough about practices and about technical rationality to support the contention that they do not consort well together – and I have done so in a way that might broadly be characterized as 'neo-Aristotelian'. But I am well aware that there are many important issues about practice that I have not dealt with and that in what I have said there is much that is problematic and contestable. I shall conclude here with a few remarks addressed to some more obvious misgivings.

First, the positive side of my analysis has concentrated on the practitioner, for example the nurse, the medic and the teacher, and on the kind of knowledge, thickly embedded in a whole background of experience and character, that she or he needs to deploy. It is right – and it is certainly Aristotelian – to emphasize that significant human goods are not achievable by any system, bureaucratic or otherwise, that would exempt people operating in that system from the need to possess and exercise a combination of intellectual and ethical virtues. While maintaining this emphasis, it is still important, however, to guard against a tendency towards subjectivism – a tendency, that is to say, to locate the construction of meaning too exclusively within individual subjects, with insufficient attention to the sociopolitical, institutional and historical matrices within which individuals themselves are located. Aristotle would have had little inclination in this direction (though, to be sure, he had significant blind spots about the wider matrices) and MacIntyre's whole analysis of practice in *After Virtue* (where subjectivism appears as 'emotivism') is explicitly aimed at rejecting it. If there is a sense in which the nurse practitioner constructs the practice, there is a stronger sense in which the practice constructs the nursing practitioner. The horizon of his or her judgements is always set by the proper ends, goods and standards of the practice and is always at least potentially directed towards, and testable by, other practitioners set within the same horizon, which establishes the practice as a collaborative and communal space.

Second, the metaphor of 'horizon' tallies well – though it shifts the sensory base from aural to visual – with my earlier emphasis on the tacit dimension of practitioners' knowledge. But this emphasis should not suggest any principled preference for the implicit over the explicit. To the contrary, the very implicitness of much that goes on in a practice should be a spur to discussion and argumentation, as judgements and their grounds are exposed to demands for discursive justification. And while the expectation will be that much of this justification can be provided within an assumed horizon it is also true that this horizon itself – with respect to the knowledge of a particular group of practitioners and even of the whole relevant community at any particular juncture in the historical evolution of a practice – is not fixed but moving. To be sure, it is hardly conceivable that any such movement could be deliberately contrived by any single practitioner (though it cannot be excluded that feats of great genius might achieve, and in particular practices perhaps on occasion achieved, this result). The important point, here, though, is that part of the repertoire of individual practitioners and groups of practitioners is a capacity not only for reflection but also, not infrequently, for articulation; any adequate conception of 'judgement' should include this capacity. Moreover, it is mainly through the critical mass of this capacity, widely distributed among practitioners, that the practice itself is kept in good order, an order that requires rather than merely tolerates some more or less steady, though never predictable, advance in its overall horizon.

Third, though I have specifically mentioned caring and teaching professions as falling under the rubric of 'practice' as I have been discussing it, a focus on the practitioner seems largely to have occluded the *patient* or *client* – there has been little reference to patients or students. Partly this is because of the generic nature of the analysis, which has not focused on any particular practice.[11] But it may need to be emphasized here that when I have spoken of the internal goods of a practice, these are mainly the goods of those whom the practice is intended to serve; and it is strictly in relation to their contribution to *these* goods that the goods of the practitioner that I have highlighted, specifically technical proficiencies and ethical virtues, are to be understood and evaluated. That all of us at some point find ourselves as 'clients' of practices is an aspect of our dependency (or interdependency). But independence, insofar as it is genuine (which implies at least that it is free of illusions of self-sufficiency and helps us to be dependable for others), is also a very great good that any of us rightly cherishes. And it goes without saying that it is a good that can be, and all too frequently has been, undermined by the ways in which people have been conscripted and treated as clients of so-called 'helping' professions. But these underminings constitute failures of the relevant professionals precisely as practitioners. For the good that is their clients' independence must be considered as internal to the practices of, for example, educative teaching, psychotherapy, medicine and nursing – a good that it is part of their end to establish or restore. This fact brings constitutive tensions to these practices and implicates them deeply in aspects of the ethics of care. Here I only acknowledge these tensions, but in doing so it serves to remind us that, in the caring and teaching professions, along with many others, *phronesis* (judgement) has an omnipresent ethical dimension.

Fourth, what are the implications for theory of the heavy emphasis on practical knowledge throughout the foregoing analysis? Technical rationality enshrines a commitment to a specific type of theory that can be seen as entirely inimical to practice. From its perspective, it can seem that practice is 'merely an expression of embarrassment at the deplorable, but soon overcome, condition of incomplete theory', or that 'to be consigned to practice means to have to make do as much as needs be without a perfect theory' (Bubner, 1981, p. 204). But the analysis of practice and of practical judgement outlined above carries no corresponding anti-theoretical commitment (it is itself indeed a theoretical exercise, of a kind first modelled by Aristotle in a series of treatises, not only the *Ethics* – *Nicomachean* and *Eudemian* – but also the *Rhetoric, Politics* and *Poetics*). Having first reiterated that this analysis did not reject technical rationality *tout court*, I want to elaborate a little here both on my reasons for distinguishing earlier between technical rationality and the modern scientific project *per se*, and on the kind of theory that I see as particularly complementary to practical rationality.

It is true that the *results* of research in the natural sciences can be exploited within a technical or instrumental frame (since they yield knowledge of the form 'if conditions a, b, c obtain, then the occurrence of x, y, z can be reliably predicted' – hence the increasing call for evidence-based practice within the caring professions). The important point, however, is that, *as practices of enquiry*, the sciences themselves cannot at all be pursued with the kind of control sought within a technicist frame. To the contrary, the generation of explanatory hypotheses – or the devising of ingenious and fruitful experiments – which lies at the heart of scientific advance, requires, for all the scaffolding of method, creative insights that cannot be reliably predicted or efficiently produced. Moreover, the most thorough demolition of that picture of the scientific enterprise (that is, 'positivism') that has made it plausible to misconstrue it in technicist terms has been effected over the past few decades not by reactionary philosophers with an animus against science but precisely by philosophers of science intimately acquainted with its history and its innermost operations and procedures. It is in their work that the affinities between research in the natural – and *a fortiori* the social – sciences and the kind of inquiries conducted in, for example, a law-court or in establishing the authenticity of an artwork have been most persuasively canvassed.[12] And it is from them that we should by now have learned the true foolishness of the 'physics envy' that has characterized so many attempts to give the prestige of 'theory' or 'proper professionalism' to upwardly aspiring practices.

What then, finally, is the role of theory in relation to practices and the kind of practical knowledge that, as I have argued here, should be at their heart? There is indeed a stock of generalizations built by research in different socio-practical domains. They do not, however, have that law-like character of established theories in natural science that ensures that – when conditions which they precisely specify are met – their (retrospective) power of explanation can be translated into a (prospective) power of prediction. Instead, they remain tied to an inductive logic and claim to establish what is the case only 'for the most part' (*epi to polu*, a stock phrase in Aristotle's *Ethics*); and from this there follows their unavoidable predictive weakness. I say 'unavoidable' because from this weakness it cannot be concluded that they *fail* by the standards of physics or biochemistry. Rather, their subject matter – that is human affairs in the variety of domains in which they are enacted – is itself permeated by an unpredictability that no theory can exorcise. This is due to the open-textured and intricate character of action-situations that I have already noted as well as to the fact that even when agents are busily trying to predict the actions of others they may simultaneously be intending to make *their own* actions unpredictable by those others. From the indefinitely reflexive character of this intention – the way in which it can recursively allow for the others' attempts to outwit it – it follows that only *after* the transaction can its outcome be reliably specified.[13]

Unpredictability, of course, is not the whole story. There are also patterns of recurrence that ground reliable expectations without which social life in general, as well as within its more specialized enclaves, would collapse into incoherence. Some of these patterns are sedimented in our habitual stocks of tacit knowledge but some may also be elucidated by social scientists in statistical regularities (of the kind, for example, used by insurance companies in calculating the risk factors associated with different categories of drivers, or indeed in epidemiology and the statistically informed identification of 'at risk' populations – the smoker, the obese child and adults of a sedentary disposition). Apart from the fact that these are *only* regularities – and so can never reliably predict in individual cases – there is another significant respect in which they differ from law-like generalizations in natural science. Whereas, the latter give us a deep-structure knowledge that is radically discontinuous from the content of commonsense, thereby opening doors to previously unimaginable technical advances, the generalizations of social science are rarely counterintuitive and so, typically, they corroborate rather than substantially reorientate the judgements of experienced practitioners. This does not of course render them valueless. But that it is to a different kind of theory that we should mainly look for illumination about the perplexities of practice may be gathered, somewhat paradoxically, from one such generalization that now seems to be a well-established finding in research on successfully innovative organizations: the inverse correlation that holds between their effectiveness and the routine predictability of their operations. Successful organizations – at least when their core tasks have a substantial degree of complexity – are ones with an inbuilt tolerance for uncertainty; an ability continually to reconfigure how problems are perceived and objectives interpreted is widely diffused in individuals and small groups, and these multiple loci of initiative are linked – and their respective contributions coordinated – through forms of communication that emphasize the exchange of information rather than the issuing of directives.

Even if this finding has itself a generalized range of application, its content – like the whole drift of the analysis in this chapter – points to a different kind of research, without generalizing ambitions. In areas such as education studies, policy studies or nursing studies (as well as in the social sciences generally) the price that generalized empirical findings must pay for their very generalizability, it would seem, is a certain thinness of content. They need to be complemented, then, by thickly descriptive studies. These will embrace a variety of narrative modes and be strongly hermeneutical in character. That is to say, they will tell stories about particular projects or episodes, for example in the history of an individual teacher or university department, and they will do so with the kind of interpretative skill that can bring out the complex weaving of plot and characters, the dense meshing of insights and oversights, of convergent or contrary motivations and interests, of anticipated or unanticipated responses from the internal environment – or irruptions from the external one – all conspiring to bring relative success or failure. If, with their deep embeddedness in a particular milieu, these studies do indeed renounce the generalizing ambitions of wider-gauge research, they are not on that account condemned to narcissism or self-enclosure. To the contrary, when they are well done – which, among other things, will require a keenly reflective awareness of their 'point of view' – they possess what might be called epiphanic power: they disclose an exemplary significance in the setting they depict so that it proves capable of illuminating other settings – without need for rerouting through abstract generalities and, indeed, with greatest potential effect for those most deeply in the throes of the very particularity of another setting.[14] Here we are reminded that the power and potentially universal import of all literary art lies in the vividness of its evocation of entirely particular characters and situations – so that any effort to create representativeness would already betray weakness. It was Aristotle himself who long ago suggested in the *Poetics* that drama and story can instruct and move us precisely because, *in* their depiction of particular cases and characters, they reveal – without necessarily stating or explaining – universal themes. And in this, as in much else, perhaps contemporary theory of the practical can still learn from 'the Philosopher'.[15]

■ Notes

1   It is noteworthy that MacIntyre's conception of 'practice' differs in connotation and denotation from Aristotle's conception of *praxis* and that this difference stems from their different ways of construing 'internal'. An activity counts for Aristotle as a *praxis* if what it achieves (that is, its end or *telos*) is internal to it, as the end of dancing transpires in the very performance, or the virtue of an act transpires in the brave or just act itself. If, on the other hand, an activity has its end external to itself, in the sense of enduring after it as a separate product or state-of-affairs – as a well-designed building or a person restored to health endure after the activities of the architect or the health care professional – then it counts as *poiesis*, a category that he explicitly distinguishes from *praxis*. For MacIntyre, however, good building and good health are internal to the practices of architecture and of nursing and health care – they are the goods whose intended achievement defines them as the particular practices that they are. Whereas Aristotle understands internality in relation to the activity of the practitioner, then, for MacIntrye it pertains to the wider practice. But here MacIntyre is still following an ancient understanding: what he has to say about practices echoes what Plato says about various *technai* and the care they have for their own proper ends (not that Aristotle disagrees with Plato on this – it is just that his own analytical angle is different).

2   The claim that teaching counts as a practice is not uncontroversial; in fact, it has been denied by MacIntyre himself. For this denial, see MacIntyre and Dunne, 2004, and for my counterargument that it *is* indeed a practice, Dunne, 2004.

3   For a fuller account of these key notions in Aristotle, see Dunne, 1997.

4   Aristotle himself employs this analogy of the rule used by builders at Lesbos (which is 'not rigid but adapted to the shape of the stone') in his discussion of the way in which equity is more flexible than the written code of law which must be amended if it is to do justice to the unique features of each concrete situation. See *Nicomachean Ethics*, 5, 10.

5   *The Tacit Dimension* is the title of a book by Polanyi, 1967; see also Polanyi, 1964.

6   Dewey, 1977 offers a succinct critical reinterpretation of contemporary dilemmas in education through appeal to a conception of experience. But for a more subtle and developed account of this conception itself, see Dewey, 2005.

7   Here I bring Aristotelian practice close to a more Eastern, and especially Zen, notion of practice as a spiritual discipline focused not only on the attainment of a specific end but, in and through this, on the achievement of mindfulness – though, conversely, mindfulness itself is achieved in and through submitting oneself to the quite specific demands of the practice. For an interesting elaboration of mindfulness as a kind of relaxed attentiveness or attunement in which there is a felicitous overcoming of dualities between 'subject' and 'object', as well as between mind and body, see Herrigal, 1971 or, in a more Western adaptation, Gallwey 1981, which describes playing golf 'in the zone', when concentration is effortless, and the golf-swing almost looks after itself. It is perhaps a similarly absorbed state that Yeats captures in the last stanza of 'Among Schoolchildren', with its concluding lines: 'O body swayed to music, O brightening glance / How can we know the dancer from the dance?'

8   For example, in the remarks on method in bk. 1, ch. 3, Aristotle writes, 'It is a mark of the educated mind to expect only that degree of exactness in a field that the field will allow – and so not e.g. to make mathematical rigour the standard for rhetoric.' Or later when he points out the need for equitable judgement to effect a 'correction of law where the latter is defective owing to its generality', he makes it clear that the 'defect' here 'is not in the law nor in the lawmaker but in *the nature of the thing*, since *the matter of practical affairs* is of this kind from the start' (bk. 5, ch. 10).

9   These examples are clearly from fields of specifically human interaction. But not too dissimilar are crafts such as navigation, hunting or (in the ancient Greek understanding of it) medicine.

10   The points I have made here are derived (I hope, recognisably) from Hannah Arendt (1998); For a much fuller elaboration of these points see Dunne (1997), chapters 3 and 4.

11   In the context of discussing educative teaching as a specific domain of practice, students have been central to my concern, see Dunne (2004, 2005).

12   Influential early examples of this work in the philosophy of science were Kuhn, 1966, Kuhn, 1977, and Putnam, 1978.

13   My discussion here is indebted to MacIntyre, 1985, ch. 8.

14   What I call here 'exemplary significance' is subtly analysed in Lovlie, 1997; for an illuminating account of the 'epiphanic' power of literature, see Taylor, 1992, ch. 23.

15   This chapter is a revised version of a paper published as 'An Intricate Fabric: Understanding the Rationality of Practice' in *Pedagogy, Culture and Society*, 13, 3 (2005): 367–389. www.tandf.co.uk/journals. In revising it, with the special case of nursing in mind, I have benefited from and am grateful for the insightful help of John Drummond.

Chapter 6

Profession and practice: The higher education of nursing

Paul Standish

■ Introduction

To educate someone is necessarily to have some sense of the good of the body of knowledge or practice that is the subject of their learning. To educate well is necessarily to act in accordance with, or to be true to, that good. This is the case whether the subject is academic or vocational; indeed it helps to weaken that distinction. To educate in, for example, history, is not merely to present or pass on a body of knowledge but to initiate the learner into the practice of historians, into the kinds of things that historians do; conversely, to educate a nurse is not merely to initiate them into a practice but to introduce them to the body of knowledge that informs that practice. The distinction between body of knowledge and practice is also blurred. It follows that to educate nurse educators or, for that matter, to research nursing education is also to relate to a practice that already incorporates the relation to the practical field of nursing. Whatever might constitute the theorization or study of nurse education is then not separable from concern with the good of nursing. It is for this reason that many chapters in this book move back and forth between the consideration of what seem to be more purely educational concerns and questions directly addressed to the matter of what it is to be a nurse. These connections are never far from the surface in what follows.

To the profession of nursing and health care education, now increasingly well established within the university and understandably eager to assert its intellectual credentials, the pressure of what Gilbert Ryle called 'the intellectualist legend' can be particularly acute. Ryle was referring to the widely held and more or less Cartesian belief that a practically competent action must be preceded – at least logically, if not psychologically – by a mental operation, and his *The Concept of Mind* was dedicated to the task of demonstrating and overcoming this false picture of mind, the idea of 'the ghost in the machine' (Ryle, 1949). If the intellectualist legend is to be resisted, two imperatives immediately suggest themselves. One is the need for alertness to the ways that the pressure to intellectualize is likely to distort. The other is that what the mind is *and* what the body is, the health of which are the objects of the professional practices in question, must be understood in different, perhaps more holistic terms. It seems clear in many respects that Ryle's lesson has not been learned. Given the nature of the connections in the fields that are our concern between vocational education and the competence it seeks to realize, how are ideas of profession and practice to be understood?

In vocational higher education today the words 'profession' and 'practice' inevitably figure prominently. In their multiple connotations, however, they are charged with a surreptitious emotive force and a disturbing lack of clarity. While much can be gained through a sociological approach to these matters, especially regarding the institutional positioning of professions and practices, the present discussion is committed to something of a different order. I propose two avenues of approach. In the first, which will constitute the major part of this discussion, I shall consider Hubert Dreyfus's widely influential and rightly celebrated account of the development of practical competence. In the professional education of nurses and health care practitioners, his work has been shown, by Patricia Benner and others, to have particular purchase (see especially Benner, 1984). Avoiding both the limitations of behaviourism and the false dichotomies of theory and practice, Dreyfus provides in many respects a rich analysis of the range of practical activity, from everyday skilled coping to expertise. In the development of these ideas, he draws especially on the philosophy of Martin Heidegger, of whose work he is a renowned interpreter. It is probably fair to say that, in Anglophone contexts, it is primarily thanks to Dreyfus that Heidegger's work has had influence amongst nursing and health care educators, as well as amongst professionals in other vocational fields. What is not well known is the fact that his reading of Heidegger developed very much out of his relationship with the American philosopher, Samuel Todes. Todes and Dreyfus had been students together at Yale, but Todes died prematurely. He did not publish widely, but the PhD dissertation he wrote was regarded as exceptional, and the influence of the thoughts that were developed there had a profound effect on Dreyfus: they undoubtedly prepared the way for, and in some ways conditioned, the reading of Heidegger that Dreyfus was later to undertake. This much is made clear in the substantial introduction that Dreyfus has written to the posthumous publication of that dissertation under the title *Body and World* (Todes, 2001). The account of embodiment in Todes's book provides a subtle yet robust challenge to the more intellectualist conceptions that have tended to shape the understanding of competence in nursing and health care, not least in education in these fields. Dreyfus's comparatively recent honouring of this text and his acknowledgement of the influence it had on him make the book a valuable guide to the thinking behind his interpretation of Heidegger and his account of practical competence. But the nature of this influence also helps to reveal what I believe to be limitations in that account, especially insofar as it relates to higher education and to the idea of a profession but perhaps also in more pervasive terms. I shall identify this weakness in terms of what I shall call the pragmatist orientation to his thought.

It is through the identification of limitations in this way that I shall move towards the second approach to the topic, which is addressed briefly as something of a coda to the main body of the discussion. This will take seriously the idea of professing suppressed in the term 'profession', with its suggestions of the profession of faith and of broader perfectionist commitments. This is by no means to dispense completely with the arguments Dreyfus provides, for these are eloquently expressed and invaluable in the avoidance of cruder understandings of practice. It is to weigh the costs, in the description of such practices, of neglecting this larger picture. I shall attempt to show the importance of that picture specifically with regard to nurse education, but the force of the argument extends also to health care education more generally and in some ways to higher education as a whole.

Let us begin by considering the emergence of the institutional conditions that have made so pressing the need for Dreyfus's account of practical competence.

■ The rise of technical rationality

As Dreyfus helps to show, in the nineteenth and twentieth centuries, the spectacular success of industrialized production, and the social structures it generated, brought new ways of thinking about the social world and about human lives. In some ways endeavouring to emulate the physical sciences and technology, the new social sciences seemed to promise an objectivity in relation to the changing social world and the possibility of freedom from subjective prejudices. Generalizability provided the means of escaping the limitations of merely local or particular contexts, while the institutionalization of procedures of replication and control suggested the possibility of overcoming unpredictability. At the same time, the emphasis on transparency and the public visibility of new developments meant that less was to be done on the strength of unspecified intentions. Transparency and accountability dovetailed with the presumption of clear-cut criteria for success and, hence, aroused the expectation of an end to ambiguous interpretations. Through all these changes there was manifest a clear tendency towards abstraction and standardization.

In comparison with the apparent machine-precision of these practices, practical knowledge, typified in the popular imagination by craft knowledge perhaps, was thought unreliable, makeshift and unaccountable. Insofar as it was characterized by adherence to traditions into which novices were initiated through protracted periods of apprenticeship, the substance of which was often opaque to outsiders and sometimes acknowledged as such by insiders, it was often disparaged as elitist. Was it not then only a matter of rationality that the *practical* should be absorbed into the *technical?* Language, it was assumed, had a primarily representational function, and so the processes in question could be rendered explicit. In an increasingly complex world, and against a background of obvious social inequality and injustice, such changes seemed eminently reasonable.

In collusion with the intellectualist legend, these factors lay the way for the model of technical competence that has progressively colonized the range of practice, for the blithe acceptance of the legitimacy of the importing from industry of quality control, and for the audit culture to which these are in service. In 1979, anticipating so many aspects of the manifestations of change in the ensuing decades, Jean-François Lyotard coined the term 'performativity', the nihilism of which is intimated in the following characterization:

> The true goal of the system, the reason it programs itself like a computer, is the optimization of the global relationship between input and output. Even when the rules are in the process of changing and innovations are occurring, even when its dysfunctions (such as strikes, crises, unemployment, or political revolutions) inspire hope and lead to belief in an alternative, even then what is actually taking place is only an internal readjustment, and its result can be no more than an increase in the system's 'viability'. The only alternative to this kind of performance improvement is entropy, or decline (Lyotard, 1984, pp. 11–12).

Lyotard is careful to draw a distinction between innovation, which occurs within the terms of the system, and invention, which involves the 'incoming' of something that breaks with or departs from that system, something at odds with the way things are. It follows, on this account, that the constant reform – the performance improvement – that besets the health service and public education, which is canonized in both managerialism and research into these practices, ends up by quickening the system but at the cost of its real sustenance and vitality.

There is no need here to detail at any length the ways in which performativity plays itself out, but it is worth recalling the missionary zeal that it sometimes exacts. Over the past 15 years, school improvement has become a veritable mini-industry. David Reynolds, for example, unabashedly celebrates the way that a technological approach to teaching can deliver more education to more people, on the strength of a 'known to be valid' knowledge base. Teachers become technical operatives, making maximal use of fail-safe procedures, in a data-rich environment (see Reynolds, 1997). Such accounts thrive on thin descriptions of practice, and these are behaviouristic in kind. The general, intellectualist tendency is towards an emphasis on procedural reasoning to the neglect of the substantive demands of the particular case and of the variety of things that are to be taught and learned. This is a suppression of the possibility of richer accounts of local practices. It is not without irony, then, that in the commitment to these practices, and in the self-conscious, no-nonsense 'rigour' of their approach, there develops a meta-language that is highly rhetorical and sometimes florid in style. Something similar is seen where Dreyfus highlights the euphoric rhetoric of the curriculum planners and managers who proclaim the possibilities of the new technology to enable 'virtually anyone who is not severely handicapped to learn anything, at a "grade A" level, anywhere, any time' (Lewis J. Perelman, in Dreyfus, 2001, p. 27). The missionary zeal here goes hand in hand with an institutionalization of ideas that simul-taneously impels their adoption and hides the extent to which they may be unclear or problematic. Thus, as one example of this, in planning, teaching, learning and research, the idea of data is naturalized. As Lyotard anticipated, 'Data-banks are the Encyclopaedia of tomorrow. They tran-scend the capacity of each of their users. They are "nature" for postmodern man' (Lyotard, 1984, p. 51).[1]

'Performativity', in Lyotard's usage, has an unremitting pejorative force. It should be noted, however, that this is apt to obscure the necessary connection between performative utterance and the establishment of institutions.[2] Whatever its descriptive or prescriptive function, language also and inevitably itself serves to enact or realize the institution it purports only to represent, and this can be for good or ill. It becomes clear that the language that is used is of central importance in determining the substance of the institutions we have. The problems noted in the previous paragraph have become endemic not only in educational research, but also in the curriculum and in assessment more generally, even in the 'official' discourse of teachers, students and other stakeholders themselves. That we stand today in need of a better, less technical, less 'spun' and more mature language of education scarcely, in the present context, needs arguing for.[3] In nursing and health care, where the need for a specialized, technical language is obvious enough, the same point can still be made. It is in this light that Dreyfus's achievement in wresting the ideas of competence and skill from the technicist and intellectualist colonization they have suffered over the past two decades is very much to be valued.

■ Competence and expertise

Dreyfus emphasizes the point that doing something well in life (in the practical world) typically involves something beyond knowing the rules and having information. Computers, he acknowledges, are exceptionally good with both rules and information, but they are apt to distract us from the fact that something more is needed. One of his most succinct expressions of his conception of practical competence is to be found in *On the Internet*, where, once again, he is at pains to show what computers – for all their amazing usefulness – still cannot do.[4] He identifies a number of broad stages in the advancement of learning, which can be set out schematically as follows (abstracted from Dreyfus, 2001):

Advanced beginner – The student is given information and instructions. She can proceed in a relatively detached, analytical frame of mind.

Competence – The student encounters a bewildering array of information and a variety of situations. She starts to orientate herself by means of a particular plan or perspective, which she adopts according to the circumstances. But this is disconcerting. She has chosen the plan herself, and so if things go wrong she knows it is at least partly her own fault. But if things go well there is a kind of elation unknown to the beginner. As we are embodied beings, and not computers, it is natural for us to become involved in this way. Resistance to involvement and risks commonly leads to stagnation and regression. Students depend very much on the kind of relation to risk that their teachers model. In the distance-learning package, this tends to be kept to a minimum.

Proficiency – Only if detachment is replaced by involvement can the student move to this stage. Situational discriminations and associated responses build up in the learner's experience. Intuition begins to replace reasoned response. The learner simply sees what needs to be done, rather than having to calculate a course of action. But she still has to decide how to do it.

Expertise – With a vast repertoire of situational discriminations, the expert sees what needs to be done *and how to do it*. As Aristotle says, the expert 'straightaway does the appropriate thing, at the appropriate time, in the appropriate way'. To reach this stage, observation and imitation of an expert can replace a random search for better ways to act.

Mastery – At this stage, it is necessary not merely to imitate an expert. One must develop one's own style, and this can be helped by apprenticeship to several different teachers. This can destabilize and confuse the learner, but the benefit is that it leads her to develop her own style or voice.

Practical wisdom – People not only have to learn a repertoire of skills. They must become initiated into the style of their culture in order to acquire practical wisdom. (What sense do skills have without this?) Like embodied common-sense understanding, cultural style is itself too embodied to be captured in a theory and to be passed on in isolation from a way of life. Barely visible to us under normal circumstances, it is the background against which our actions have their sense. Practical wisdom cannot be divorced from it.

There is obviously scope for questioning the detail of these categories, just as there is for considering their pertinence to practices of different kinds, but I do not propose to examine the stages of development that Dreyfus delineates in any detail. More important for present purposes is the power of such an account to disturb the kinds of assumptions that otherwise acquiesce in technicist ways of thinking. And probably no one has done more than Dreyfus to advance the understanding of the skilled coping at the heart of human practices. He has done this in such a way as to cast light on critical aspects of the postmodern world (on what computers can and cannot do, on expertise and entrepreneurship, on the Internet and teaching and learning, and on changing technology and community), the authority of this 'applied' work deriving in no small measure from his research into Husserl and Heidegger, and especially from his perspicuous reading of Division I of *Being and Time* (*Sein und Zeit*). His introduction to Todes's *Body and World* reveals a thinker who is far less well known but who, it is Dreyfus's clear belief, is badly underrated. It is a book that in many respects provides the background thought to the account of competence presented above, elaborating a theory of skilled coping in relation to perceptual judgement. It is because this book has so much influenced Dreyfus and because of its limitations that I want now to examine it directly.

■ Skilled coping, perceptual truth and satisfaction

Body and World is a powerful book and in some ways an eccentric one. Its central claim is that the 'failure to understand perceptual judgement opens an unbridgeable gap between knowledge and feeling' (Todes, 2001, p. 261). What we encounter here are, to be sure, difficult arguments, but if we are to gain insight into the limitations of Dreyfus's work, and the significance of these limitations in professional education, they will repay some examining. Let us begin by considering some representative passages from the book, which I propose to quote in some detail.

Our being in the world involves, according to Todes, first of all a skilled bodily comportment, through which we, for example, move to sit in a chair or switch on a light. There is a natural 'fit' between things and our bodies, between body and world, and this is realized in perceptual judgement of this kind, through 'the umbilical cord of bodily movement' (p. 53). Todes uses the term 'poise', which he contrasts with the will, to capture 'the *perfect fit* of me in my circumstances' (p. 70). It is only in moments of breakdown – say, where the light-switch fails to work – that we become cognitively aware of what is happening: 'Thus, when one fails in what he is attempting to do, one necessarily loses his poise and is, at least, momentarily, thrown off balance, however quickly one may recover his balance and poise. To be poised is to be *self*-possessed by being in touch with one's circumstances' (p. 66). The effect of the intrinsically habit-forming character of perception is to stabilize our experience (p. 80): 'Our poise is sensuous proof that the perceptual experience of our immediate future conforms to that of our immediate past, and without poise no determinate perception is possible' (p. 79). The structuring indicated in this and similar statements is elaborated in architectural terms: Todes refers recurrently to the natural philosophy of the body as providing a first floor for the development of understanding concerning higher levels of experience – 'I will attempt to show that there are no "pure" forms of conceptual imagination by showing that the whole *level* of our conceptual imagination (form as well as content) makes sense only in terms of a primordial level of perceptual experience' (p. 156). The inactively regarded object is derivative from the object that is actively felt: 'The human body is the material subject of the world' (p. 88).

This much, I believe, is powerful enough, but further dimensions of the picture need to be revealed. A critical factor in this account is its ethical naturalism, in which desire finds fulfilment in satisfaction: 'The human body is first prompted to be a moving body at all, and thus to generate the spatiotemporal field of appearances (which is the apparent world of our needs), only by its needs that, literally, move the body to find pleasure (satisfaction of its needs), and to avoid pain (dissatisfaction of its needs)' (p. 73). In fact, the vocabulary of fulfilment, harmonizing with the elaboration of the 'fit' between body and world, which is the ground floor of our experience, is strongly evident throughout the book:

> Satisfaction involves a relation not just between ourselves and the satis-
> fying object, but also between both of these and the world of experience
> that is to some extent closed and completed in the satisfaction . . . To be
> satisfied is to be content; it is to be full-filled with the given content of
> the world of our experience, so that our world no longer seems open,
> empty, still-to-be-satisfactorily-filled (p. 59).

This naturalism is more or less pervasive: 'A degree of pleasure and of pain, of satisfaction and of dissatisfaction, thus pervades every possible experience in virtue of its being in the world of experience' (p. 73). The moderation of pleasure and pain, understood in terms of needs, suggests a kind of homeostasis in which a certain conception of health is modelled.

Leading influences behind Todes's thought are Maurice Merleau-Ponty and, especially, Immanuel Kant, but this brief excursion into the eloquent language of this text may well prompt in the reader a sense of the prox-imity of these thoughts to the phenomenological analyses developed in Heidegger's *Being and Time*. While the central claim regarding perceptual judgement provides a sound thematic basis for the argument, and while the detail of the analysis is fascinating, I am less persuaded than Dreyfus of its originality, and there are central aspects of the position that is advanced that remain unconvincing. On the strength of these doubts, I shall in what follows raise questions for Todes's account concerning, first, the relation of perception to the social world, and, second, the prominence of the idea of satisfaction. On the strength of this I shall then turn to aspects of Dreyfus's position as elaborated elsewhere.

In his own introduction to *Body and World*, Todes makes clear what he is not setting out to do. This is not a study in the social philosophy of the human body (concerning the body's role in our knowledge of persons), nor in what he calls its theology (concerning our sense of death and intimations of mortality). It is a study in the natural philosophy of the human body. Todes concedes that the social questions are both more obvious and of more general interest than the natural ones, but their solution, he claims, turns out to presuppose a solution to the natural ones, and the theological issues in turn depend on the natural and the social questions. As we saw above, Todes refers recurrently to the natural philosophy of the body as providing a first floor for the development of understanding concerning higher levels of experience.

While it seems correct to say that the social philosophy of the human body (say, concerning gender roles or our relation to childhood, or perhaps in the construction of the idea of 'the patient') depends upon the natural philosophy of the human body, there are problems with the suggestion that there could be such a natural philosophy, especially where this concerns perceptual *knowledge*, in the absence of acknowledgement of the social world. In the context of the *social* world it is indeed possible to provide an account of the ongoing satisfaction of the anticipations of poised perceptions. The absence of an attempt even to consider this in Todes's account is remarkable, for without it the claim that ongoing coping gives us perceptual knowledge is hard to sustain. In short, there can be no account of driving a car or dribbling a basketball or sitting on a chair or picking up a box in the absence of rule-following. Todes's discussion of rule-following is tied very much to his notion of habit and to what makes the world 'habit-able'. But the crucial point, if Wittgenstein is right, is that rule-following presupposes the existence of a social world. Wittgenstein's so-called Private Language Argument depends upon the idea that rules logically presuppose the possibility of mistakes, and mistakes presuppose the possibility of correction, which in turn requires the existence of norms of practice within a social group. Moreover, it is not just that the practices cited here are particularly complex social practices: in human activity rule-following goes all the way down.

In the absence of the acknowledgement of the social world on the same 'floor' of the building, as it were (indeed in the same rooms), Todes's perceptual knowledge claim looks decidedly unsteady, if it does not smack of anthropomorphism. The claim would be anthropomorphic to the extent that the account of perceptual knowledge depends upon full-blown human nature in ways that it is not prepared to acknowledge. He guards against some of the difficulties here with the use of inverted commas – for example, in referring to non-conceptual perceptual 'beliefs' – but one wonders to what extent this textual device merely serves to hide the problem. Todes's architecture persistently gives the impression that there can be perceptual knowledge in a human being in the absence of initiation into the social world. So the following questions arise: Does such knowledge extend to the experience of animals? If not, why not? And does it extend to infants?

Wittgenstein's account of something like the primordial, of 'forms of life', seems in part to draw attention to differences between cultural practices, but it is important to emphasize the greater prominence it gives to the bodily aspects of human beings – to the ways in which forms of life develop in relation to physiological needs. The idea of a form of life is closely tied to what Wittgenstein calls 'agreement in judgements'. With this phrase, he has in mind not the kind of agreement that might be reached as the result of a debate, say, but rather the fact that human bodies condition people to find things the same – for example, that some things are edible and some not, or that a particular atmospheric temperature range is tolerable. His enigmatic remark, 'If a lion could speak, we could not understand him' (Wittgenstein, 1958, p. 223), testifies to the essential role of the *human* body in the nature of our thought. These remarks demonstrate not only the ways in which human thought is tied to the particular configuration of the bodily features of human beings, a point that Todes richly develops, but also the fact that such thought is not generated by the individual alone, a point to which Todes seems blind.

None of this is intended to defend the idea that Todes is attacking: that ongoing successful coping must involve conceptual identification. On the contrary, Todes is right to say that such (smooth, ongoing) coping excludes cognitive activity of this kind. But it *is* to emphasize that coping cannot be understood in the absence of the background of the social world.

An essential feature of this social world is language, which in human experience also goes 'all the way down'. To recognize that this is so is to foreground not abstract conceptual thought but rather human activity understood as rule-following practices. (Wittgenstein will speak of language-games, of course.) While there are forms of human activity that do not directly involve language, they are nevertheless characterized by a background that is linguistic. It is in the light of that background that it does indeed become plausible enough to speak of non-conceptual perceptual knowledge. But a further point follows from this to the effect that while the infant has the same bodily configuration as the adult, any claims to perceptual knowledge on her part must be severely constrained by the fact that she is not (yet) a participant in the linguistic background that is the condition for such knowledge. In other words, perceptual knowledge in its mature forms cannot develop in advance of social and linguistic initiation, and so to speak of the perceptions of the infant does indeed involve a degree of anthropomorphism. This is not to say that language must come first: light dawns gradually over the whole. But Todes's argument seems to proceed as if the linguistic turn had never happened. In sum, this brings me to the conclusion that Todes's account of this first floor of our experience cannot stand up in the absence of the acknowledgement of the social world.

The second, more qualified question that I raise has to do with how far Todes's thought is constrained by the limitations of the economies of satisfaction that are central to his argument. I referred to these above in terms of his ethical naturalism. How far do these fail to do justice to the body and to perception?

Todes draws a distinction between objective and subjective satisfaction. A sentence such as 'I am satisfied that she is dead' is ambiguous, in the absence of any determining context, between my having evidence that she is dead and my being pleased or relieved by this fact. In the former case, I am satisfied *that* something is so, while in the latter I am satisfied *by* its being so. In other words, objective satisfaction relates primarily to conditions of truth, while subjective satisfaction refers to conditions of desire.

This economy has a bearing on how truth and desire are conceived. Thus in objective satisfaction, it becomes apparent that truth is understood in terms of correctness (or adequation) and not *aletheia* (that is, truth as revealing). (Of course, the vocabulary of correctness belongs to propositional rather than perceptual knowledge, but I am suggesting that in the account of perceptual satisfaction it comes to shape the understanding of perception also.) How, it needs to be asked, might an account of perceptual knowledge that derived from notions of *aletheia* be different? In subjective satisfaction, desire is understood in relation to lack. Hence both are tied to economies of thought that, on certain arguments (say, those of Deleuze or Levinas, or Kierkegaard or Nietzsche, or for that matter Heidegger himself), close off possibilities of understanding the human condition – mind and body – and that constrain the ways in which the possibilities of life might be conceived. Ethical naturalism along these lines amounts to a constriction of the very idea of the ethical.

It will be recalled that Todes insists that his concern is not with the theology of the human body. He uses this phrase, let it be remembered, to refer not to matters of theistic belief but to our sense of death and intimations of mortality. What is noticeable, however, is that there are points in Todes's text at which something seems to break through, something beyond any simple economy of need and satisfaction. Todes acknowledges that satiation, like apathy and frustration, can make one 'incapable of responding to anything through felt want' (p. 69). And recognizing the role of affect in both subjective and objective forms of satisfaction, he draws attention to an interesting asymmetry between the way that the former tends to be characterized by relief from distress, or the gratification of desire, and the way that the latter encompasses not only some sense of relief but also a positive pleasure at the original stimulation – a pleasure prompting us to similar exertion in the future, making us keener for experience and heightening our sensitivity. In the light of Todes's valuable observation here, I want to draw attention also to a perhaps muted but nevertheless welcome irruptive element in his language. He speaks more than once in almost Dionysian terms of the 'clamorous chorus' of needs (p. 67); the boy who looks up at the hills of the valley in which he has grown up finds the 'beckoning' horizon, calling him to give what lies beyond it 'the determination of place' (p. 57); more bleakly he acknowledges Auschwitz as a 'break-out-from the world' (p. 62). It is language such as this that intimates momentarily something beyond or other than the satisfaction of needs, though the extent of the importance of this for Todes is difficult to fathom.

Moments of insight these may be, but the significance of the present discussion remains very much with the question of the kind of place that is given to ongoing skilled coping in the living of our lives and, hence, in the understanding of body and mind. Todes's architecture gives it foundational importance. For Dreyfus the significant metaphor is the centre. The nature of this placing opens up interesting questions, I believe, regarding Dreyfus's relation to Heidegger but also in connection with a kind of restraint that is evident in his introduction to *Body and World*.

■ Dreyfus and Heidegger

As Dreyfus has recently put this in a reply to John Haugeland, in *Being-in-the-World*, his commentary on Division I of Heidegger's *Being and Time* (Dreyfus, 1991), it was in part his purpose to demonstrate (and celebrate) Heidegger's shifting of the philosophical tradition's emphasis 'on getting our descriptions of objects right to Dasein's absorption in unimpeded coping with equipment' (Dreyfus, 2000, p. 313).[5] The roughly pragmatist reading towards which Dreyfus was then inclined tended to see this coping as in service of yet more ongoing coping, a figure in which the modelling of health as homeostasis is tacitly reinforced. This was the product, he has come to concede, of 'more or less ignoring Division II of Heidegger's book as something of an existentialist embarrassment' (ibid.). The correction of this neglect has led Dreyfus to the view that Dasein 'copes with equipment and pursues truth not merely for the sake of understanding entities but ultimately for the sake of taking a stand on *its own* being' (p. 314). Admirably clear though *Being-in-the-World* is, this later realignment suggests a deeper reading. But at this point two crucial questions arise. The first is the question of how ongoing coping is *placed* with regard to the 'fantastic exaction' of being towards death that Division II identifies? Such an exaction would surely lead beyond the economies I have discussed. The second is the obvious one: how can an account of practical competence that 'more or less' ignores our sense of death and intimations of mortality be adequate to the profession of nursing and nurse education?

The question of the placing of ongoing coping should also be raised in connection with Dreyfus's equally clear but still somewhat secularized reading of the later Heidegger. The centering that is to the fore here is found in the idea of focal practices. As an example, in 'Highway Bridges and Feasts: Heidegger and Borgman on how to affirm technology', Dreyfus and Charles Spinosa ponder the kinds of focal practices that can exist in conditions of contemporary technology, seeking to understand such practices in terms of Heidegger's 'fourfold' of earth, sky, gods and mortals. The relation between these forces or conditions is to be understood in the form of the intersecting lines of a cross, in the necessary tensions of which human beings live out their lives and through which their practices are constituted. 'Earth' implies the fruitful yet retiring source of sustenance, 'sky' the cycles of time and changes in atmosphere and mood, 'gods' our orientation by aspiration and vocation, while 'mortals' suggests our flickering awareness of our own finitude as the place of revelation. In relation to the gods, Dreyfus and Spinosa write,

> When a focal event such as a family meal is working to the point where it has its particular integrity, one feels extraordinarily in tune with all that is happening, a special graceful ease, and events seem to unfold of their own momentum – all combining to make the moment more centered and more a gift. A reverential sentiment arises; one feels thankful or grateful for receiving all that is brought out by this particular situation (Dreyfus and Spinosa, 1997, p. 167).

These are moments that are constantly threatened by the dispersal of modern technological practices – as found *par excellence* in the institutions of health care and education – through which we are converted into nothing more than flexible resources. Dreyfus and Spinosa's response to this threat is to suggest that we should see ourselves as mortal disclosers of plural worlds, finding our integrity in our openness to dwelling in many worlds, with the capacity to move among them.

For many people scenes of the kind depicted here may truly consti-tute heightened moments in their lives, and one should be cautious about casting doubt on their value. But in Dreyfus and Spinosa's emphasis on attunement and sentiment, and in the general dampening of the reli-gious (including the Christian) resonances of Heidegger's vocabulary (the intersecting lines of the cross), it is difficult not to see once again a centering, perhaps naturalizing movement – one that may render the distance between these thoughts and the economies of satisfaction iden-tified above less problematic. For Heidegger, early in *Being and Time*, a vivid example of the ready-to-hand (*Zuhandenheit*), which apparently corres-ponds well with Todes's perceptual satisfaction, is the action of hammering a nail into wood. But can such a practice, understood holistically in terms of the micropractice of which it is a part, make sense without taking in, full-blown, as it were, the social world of the building of the house or the barn, or, for that matter, the building of the church itself – its social philosophy, its theology?

A vivid cinematic realization of this is to be found in Peter Weir's popular film *Witness* (1985), where the hardened city cop is investigating a brutal murder, in the toilet of a big city railway station, which has been witnessed by an Amish boy, who is travelling with his mother. He finds himself the victim of police corruption, is wounded and, with the mother's help, escapes to the Amish community, where he is sheltered and nursed. During the time of his recovery, he becomes partially absorbed into the Amish way of life. He acquires the carpentry skills upon which they depend, entering into the daily round of the community's life and work. Just as the opening of the film crosscuts the peace of the Amish farmlands with the sordid and frenetic life of the big city, so now the community's building of the new barn, its mainframe hoisted magnificently against the sky, stands as an expression of the good in stark contrast to the predatory corruption of the police department. The micropractice of carpentry, hammering the nail into wood, has its place in something that exceeds economies of satisfaction. The health of the community, its raising of the barn, bears witness to the greater glory of God.

It is plainly the case that, in his later essays, Heidegger draws upon an evocation of the rural world of the Black Forest and that this, especially in the context of his account of the colonizing effects of technology, is vulnerable to the charge of nostalgia. The same charge applies, with greater force perhaps, to the evocation of the Amish community in *Witness*. If this is to be avoided, it is vitally important that the fourfold is understood also in terms of such ordinary contemporary practices as cruising along the intersections and cloverleafs of city highways, a telling example for Dreyfus, and, an example more germane to the theme of the present essay, as working in a busy hospital ward.

It was said above that the moderation of pleasure and pain, understood in terms of needs and their satisfaction, suggests a kind of homeostasis in which a certain conception of health is modelled, and this is a conception that the culture of accountability can readily recognize. The health of the body as the ground floor in the architecture of our being has an apparent plausibility, and separation of mind and body is convenient for thinking in these terms. But, as William James remarked, foiling the imagery of satisfaction as well as the sanctimonious call to something 'higher', man lives by bread alone only when there is no bread. Restoring a sick person to good health is the restoring of a being who will *not* succumb to the satisfactions of this homeostasis, or who will do so only through a kind of tranquilization. To fail to acknowledge this 'theology', as Todes puts it, or the conditions of the fourfold, as Heidegger puts it, on the ground floor of our being is to misunderstand the architecture of health.

Heidegger can surely never have been far from Dreyfus's introduction to Todes's work. The question that my discussion opens up is this: How far does Dreyfus's partial secularizing of Heidegger incline *him* towards accepting the economies of satisfaction in Todes's account and away from ways of thinking – including Heidegger's thinking about skilled coping – that exceed such bounds? The price of ignoring the existential embarrassment of death is reflected in the attunement of focal experience and the seductions of satisfaction. This skews the context of practice towards a kind of homeostasis, which is of a piece with the underlying ethical naturalism and which is ultimately tranquilizing. This is, one might say, a Californian Heidegger, conditioned, as I have tried to show, by Todes's *Body and World.*

■ Practice and profession

This perfectionist critique of Dreyfus brings me to the second approach to the topic, the coda to the main body of the argument. In working through these accounts of the nature of the body and of perceptual satisfaction, we have circled around the idea of profession in relation to practice. In the light of the preceding attack on ethical naturalism, it is time to take seriously the idea of professing suppressed in the term 'profession', with its suggestions of the profession of faith and of broader perfectionist commitments. The account of competence and expertise that Dreyfus offers is immensely more rich than technicist conceptions of professional competence and practice, and it provides the means of a powerful critique of them. But in its concentration on the holistic coherence of particular practices, it misses the ways that these are riven by something that exceeds their terms.

In nursing this is felt with special poignancy. While all human experience is exposed to the irruption of the event, the proximity in nursing of death itself gives this a particular urgency, casting light on the object of the practice (the patient's health) but extending back into the nurse's embodied involvement in the scene of care and to her own mortality itself. It is not just that nurses need to be ready for the emergencies and other unexpected happenings that will undoubtedly arise, for such contingencies can be planned for. It is rather that mortality and human vulnerability always exceed anything that admits such preparation: this is the irruption of the event. To appreciate this is to understand better the human condition and better to be able to care for the sick. Nursing inevitably involves more than technical competence, then, but one might go further and say that the implications of this for nursing are more far-reaching than for doctors themselves. The nurse is the one who stays when nothing more can be done.

It was said at the start that the theorization or study of nurse education is not separable from concern with the good of nursing. It follows that the credibility of the profession of nurse education must depend less upon its intellectualization than upon its proper acknowledgement of and engagement with the nature of the practice of nursing as indicated in the preceding paragraph. Can any further light be cast on what profession in such circumstances might amount to or require?

In 'The Future of the Profession or The Unconditional University (Thanks to the 'Humanities', What *Could Take Place* Tomorrow) Jacques Derrida sets out what he claims is 'less a thesis, or even a hypothesis, than a declarative engagement, an appeal in the form of a profession of faith: faith in the university and, within the university, faith in the Humanities of tomorrow' (Derrida, 2000, p. 1). Derrida here once again revisits J.L. Austin's celebrated distinction between the constative and the performative in order further to unsettle the distinction between theory and action. The effect is altogether to alter the stakes, in any questioning of the idea of profession, from the preoccupation with status that typically characterizes the mobilization of that term. The questions raised by Derrida's remarks can strike one habituated to such preoccupations as little short of an embarrassment: How far does profession (as of faith) characterize the work in which the professor should rightfully be engaged? How might this indicate something of the future of the profession?

Derrida explores ways in which the idea of profession requires something tantamount to a pledge, to the freely accepted responsibility to profess the truth. Let us expand on this, in the context of vocational education, to say that there must be professed a commitment to the good of the practice, where profession cannot be simply a matter of signing up to agreed precepts or to a professional code but must involve also the continuing, responsible projection of that good. The professor enacts this performative continually in her work: what she says is testimony; as *work* it is necessarily an orientation to a to-come. The academic work of professing must then be something more than the (purely constative) statement of how things are.

The social sciences, no less than the humanities, are not to be understood without reference to questions of mind and body, and of body and world. They relate to a certain conception of public space. That public space is now undergoing fundamental changes with a new virtual topology, with the puzzling contemporary preoccupation with an array of cognate performatives, involving profession or confession: perhaps in the muddled obsession with procedure in the (often over-anxious and unconvincing) definition of various 'professions' and in the sometimes uptight 'rigour' of codes of practice; perhaps in the sometimes narcissistic tendencies of confessional psychotherapy or the self-display and voyeurism of 'reality TV'.

This role of education for nursing and health care cannot be properly played if it is restricted either to the description of what is, or to a training in practical competencies or proficiencies. The emphasis on the performative entails a change of modality: if the description of the world relates to the way *it is*, the work of profession involves always some attempt to see it *as if. . .* ; profession involves the performative putting to work of the *as if.* The responsibility of the professor extends to an openness to the event. It must extend beyond the 'masterable possible', which is the result of conventions and legitimate procedures, to the surprise of the impossible possible, which has the character of the *arrivant*. Openness to the impossible possible, something beyond the range of predetermined categories or a purely autonomous control (certainly beyond measures of effective performance), is essential to the exercise and growth of the imagination that this professing requires. The alternative to this perform-ative professing would be to rest complacently within the settled ways of one's thought, with the presumption that one could simply represent what is or contain the practice in a finite series of competencies, in what amounts to a relinquishing of the very responsibility the university must require. This, surely evoking an older resonance of the term, extends to its *voca-tional* education. I have tried to show the ways in which the very character of nursing and health care make this especially pertinent.

I began by mentioning the ways in which the pressure of 'the intellec-tualist legend', in Ryle's phrase, might have its bearing on a profession eager to establish its intellectual credentials. Ryle is commonly thought of as a central figure in Anglophone, analytical philosophy. What is less well known is that he was influenced by Heidegger. He had reviewed Heide-gger's *Sein und Zeit* in 1929, and he was critical but acknowledged that he was deeply impressed by the book's originality and the power of the mind of its author. A close reading of *The Concept of Mind* reveals remarkable parallels with Heidegger's text. Shortly before he died, when asked about Heidegger's influence on him, Ryle admitted that there may have been an influence that he had been reluctant at the time openly to accept.[6] One critical difference between Ryle and Heidegger, which is relevant to the development of the present discussion is Ryle's tendency towards the kind of ethical naturalism that is in part the target of this chapter – a naturalism in which ideas of body and mind are, in my view, contained and constrained. In view of the political circumstances of the time, and of Heidegger's notorious actions, Ryle's failure of acknowledgement may seem less culpable, but it is reasonable to speculate that it reflects also what must have been his own, perhaps characteristically Anglophone aver-sion to the 'existential embarrassment' of the theme of death. In terms of the philosophy of mind, body and practical competence, this failure of acknowledgement skews the whole picture. Parallel failures of acknow-ledgement in technicism also conspire to subdue understanding of the ordinary, existential and embodied experience of nurses. They prevent the realization of a better professional education in nursing and health care.

■ Notes

1   For a discussion of the idea of data in educational research, see my 'Data Return: the sense of the given in educational research' (Standish, 2001).
2   I draw here more on the thinking of J.L. Austin, whose account of the difference between constative and performative utterance was partly adopted by Lyotard.

The performative nature of the language of institutions is central to the work of Judith Butler. This applies both to formally established institutions such as hospitals or, more generally, the Health Service and to such institutions as racism or indeed gender. The depth of the significance of the distinction in Austin's work has been a sustained preoccupation of Stanley Cavell (e.g., Cavell 1979, 1995, 2005) as well as the subject of the infamous exchange between John Searle and Jacques Derrida recorded in *Limited Inc.* (Derrida, 1988).

3 For an attempt to demonstrate that this is so, see Richard Smith and Paul Standish, ' "It lifted my sights": revaluing higher education in an age of new technology' (Smith and Standish, 2001). For a more developed discussion, relating the degenerative tendencies evident in the modern language of education to the philosophy of Nietzsche, see *Education in an Age of Nihilism* (Blake *et al.*, 2000).

4 For a review symposium based on this book, see *Educational Philosophy and Theory*, 34.4 (2002).

5 In *Being and Time*, Heidegger avoids using the terms 'man' or 'human being' on the grounds that these have become irrevocably burdened with the assumptions of modern metaphysics, preferring the term *Dasein*, which literally means 'being-there' or 'there-being'.

6 In a letter to Michael Murray in 1973, Ryle acknowledges that in respect of Heidegger there may have been 'an indebtedness that I wanted to keep dark' (Ryle, in Murray, 1978, p. 290). For a more detailed discussion, see Murray's 'Heidegger and Ryle: Two Versions of Phenomenology', also in that volume.

Part 3

Curriculum and Expertise

Chapter 7

The myth of the golden mean: Professional knowledge and the problem of curriculum design

Gerard Lum

■ Introduction

In recent years there have been increasing tensions between two conceptions of nursing education: one centred on higher education, on theory; the other centred on work-based learning, on practice. Each has its own advocates who, whatever other differences they might have, would seem to differ first and foremost in their conception of what practitioners need to know. Attempts to reconcile these two positions characteristically take the form of conceding a place for both theory and practice, hence reinforcing the idea that professional capability consists of two fundamentally different kinds of knowledge. And it is thus that the role of the curriculum designer comes to be perceived as one of achieving an appropriate balance between these ostensibly disparate components of knowledge, of seeking out a 'golden mean' such as will delineate the ideal proportions of the theoretical and the practical. Often, to judge by so much discussion in the literature, it is as though all the perceived ills of nursing education could be remedied if only it were possible to somehow strike the correct balance between theory and practice. It is with this that I wish to take task.

■ The problem with the golden mean

From the outset, there are reasons to doubt whether this ambition to achieve the 'golden mean', to strike the correct balance between theory and practice, could ever properly be realized. At the very least, we might question whether the task could ever be approached in the spirit of open-mindedness that might be hoped for. For it would seem that invariably we come to such a task predisposed, as it were forearmed with our own prior conceptual commitments and predilections. The very language we choose to describe the supposed twin components of professional capability often betrays the prejudices we bring to the task. To speak, for example, of some combination of 'knowledge' and 'skills' is at once to intimate that the main thrust of what needs to be *known* is theoretical, supplemented here and there by some appropriate physical or manual dexterity. Conversely, to adopt the current vogue for 'competencies' or 'standards of proficiency' (Nursing and Midwifery Council, 2004b) and 'underpinning knowledge' is to suggest that theory, if not entirely extraneous to the issue of occupational competence, is certainly of secondary importance.

Expressing the distinction in terms of theory and practice may sometimes conceal such differences but does nothing to resolve them. At root is a dissension which is as fundamental as it is familiar. On one side, there are those who see theoretical understanding as the very fountainhead of human action and would regard practice devoid of such understanding as nothing more than brute mechanical behaviour – the very antithesis of professional capability. On the other side there are those for whom the first priority of a vocational preparation must always be the facility for action, the ability to 'do the job'. For theory to be elevated beyond the role of handmaid to practice is, on this view, to slide inexorably towards curricular irrelevance and a preparation less likely to provide that which is necessary for effective performance.

Amidst the discord there is one point of commonality, an issue upon which there can be found almost universal agreement, *viz* the idea that professional capability consists of two logically distinct kinds of knowledge and that the trick is simply a matter of achieving the right balance. It is an idea that runs through every level of thinking and policy-making in vocational education in the UK, not least in nursing education. However, against this tide of assent, I want to propose that the theory–practice distinction, understood as indicating two forms of knowledge, is fundamentally incoherent and the prospect of finding some ideal balance of theoretical and practical knowledge is illusory. I want to suggest that the quest to achieve such a balance not only is futile but can be seen to have profoundly detrimental effects on the entire enterprise of nursing education – that merely conceiving of knowledge in these dichotomous terms is deeply inimical to meaningful curriculum design and effective educational provision.

A suggestion such as this is likely to be met with considerable resistance if not incredulity; yet even those with the strongest affinity for this dual conception of knowledge will admit to some crucial tension between the notions of theory and practice. In the context of nursing education, this most commonly finds expression in references to a theory–practice 'gap'. The phrase 'theory–practice gap', as an articulation of something essentially problematic, has long been part of the vernacular not just within nursing education but within the nursing community at large. Whatever the exact nature of this supposed 'gap' – and we shall examine this in due course – it is clearly something that continues to exercise those concerned to ensure the effectiveness of nursing education. As Hewison and Wildman (1996) acknowledge, 'the existence of a theory–practice gap in nursing in the United Kingdom has been an issue of concern for many years' (p. 754). It is a notion that has come to be 'well known within nursing education' (Ekebergh *et al.*, 2004, p. 622). Similarly, Gallagher (2004) confirms that the notion of a gap between theory and practice has come to be 'firmly established in nursing education' (p. 263).

The issue is generally perceived to be one of integration, a matter of closing the gap, of 'integrating theory in praxis' (Ekebergh *et al.*, 2004, p. 622). And it is one which would seem to have official recognition: the UKCC (The United Kingdom Central Council for Nursing, Midwifery and Health Visiting) Commission for Education's express remit in recommending improvements in the education of nurses and midwives was, in part, to have due regard for the 'sound assessment of practice and its integration with theory' (UKCC, 1999, p. 6). As might be expected, there has been no shortage of suggestions as to how such a gap might be closed, how theory and practice might be reconciled. For some, the essential difficulty lies with the educators: there has been the suggestion, for example, that tutors should be required to have greater involvement in or exposure to clinical practice (e.g. Northcott, 1988). For others, the problem lies in the manner in which students learn, the solution perhaps being seen as the adoption of more appropriate educational strategies such as 'reflective practice' (Proctor and Reed, 1993).

We might note that belief in this fabled schism is not universal for there is occasional dissent in the form of a somewhat different characterization. There is a suggestion that the theory–practice gap should be regarded as a theoretical construct, as a 'metaphor' as one commentator has put it (Gallagher, 2004), that in some sense has mistakenly or inappropriately been applied to nursing education. As we shall see, such characterizations are not without significance; the difficulty is that without some *explanation* of why the notions of theory and practice dominate so completely our thinking about the vocational these will seem simply to fly in the face of hard reality. The claim that the theory–practice gap is merely a 'metaphor' is belied by the personal experience of a good many practitioners who not only can vouch for the existence of some such gap but can testify to its pernicious consequences.

Part of the problem here is a lack of clarity as to what exactly is meant by 'theory–practice gap', or, more precisely, there is a tendency to conflate two very different meanings. First of all, to speak of a theory–practice gap is to draw attention to a perceived shortfall between training provision and the substantive knowledge requirements of an occupation; that is, a discrepancy between what is taught and what is actually needed in order to perform effectively in the workplace. Understood thus, 'theory–practice gap' is roughly equivalent to 'training–work gap' or 'preparation–performance gap'. The issue is essentially one of ends and means, about the relevance and sufficiency of what is learned. Certainly, there is evidence to support the view that there is a gap of this kind. The UKCC (1999), for example, reported 'concern that newly-qualified nurses, and to a lesser extent midwives, do not possess the practice skills expected of them by employers' (p. 4). Clearly, such findings should be of as much concern to nursing educators and those tasked with curriculum design as they are to the employers and the many practitioners who have long had reservations about the relevance and sufficiency of nursing education and for whom such findings probably come as little surprise. The UKCC report goes on to cite the words of a theatre sister:

> More clinical experience is required pre-registration than is currently being provided – there appears to be an over-emphasis on the academic area at the expense of clinical experience. A good nurse should be able to use her hands as well as her brain (UKCC, 1999, p. 39).

Here, again, there is the clear implication that what is taught falls short of what is needed, that the means are somehow insufficient to achieve the desired end. Importantly, however, there is a further, different kind of distinction very much in evidence here, a distinction couched in terms of the academic and the clinical, that is, a distinction between theory and practice understood not as means and correlative ends but as two competing means, ostensibly two alternative ways of achieving the end of effective performance. The distinction between theory and practice in this sense thus cuts across the distinction of theory and practice understood as ends and means. Now I want to suggest that in much talk about theory and practice there is a tendency to conflate these two very different distinctions. It is a tendency facilitated in large part by an ambiguity in the use of the word 'practice', which can be used both to convey the idea of occupational performance in its most general sense, and also to indicate the application of specifically practical as opposed to theoretical capabilities. Indeed, to return to the earlier quotation from the UKCC report, to say that a person does not possess 'practice skills' is to blur the substantive issue of whether it is being claimed that they do not have the wherewithal for practice, or more specifically that the shortfall in their capabilities, the kind of capabilities they lack, is of a particular type, that is, practical as against theoretical.

What makes the rhetoric of the theory–practice gap so powerful, and at the same time so difficult to deal with, is that it merges a general claim about the relevance and sufficiency of vocational provision – a claim which demands and deserves our attention – with a whole range of deep-seated assumptions about the nature of knowledge, teaching and learning. And the distinguishing feature of these assumptions is that they emanate from a starkly bifurcated perspective according to which the entire educational enterprise is perceived as consisting of two opposing camps into which any and every educational consideration might be conscripted and set one against another: theory–practice, thinking–doing, academic–clinical, education–training and so on. To express doubts about the adequacy of nursing education in terms of a theory–practice gap is to become ensnared in any number of such oppositions, the most fundamental being the idea that professional capability consists of two logically distinct forms of knowledge.

This dual conception of knowledge is such a familiar part of the educational landscape that many would find it difficult to conceive of knowledge in any other terms. It not only figures in ordinary discourse about the vocational but is reflected in many of the formal arrangements for nursing education and, indeed, vocational education and training generally. And this is no mere contingent feature of current policy-making. The idea that there are essentially two fundamentally different kinds of knowledge is a perennial theme throughout the history of Western philosophy, and there is a long and distinguished philosophical provenance associated with the dichotomies of theory–practice, thinking–doing, etc. The origins of these and related dualisms can be traced all the way from ancient Greece and the Aristototelian notions of theoretical and practical reason, through Descartes' seminal separation of mind from body in the seventeenth century, to Gilbert Ryle's famous distinction between knowing-how and knowing-that in the mid-twentieth century. This is not, of course, to suggest that there is any common purpose to be found in Aristotle's cataloguing of the intellectual virtues, Descartes' search for secure epistemological foundations or Ryle's positivistic account of mental concepts. But the fact that these intimately related dichotomies should figure in such diverse philosophical projects demonstrates the extent to which they have long permeated thinking about knowledge and the mind. That Ryle, the celebrated arch-opponent of ontological dualism, should leave as his most enduring legacy a dual conception of knowledge is testimony to the resilience of this tradition.

There are other reasons why Ryle may be significant here. For one thing, the distinction between knowing-how and knowing-that, as Ryle presents it, is not a particularly technical or philosophical distinction but one grounded in the ordinary use of language. Of course, the fact that it is our habit in everyday language to speak of two kinds of knowledge does not make it true that there are two kinds of knowledge – a point arguably overlooked by Ryle. But what is useful about Ryle's formulation is that in reminding us that such notions have their roots in ordinary discourse, our attention is drawn to the question of why, in what contexts or circumstances, we find it necessary or useful to make a distinction between knowing-that and knowing-how – or indeed, between theory and practice. For whatever philosophical weight might be thrown behind the claim that there are two forms of knowledge, our reluctance to abandon the theory–practice distinction tends to derive from reasoning of a more prosaic kind – though not any less cogent for that. It will be insisted that we can *see* plain instances of theory and practice, we can easily distinguish them; we can readily determine whether a person knows the theory or whether they know the practice of something; we *know* when we are teaching theory and when we are teaching practice and so on. Observations such as these lie at the heart of our commitment to the theory–practice conception of knowledge.

Yet I want to suggest that when we examine these and similar allusions to theory and practice more closely, it can be seen that they are shot through with conceptual vagary and philosophic confusion. Far from there being any single coherent focus to our use of the theory–practice distinction, something possibly constituting *prima facie* evidence of two forms of knowledge, there is instead a disparate array of uses connected often by only the most tenuously associated meanings which beg rather than answer the substantive question of whether there are two logically distinct kinds of knowledge. The first task here then is one of unravelling this complex and multifarious distinction. For it is only by getting clearer about exactly *what* is being referred to when we talk of theory and practice that we can begin to shake free of this dichotomous view of knowledge and come to recognize its damaging effects.

When we scrutinize our use of these terms, when we consider what it is exactly we are referring to when we speak of theory and practice, it is clear that, although presuming to delineate two kinds of knowledge, often the focus of our attention is explicitly on things that are ontologically distinct from the epistemological. For convenience we can group these into two broad categories. First, the distinction is used to highlight differences in what we might call the conditions *antecedent* to knowledge; differences, that is, in the forms of learning or sources of knowledge. It is not at all controversial to distinguish learning that takes place in a formal situation from that which may occur more informally in the workplace – to distinguish what in some occupations is termed 'off-the-job training' and 'on-the-job training'. Similarly, it is not unreasonable that we should want to acknowledge that learning from a text is a different thing from learning by means of a practical exercise. Often, when we make a distinction between theory and practice it is to draw attention to differences of this kind. And by the same token we can see how differences in styles of learning or techniques of presentation, for example passive/active, listening/doing, representational/actual, and so on, might similarly come to be associated with the terms 'theory' and 'practice'.

Secondly, the theory–practice distinction is often used to indicate differences in what we might term the *consequent* conditions of knowledge, that is, differences in the ways in which knowledge manifests itself. Perhaps the most common example of this is where we wish to contrast the ability to do X with the ability to recite certain facts about X. Again, it is entirely reasonable that we should sometimes want to make this kind of distinction. There is clearly a difference between, say, someone who is able to ride a bicycle and someone who can say a lot about cycling but cannot ride a bicycle. This kind of difference is not always clear in statements to the effect that a person 'knows X' or 'knows about X', and in such cases we find it useful to make a distinction between theory and practice or, following Ryle, between knowing-that and knowing-how. In saying that someone 'knows the theory but not the practice', or vice versa, by indicating how that person's knowledge manifests itself, we are able to communicate more clearly what it is they know. And in this sense we can see how it is entirely appropriate to distinguish between having a practical involvement in something and theorizing about it.

None of this, of course, settles either way the issue of whether there are two kinds of knowledge. But what it does do is explain why we are so reluctant to relinquish the theory–practice distinction. Undeniably, there are real and valid distinctions to be made as regards the antecedent and consequent conditions of knowledge – what might crudely be described as the inputs and outputs of learning. Importantly, however, such differences neither entail nor logically necessitate any corresponding epistemological distinction: it is one thing to acknowledge these differences, it is quite another to claim that there are two forms of knowledge. Yet there is a widespread and pervasive tendency to confuse the conditions associated with knowing with knowledge itself, thus conflating two very separate issues. For example, to say that a course of study consists of 50% theory and 50% practice is to suggest not just that there are two distinct modes of provision but that related to these modes of provision are two distinct kinds of knowledge. Likewise, to speak of identifying 'outcomes for theory and practice' (the UKCC has proposed that 'standards required for registration as a nurse . . . should . . . be constructed in terms of outcomes for theory and practice' [UKCC, 1999, p. 57]) is to intimate not just that the outward, evident manifestations of professional proficiency can meaningfully be categorized in this way, but that the knowledge that gives rise to such manifestations is such as can similarly be divided. For the moment it is sufficient to note how, in distancing ourselves from the presumption of two corresponding forms of knowledge, such distinctions appear more arbitrary, potentially even trivial. This is not to suggest that either the manner of learning or the consequences of knowledge are unimportant; it is rather that such considerations leave the most important questions unanswered. We are prompted to ask what is gained by learning being divided between contrasting modes of provision; we become less concerned with the attainment of 'outcomes' than with the question of what the student needs to know in order to manifest such outcomes. But the essential thing here is that we can see how the tendency to disregard this basic ontological distinction, between knowledge and its contingent conditions, causes knowledge to be *identified* with those conditions, either with those antecedent to or those consequent to knowledge.

Of the two, the identification of knowledge with its antecedent conditions is manifestly the less plausible. There are obvious difficulties with the idea that it is possible to categorize knowledge according to its sources: not only might the 'same' thing be learned from different sources but, conversely, different learners might be said to learn different things from the same source. Accordingly, few would advocate with any seriousness categorizing knowledge according to its antecedent conditions – even though, as we have seen, in ordinary talk about theory and practice there is often an implicit assumption that this is appropriate.

It is a very different matter, however, when we consider the tendency to identify knowledge with its consequent conditions. The assumption that knowledge can be described in terms of its outward manifestations – that knowledge effectively *is* those manifestations – has come to permeate almost every area of education over the last two decades. It is the explicit and unquestioned assumption behind every educational procedure that is centred on 'outcomes' or 'competencies', or styled as 'evidence-based'. And it is not difficult to see why an account of knowledge expressed entirely in terms of what it enables someone to say or do should have taken such a hold. In addition to its overt instrumentality, it is completely and utterly at one with the colloquial representation of knowledge and the assumed duality of knowing implicit in the everyday use of terms such as 'knowing how' and 'knowing that'.

Yet, logically, there is no more justification for the identification of knowledge with its consequences than with its antecedent circumstances. Any claim to the effect that knowledge is equivalent to its outward manifestations is controverted by the simple fact that such manifestations are neither necessary nor sufficient conditions for knowledge. Not necessary because it is conceivable that a person may know something whilst being unable to produce any outward manifestation of that knowledge – paralysis being an extreme case in point – and we would not want to deny knowledge in such cases. Not sufficient because such manifestations can obtain in the absence of knowledge – as with the parroting of facts or the mechanical performance of tasks. The logical space that exists between knowledge and its outward manifestations is of huge significance in the context of assessment where disparities of this kind are of very real consequence. But the main point here is that there is not only a clear ontological distinction but an important logical distinction between knowledge and its consequences that prevents any straightforward identification of the one with the other. The hypothesis of two kinds of knowledge on the basis of such an identification thus fails.

Now it might be argued that the presumption of two forms of knowledge is justified not because knowledge is to be identified in any strict sense with its consequences but by virtue of there being a causal or quasi-causal relationship between the two. In other words, it might be thought that since the consequences of knowledge can be categorized as either theoretical or practical, and since knowledge is causally connected to those consequences, then we can similarly categorize the knowledge from which those consequences flow. However, there is a fundamental difficulty with this way of thinking. On the one hand, if we take it that the relationship between knowledge type and outcome type is exclusive, that is, theoretical outcomes derive only from theoretical knowledge and practical outcomes from practical knowledge, then it would be impossible for theory and practice ever to impact on each other: theory and practice would in effect comprise two closed systems, each isolated from and without any means of influencing the other. It is difficult to see how anyone could or would want to defend a conception of professional knowledge such as this. On the other hand, to admit that practical outcomes might sometimes be informed by theoretical knowledge, or theoretical outcomes by practical knowledge, is to undermine the very rationale upon which the presumption of two forms of knowledge is based. We are obliged to question the sense in which knowledge can be said to be theoretical or practical if either kind of knowledge can give rise to either kind of outcome. Again, the fact that we can make reasonable and uncontroversial distinctions in the outward manifestations of knowledge does not entitle us to infer any corresponding epistemological division.

We begin to get a sense here of how the theory–practice distinction only has any coherence, any substantive meaning, when used to signify the conditions contingently associated with knowledge. When removed from that context, when we try to conceive of theory and practice as epistemological categories, there is simply nothing to sustain the distinction: we are at a loss to articulate what we mean by theory and practice except in terms of those conditions. It would seem that any attempt to conceive of the theoretical or the practical necessitates a turning away from the epistemological, a shift in our attention *away* from knowledge towards either its sources or its effects. The crucial point here is that the demand for a curriculum couched in terms of 'outcomes for theory and practice' effectively requires the educator to relinquish knowledge as their first and overarching concern. However disquieting we may find this prospect, there are many who would not be at all perturbed by the idea that education should abandon its traditional preoccupation with knowledge to give priority to knowledge's outward manifestations, and they would be quick to explain why. Surely, they would say, what matters *is* how knowledge manifests itself – particularly in the context of a vocational education. Whatever philosophic interest we might have in the nature of knowledge, ultimately, common sense dictates that our prime concern must be with the consequences of knowledge, and these consequences are essentially of two kinds: what people can say and what they can do – in other words, theory and practice. Moreover, they will insist, there is no inconsistency in describing knowledge in terms of such consequences because when we speak of a person having knowledge or being knowledgeable that is precisely what we mean – we mean that they are able to make certain kinds of utterances or do certain kinds of things. Clearly, we cannot look inside someone's head to see what they know. And even if we could, how could we possibly describe what we found? How else, it will be asked, are we to describe knowledge if not by its consequences, by what it enables a person to say or do?

Now not only will many find this kind of reasoning extremely persuasive but it is a way of thinking implicit in many of the formal arrangements currently employed in nursing education and, indeed, vocational education generally, especially in the UK. Moreover, there are important philosophical precedents for such a position. Gilbert Ryle is again significant, for *The Concept of Mind* provides us with what is probably the most cogently argued defence of just such a position. Ryle's intention was to show that although we may presume to be describing characteristics of the mind when we use mental predicates such as 'competent', 'knowledgeable', 'intelligent', 'stupid' and so on, this simply cannot be so:

> When we describe people as exercising qualities of mind, we are not referring to occult episodes of which their overt acts and utterances are effects; we are referring to those overt acts and utterances themselves. (Ryle, 1949, p. 25)

Ryle's complaint, then, is primarily about our use of language, and his point is twofold: first, about the kind of access we have to the mental, and, second, about what it is possible for us to mean when we use mental predicates – the 'concept of mind' it is logically possible to delineate given the kind of access we have. In one respect, his argument is compelling: clearly we do not have access to the inner workings of other minds; the evidence we have of such workings does indeed, on the face of it, appear to be profoundly limited. The problem with this, as Ryle himself recognized, is its apparently inescapable behaviourist consequences. It leaves us incapable of explaining, for example, how we are able to distinguish different mental states that may manifest themselves in the same or similar behaviour. To take Ryle's own example, we need an explanation of how it is possible for us to distinguish the trippings and tumblings of a skilful clown from the 'visibly similar trippings and tumblings of a clumsy man' when there is no discernible difference in the evidence before us. Ryle's solution was to introduce the notion of 'dispositions': he proposes that we are able to distinguish the actions of the skilful clown from those of the clumsy man by virtue of the former being *disposed* to behave that way. It is of interest to note the way in which this corresponds with the notion of having a 'sufficiency of evidence' in competence assessment procedures. The main point here, however, is that Ryle's notion of dispositions clearly will not do, neither as an explanation of how we arrive at such judgements nor as a way of avoiding the slide into behaviourism. What Ryle misses is that it is not the clown's dispositions but the dispositions of the *spectator* that are crucial

(Lum, 2004). We are able to distinguish the actions of the clown from those of a clumsy man by virtue of being predisposed by *our* previous experience of the kinds of things that happen in circus tents, the way clowns tend to dress and so on. We are predisposed to interpret behaviour in the light of its context and in so doing we are sensitive to a potentially vast range of clues, many of which we may not even be aware are influencing us in our judgement that the behaviours we witness are, say, intentional rather than accidental. The difficulties faced by Ryle's account – its ineluctable behaviourism and its failure to capture the processes substantively involved in our interpretation of the world around us – are a corollary of his essentially positivistic stance (see Rorty, 1980). But for our purposes the most crucial thing is that in *The Concept of Mind* we have a clear illustration of the profound shortcomings of an evidential conception of knowing, that is, a conception of human capability circumscribed and delimited by what it is possible for us to observe and describe.

Clearly, this is not the only way we might approach the question of knowledge and mind. We can usefully contrast this with a phenomenological approach, that is, one based not merely on the evidence accessible to some supposedly detached, impartial observer but, rather, on own experience of what it *is* to have certain kinds of knowledge or capabilities. Martin Heidegger's (1962) famous account of *Dasein*, the 'there-being' of human existence, for example, shows just how wide-ranging our understanding of human knowledge and capability can be when it is not confined to the 'overt acts and utterances' that characterize Ryle's account. An account in these terms suggests a far richer notion of professional capability (Lum, 2003), one that consists first and foremost in being able to perceive and make sense of a 'world' of interconnected meanings and involvements unique to a particular occupation, a 'world' that is in effect constituted by such understandings and given coherence by virtue of the purposes and priorities held in common with a wider community of practitioners. It would be a mistake to regard such understandings as either theoretical or practical for our ability to manipulate propositions or to perform in practical ways is both derivative of and secondary to these more basic understandings. Moreover, such understandings are fundamentally non-discursive; it could hardly be otherwise given that our capacity to use language is itself dependent upon them.

This last point turns out to be quite critical. The last two decades have seen an increasing political and managerial preoccupation with educational strategies centred on 'standards', 'competencies' and 'outcomes', the characterizing feature of all of these being the assumption that it is possible to describe or specify occupational capabilities in statement form (Lum, 1999). Motivated less by any particular educational consideration than by the bureaucratic imperative for 'objective' and unambiguous specifications, the focus of such strategies invariably gravitates towards that which lends itself to precise description whilst neglecting the kinds of understandings substantively at issue. Just as Ryle's 'concept of mind' is limited to an account of overt, accessible 'acts and utterances', similarly, the conception of professional capability implicit in these strategies is one circumscribed by what it is possible to observe and describe, that is, the outward manifestations of knowing – the sayings and doings identified variously in terms of 'theory and practice', 'knowledge and skills' or some such similar locution.

The difficulty is not just that specifications couched in these terms are insufficient, that they fall short of capturing the more obscure or intangible features of human capability; to suggest this would be to hold out the false hope that they at least suffice as regards the more basic capabilities. It is rather that an account in these terms fails to capture the essence of *any* capability. The idea that it is appropriate to equate a person's knowledge with the evidence it is possible to have of that knowledge, that we can account for such capabilities in terms of theoretical and practical outcomes, is fundamentally incoherent and runs counter to all our best intuitions about curriculum design.

On the one hand, it is difficult to ascribe *any* useful role to theory conceived as an outcome: as Ryle rightly recognized, people rarely preface their actions with a recital of relevant propositions. When we think of knowledge in this way there does indeed seem to be little value in learning 'bucketfuls of facts' (Wolf, 1989, p. 41); we are obliged to acknowledge that 'even in the most professional occupations the proportion of "knowledge-heavy" competences is quite few' (Moran, 1991, p. 8). A still further difficulty arises when we consider what possible relationship there could be between theory and practice thus conceived, how theoretical outcomes could be said to inform, underpin or support practical outcomes. On the other hand, the role of practical outcomes in the curriculum is also problematic. Professional occupations often demand little by way of physical or practical deftness, and even where such skills are required it will generally be recognized that it is not so much the skill but the understanding behind the skill that is key. The only conclusion to draw from all of this is that *any* account couched in terms of theoretical and practical outcomes will necessarily and quite seriously underdetermine what it is to be competent or professionally capable, with the consequence that the extent of what is needed by way of a preparation stands to be radically underestimated.

■ Conclusion

It is significant that when pressed to say what is missing from such accounts or to explain what new trainees lack, experienced practitioners will often resort to such phrases as 'being streetwise' or being able to deal with 'difficult situations' (NHS Confederation cited in UKCC, 1999, pp. 40–41). In common with such terms as 'judgement', 'initiative', 'imagination', 'leadership' and so on, such notions defy precise explication; they are simply not amenable to being cashed out in terms of outcomes. But the fact that the substantive ends of a vocational preparation do not lend themselves to precise explication does not mean that we lack the means to achieve such ends. On the phenomenological account outlined above, the competent practitioner has, by definition, a tacit understanding of what is required for effective performance. It is the special and additional role of the curriculum designer, the lecturer and the mentor to conceive of the means likely to bring about those capabilities in others, to devise strategies likely to promote those capabilities. And in being no longer bewitched by the false representation of knowledge as outcomes it is possible to appreciate the sheer complexity and extent of what is required.

Accordingly, it is only right and proper that we should wish to draw upon any and every educational means at our disposal in order to achieve these ends, both the academic and the clinical. Between the academic and the clinical there will, of course, be differences in modes of learning, sources of knowledge and so on, that is, differences in what has been referred to here as the conditions antecedent to knowledge. And though it is not unduly problematic that these differences should be characterized in terms of theory and practice, there is a potential danger. For if we lose sight of the fact that what we characterize as theory and practice are merely the means to our tacit ends, if we mistake the antecedent conditions of knowledge for knowledge itself, then we run the risk of a curriculum detached from such ends. When this happens, the 'world' of meanings, purposes and priorities adopted by the student may come to be those of the academy rather than those of the profession. The result is a not just a crisis of relevance but a conflict of cultures:

> Nurses who are theorists and educationalists, and nurses who are engaged in nursing practice tend to use different vocabularies, to have different perceptions of patients and of nursing, and to value different kinds of nursing knowledge . . . [P]ractitioners undertaking academic courses in particular encounter difficulties in reconciling nursing theory with nursing practice . . . [O]ne suspects that they either develop mild schizophrenia, or, if they absorb very large doses of nursing theory, they become so deviant that it is difficult for them to function adequately as practitioners (Miller, 1985, pp. 417f).

But by the same token, we can recognize that the pressures and contingencies of work continually conspire to divorce clinical practice from the profession's overarching rationale and values, and that the university can have an important and valuable role in helping to consolidate clinical aims and unify the profession. What is clear is that such difficulties are not countered by merely giving priority to one mode of provision rather than the other. Neither does the remedy lie in striving for some 'golden mean' or ideal proportioning of theory and practice; as we have seen, the idea of a perfect epistemological equilibrium is illusory. Rather, it lies in the willingness of educators and policymakers – on both sides of the academic–clinical divide – to get clearer about what it is to be vocationally capable, perhaps even to have a *philosophical* understanding of professional knowledge. Given the misguided and naïve preoccupation with 'standards', 'outcomes' and latterly 'proficiencies' that presently dominates, this is, for the time being at least, perhaps unlikely. Sadly, rather than plumb these philosophical depths many will be content merely to proclaim the perils of a preparation either 'too theoretical' or 'too practical' as they set out to steer a course between irrelevance and ignorance, like ancient navigators venturing the waters between Scylla and Charybdis.

Chapter 8

Distributed cognition and the education reflex

John Paley

■   A very brief introduction

A very common response to the recognition that things-are-not-working-very-well is the assumption that Somebody Needs Educating. I call this the education reflex, and observe that it persists despite persuasive evidence that, without a substantial and expensive investment on the part of both teacher and learner, the usual forms of continuing professional development (CPD) are ineffective. In view of this, the persistence of the education reflex deserves an explanation; and, in this chapter, I argue that it reflects a residual form of Cartesianism, specifically the belief that cognitive processes can only be attributed to the individual knowing subject. This residual Cartesianism is maintained even by authors who are critics of classic Cartesian thought. I contrast it with distributed cognition, a perspective which has recently emerged in cognitive science, and which ascribes cognition not to individuals, but to cognitive systems (in which individuals may play a part). This perspective opens up an alternative way of responding to things-not-working-very-well: changing other components of the cognitive system, rather than tinkering with what is inside people's heads. The chapter makes use of four health care scenarios: they are introduced at the beginning, and I return to them at the end in order to illustrate the strategies that a distributed cognition perspective might suggest.

Here is a very important observation. 'All over the world, in great metropolitan centers as well as in the remotest rural backwaters, in sophisticated electronics laboratories, and in dingy clerical offices, people everywhere are struggling with a Problem: *Things Aren't Working Very Well*' (Gall, 2002, p. 5). Health care organizations are not specifically mentioned by Gall, but they would not be out of place on the list. In this chapter I would like to consider four examples of 'things that were not working very well', and say something about how they could be put right. They are all 'micro' examples – I will not be discussing large-scale health policy or financial matters – but they are still of great clinical significance because, in each case, patients were missing out on expertise that was available, but not being delivered.

They have one further feature in common which makes them relevant to this book. In all four situations, once it had been recognized that *Things Aren't Working Very Well*, there was the same initial reaction, despite the fact that they occurred in different health care sites, and concerned different people. The reaction was, *Someone Needs Educating*. When problems arise, this reaction is so familiar, so apparently automatic, that I will call it the 'education reflex'. As that label is intended to suggest, I think it is something to beware of; and, as often as not, I think it is misconceived. Let me begin by introducing the four health care scenarios, each of which is presented in the form of a problem.

■ Four problems

☐ Administering the wrong medication

Many drugs have at least two different forms: one which releases chemicals gradually over a period of time, and another which delivers an instantaneous 'hit' shortly after being administered. One such drug available in both forms is Oxycodone, a strong semi-synthetic opioid used in the relief of severe pain, either postoperatively or in cases of cancer. The prolonged release version is called OxyContin, and the immediate release version, used for breakthrough pain, is OxyNorm.

A palliative care clinical nurse specialist (CNS) in a Scottish hospital was alerted by the hospital's Clinical Development Manager (CDM) for medical services to the fact that, on three occasions during a single month, the wrong form of Oxycodone had been administered. As no other directorate had reported comparable problems, the CNS contacted Napp Pharmaceuticals Limited, the drug's manufacturers. She was told that similar errors had occurred throughout central Scotland, so this was not just an isolated series of mistakes (Kerr, 2004).

The company had a standard response to such reports, which was to regard them as symptomatic of an educational problem, and to propose that a representative should visit the wards concerned to hand out literature. This reaction was certainly consonant with that of the CDM; for, when she had approached the CNS, it was with some form of educational initiative specifically in mind. In both cases, then, it was assumed that nurses making the errors were unfamiliar with the drug, and that (therefore) they needed educating.

☐ Referral to cardiac rehabilitation

A cardiac rehabilitation unit in Scotland was receiving very few referrals from the cardiology ward – I shall refer to it as Ward C – and many of those it *was* receiving were post-discharge. The background to this problem is outlined below.

Ward C was for many years a cardiology and respiratory ward. Its nursing staff were experienced, had worked together for a long time, and had excellent working relationships with the coronary care unit. However, both the respiratory consultants and the cardiologists felt that they required more beds than could be managed in a single ward; and the ever increasing number of medical admissions meant that another ward had to be opened to cope with the numbers.

Ward R was originally created as a short-term measure to deal with the crisis in the winter of 2000. Its staff were therefore employed on short-term contracts. Many were newly qualified or unfamiliar with the hospital. A staff nurse with six years of experience in high dependency and acute admissions was appointed as the new ward manager. It soon became clear that this new ward would need to stay open, and a decision was taken in to rationalize the medical unit beds according to need. It was decided that Ward R would become a respiratory unit and that Ward C would remain the cardiology unit with some beds allocated to gastroenterology.

'This had implications for staff in both wards. The staff in Ward C were permanent staff, and they were given the choice of which ward they wanted to work in. A large number elected to move to Ward R and the new respiratory unit. This meant that many of the staff now employed in Ward C had very limited experience, and that the ward sister had no cardiology experience at all. Only the senior staff nurse and another staff nurse elected to stay behind. This left a total of 28 staff, of whom only two had cardiology experience' (McKay, 2003, p. 7).

We can now return to the problem, which became evident some time after the wards were reorganized. The question is, why were referrals (in the words of the cardiac rehabilitation CNS) 'late or not at all'? Given the history of the cardiology ward, the answer was obvious. The inexperienced staff in Ward C did not appreciate the clinical significance of rehabilitation. Clearly, they needed to be educated.

☐   Miscalculating the dosage

Photofrin is a photosensitizing agent administered to patients who suffer from various forms of cancer, particularly oesophageal cancer, in preparation for photodynamic therapy. During a 48-hour period, the drug concentrates selectively in cancer cells (because of lymphatic deficit and the increased pH), but is largely cleared from healthy tissue. After 48 hours, a red laser is directed at the tumour, damaging the mircrovasculature by destroying proteins and cell membrane, so rendering it ischaemic and causing cell death. The depth of destruction is usually 2–5mm. However, light exposure must be timed carefully to ensure that the photosensitizing agent has cleared from the healthy cells, while remaining in the cancer cells.

Photofrin dose calculation, reconstitution and administration is relatively complex, involving a certain arithmetical skill. The calculation is based on the patient's weight, according to the following formula: patient's weight (in kilograms) x 0.8 = millilitres (mL) to be administered. The drug is supplied in 75 mg vials, and each vial is reconstituted with 31.8 mL of 5% dextrose solution. The volume to be given, therefore, is divided by 31.8 to determine how many vials should be reconstituted (UK Clinical PDT Study Group, 2002). In summary, the number of vials needing to be reconstituted is weight (kg) x 0.8/31.8. Photofrin is an expensive drug, which costs £750 per 75 mg vial, making an average of roughly £1500 per dose. For both economic and health care reasons, then, this is not a calculation one wants to get wrong too often.

However, a case-note audit, carried out in a large Scottish hospital, revealed a worryingly high level of drug administration error with Photofrin, 47% of doses being wrongly calculated. While many of the errors were within a fairly narrow range, some were not. In one case, for example, the patient received half the correct dose, in another case it was double the correct dose. Moreover, it is very likely that the 47% figure is an underestimate, as the calculations could be checked in only 51% of cases; in the remainder, either the weight or the dose had not been recorded. In several instances, neither of them had (Hodgson, 2004).

This is not, in general, an unusual situation. It is well known that a proportion of drug administration errors are the result of miscalculations (O'Shea, 1999; Armitage and Knapman, 2003), whether by nurses or junior doctors (Rowe *et al.*, 1998). Nor is the reaction to this kind of problem unfamiliar, in that the crux of it is assumed to be the mathematical skills of nursing and junior medical staff. Indeed, there is a considerable literature on the subject, with various forms of pre- and post-registration mathematical education being proposed and discussed (Hutton, 1998; Starkings, 2003; Sabin, 2004 is a good review). As before, then, it is concluded that someone needs educating.

☐   Diagnosing malignant spinal cord compression

Malignant spinal cord compression (MSCC) is an oncological emergency, occurring in about 5% of cancer patients. It can cause sensory impairment, loss of motor function and significant disability. It is usually the result of a metastatic cancer in the epidural space compressing the spinal cord and is most commonly treated with steroids and radiotherapy. Early diagnosis and swift treatment of the condition is essential to minimize the damage to the spinal cord, and to prevent consequent loss of function and mobility. The later the diagnosis, the more likelihood there is of a poor outcome following treatment (Loblaw and Laperriere, 1998).

The signs and symptoms of MSCC are well known, including pain (usually in the back), sensory loss, motor weakness and autonomic nervous system problems. For any cancer patient (but especially in the case of cancer of the breast, lung or prostate), there is a distinct risk that such symptoms are indicative of the onset of MSCC. Nevertheless, an audit carried out by the Clinical Resource and Audit Group in Scotland (CRAG) revealed that even when patients had a long history of painful symptoms and a past diagnosis of cancer, the diagnosis of MSCC was being made late, and in most cases too late to prevent paralysis. Survival time was also poor, and associated with ability to walk at time of diagnosis. The median time from onset of symptoms, as recalled by the patient, to a diagnosis of MSCC being made, was 90 days (18 days for the patient to tell their GP). Delays were attributed to both a lack of recognition (by GPs and hospital doctors) of the early symptoms and the absence of an efficient referral pathway (Clinical Resource and Audit Group, 2001). The results of the audit, it should be observed, are consistent with previous reports (Byrne and Waxman, 1990; Johnston, 1993; Husband, 1998).

Not surprisingly, the CRAG report recommended improving awareness of MSCC and knowledge of the early signs through a national education programme, although there were also suggestions about how to reduce delays in the diagnostic and referral process (a complicated process since there were at least four different referral pathways leading to the specialist cancer centre). However, it was clear to all concerned that the education programme would have to be extensive, as both nursing and medical staff in primary care, in the district general hospitals and in the cancer centre were all implicated. In this example, then, there were a *lot* of people who needed educating (Hutchison, 2003).

■ The limits of the education reflex

I am sorry to have taken up so much space, in a book of philosophy, with local empirical detail. But I want to show how pervasive – and, I suppose, how natural – the education reflex is. If we were to act on all the impulses to educate someone as a result of problematic situations, health care organizations would be awash with professionals educating other professionals. Examples of the referral-to-cardiac-rehabilitation type (broadly speaking) are especially common. It is not at all unusual to come across a professional group – let us call them PGs – who are not getting the referrals they think they should, and who believe that the solution is to 'educate' the potential referrers, specifically about the 'role' of PGs. Make this clear, the story goes, and suitable referrals will naturally follow.

But how plausible is this? How well founded is the education reflex generally? To illustrate part of my response to this question, I will develop the Oxycodone scenario a little further. The first instinct of the CNS, as she later reported (Kerr, 2004), was the same as the CDM's and the company's: that there should be some kind of educational initiative, a proposal the company was happy to support. To this end, dates were fixed, literature was provided, and posters were stuck to the CD cupboard door – in all wards, in two hospitals. The CNS visited every ward, explained the proposal, and asked each nurse in charge to inform other staff of the training events. She also organized several drop-in sessions. The same information was emailed to all medical consultants and ward managers. Result? Almost nothing. Very few staff attended the sessions and, in particular, the wards where the errors had actually occurred were unrepresented. It was, in her own words, a waste of time.

One might, of course, feel sceptical about any particular case. Perhaps the training was not marketed in a very effective way. Perhaps it could have been organized differently. However, this story is far from atypical. Systematic reviews of research on continuing professional development (CPD) show that it is minimally effective unless it is highly interactive; provides opportunities for health professionals to use new ideas and practise new skills; targets measurable changes in participants' clinical behaviour; offers positive feedback subsequently when good outcomes are achieved; and is supported and reinforced by the learner's work environment (Oxman *et al.*, 1995; Bero *et al.*, 1998; Berwick and Nolan, 1998; Davis *et al.*, 1999). Didactic sessions and educational literature are largely ineffective in changing behaviour, especially when there is no prior motivation to learn, or any particular incentive to attend. This is true, for example, in the context of implementing clinical practice guidelines (Dodek and Ottoson, 1996; Davis and Taylor-Vaisey, 1997); and similar findings have been reported across a wide range of specialities in nursing, from intensive care (Tennant and Field, 2004) to cancer care (Blunden *et al.*, 2001). So it is not surprising that a modest initiative such as the series of Oxycodone sessions should fail to achieve much in the way of positive results, however well prepared it may have been.

Educating somebody, then, takes a lot of time, energy and expense; and, without a great deal invested in it on the part of both teachers and learners, it is quite likely to be ineffective. This is not, of course, a universal truth, and I am a long way from saying that the education reflex is always inappropriate. But to assume that *Someone Needs Educating* is the solution to every clinical and organizational problem is obviously to invite disappointment. It is to place more faith in routine educational experiences, such as lectures, seminars, small groups and workshops, than is justified by the actual evidence.

And yet, as I have suggested, this response to things-not-working-very-well is habitual. We might ask why. Why is the 'education reflex' a reflex?

Why are we so quick to assume that problems of this kind can be tackled by educating somebody? In the next few pages, I will sketch an answer to this question, incorporating a number of significant philosophical and psychological ideas; but here is the bullet point version.

- The four situations I have described, in common with many others, are cognitive problems. They involve knowledge, assessment, calculation, perception, thinking, and decision-making.
- Cognition is assumed to be a process that happens inside the heads of individuals. So dealing with cognitive problems must be a matter of intervening in heads, in order to extend, improve or upgrade what is inside them.
- This assumption is a type of residual Cartesianism: knowledge gets stored in individuals – solo minds or, on some accounts, solo bodies – either as a result of information explicitly acquired, or as the implicit consequence of experience.
- But there is an alternative way of looking at cognition and, consequently, expertise. Cognition is a property, not of the individual, but of cognitive systems, extending well beyond brains and bodies, and incorporating inanimate objects. It is *distributed* across those systems.
- So delivering expertise, solving cognitive problems, is not just about trying to put new stuff in brains and bodies, or amending what is already there. It's also about fixing other parts of the system.

In the rest of this chapter, I will develop the notion of residual Cartesianism a bit more, and argue that (despite some fairly ferocious Descartes-bashing in the nursing literature) it underlies the best-known accounts of nursing expertise and nursing knowledge. As the bullet points imply, the account involves a crucial contrast between residual Cartesianism and distributed cognition, a theoretical approach I will explain by drawing on sources in cognitive science, human–computer interaction, and the design of everyday things (Norman, 1998). Later, I will return to the four problem situations already described, and show that they are more amenable to solutions based on distributed expertise than they are to the (residually Cartesian) education reflex.

■ Distributed cognition

Let me begin with a very simple example. Consider two different ways of remembering which page of a book you have reached. The first is just to note, and then remember, the page number. It may not be fully clear exactly how we do this without resorting to psychology textbooks (Baddeley, 1997); but the process is familiar enough, as is the subsequent process of trying to retrieve the number from memory when we want to continue reading. Equally familiar is the unreliability of this method, at least after a significant lapse of time. The second method is simply to crimp the page, or insert a bookmark. Then, when we pick up the book again, all we have to do is open it at the crimp. The difference between the two methods, from a user's point of view, is that the first recruits only individual resources (perception and memory), while the second recruits the book itself, or some other artefact (bookmark), and offloads the potentially difficult bit on to them.

Here, then, is a modest cognitive task (retrieving the page number) approached in two distinct ways. In the first case, the relevant cognition is confined to the reader's head; in the second case, it is distributed across what we can call a cognitive system, consisting of the reader, the book and (if it is used instead of a crimp) the bookmark. The reason for referring to this second method as an example of *distributed cognition* is simply that no single part of the system can be said to remember the page number. Clearly, the reader doesn't: inserting the bookmark is, precisely, a way of not *having* to remember. And neither the book nor the bookmark can be said to know, or remember, anything. It is the cognitive system as a whole – reader, book and bookmark – which retrieves the right page when the system is activated (that is to say, when the reader picks up the book, and turns to the one with the crimp or bookmark in it). The information required to do this is not coded in any one component individually; it is rather a function of the system in which it is distributed.

This idea can obviously be generalized, and it rapidly becomes apparent that distributed cognition is in everyday use. Sometimes this involves improvization, in the sense that we make use of generic bits of the world to carry out cognitive tasks. For example, pencil and paper are used to create a shopping list, multiply large numbers, draw a map or diagram (Paley, 2004). As a diabetic, I place clusters of tablets at strategic locations in the kitchen in order to remind myself to take medication at certain times of the day. But other cognitive tasks are performed by specially designed artefacts: bookmarks, calculators, monitors, post-it notes, various dials and switches, and of course computers. These instruments are so completely woven into the fabric of life that we cease to notice them, cease to appreciate the cognitive functions they perform. However, research during the last 10 years has identified 'a host of ways that embodied agents enlist the world to perform computation for them' (Hollan *et al.*, 2000, p. 191). There have been studies of distributed cognition in nuclear physics (Giere, 2002), airline cockpits (Hutchins and Klausen, 1996), shipboard navigation (Hutchins, 1995); classrooms (Brown *et al.*, 1993); cooking, bicycle maintenance, shopping, doing jigsaw puzzles, playing Tetris (all in Hollan *et al.*, 2000); waitressing (Stevens, 1993); and bartending (Kirlik, 1998). We are constantly devolving cognitive tasks and processes to systems which include ourselves, but which are not 'bounded by the skin or the skull' (Hutchins, 1995, p. 292).

The literature on distributed cognition, it is worth adding, intersects with several others, particularly in education (Salomon, 1993), and the fields of human–computer interaction (Hollan *et al.*, 2000; Dourish, 2004), artificial neural networks (Clark, 1997; Bechtel and Abrahamsen, 2002) and design (Winograd and Flores, 1986; Norman, 1998). For example, neural nets model the brain in a manner which implies that *all* cognition is distributed, since 'items of knowledge that the network can be described as possessing are inextricably interlinked and *distributed* across the network as a whole' (Bermúdez, 2005, p. 129). If these models are viable, then there is no part of the brain, no specifiable population of neurons, that can be identified with any particular belief, concept or memory. This is comparable to the idea that when a bookmark is used to retrieve the page number, no single component of the cognitive system – whether reader, book, page or bookmark – can be said to 'know' what the page is. This is an item of knowledge which is distributed across the network as a whole. So in constructing distributed cognitive systems out in the physical world, it is as if we are reproducing (in massively simplified form) the kind of network processing that is characteristic of the brain.

In a similar way, the literature on design recognizes that 'not all of the knowledge required for precise behaviour has to be in the head... [it] can be distributed – partly in the head, partly in the world, and partly in the constraints of the world' (Norman, 1998, pp. 54–55). The principles of good design – when we choose to offload cognition onto the world, through cognitive systems – are, according to Norman, universal. One of these principles is transparency: by looking, a user should be able to tell the current state of the system, and what can be done with it. Another is good mapping: there should be a visible correspondence between the system's controls and the effects for which they are variously responsible. Think, for example, of the way in which the arrangement of controls on a stove may, in itself, indicate which hob each dial turns on and off. And contrast that sort of arrangement with an entirely arbitrary one, in which there is no relation at all between the geometry of the controls and the geometry of the hobs. In the latter case, the user is obliged to remember which control corresponds to which hob. In the former case, this cognitive function is successfully offloaded on to the controls themselves. I shall consider one further example of the principles of design when I return to the four health care scenarios later on.

■ Residual Cartesianism in nursing

The concept of distributed cognition represents a final, decisive break with Cartesian epistemology. To recognize that, at the very least, a great deal of cognition is distributed is by definition to abandon the notion of a Cartesian subject to which the predicates of knowledge and belief are applied. In this sense, distributed cognition is the last in a series of shifts away from the classic picture of an immaterial mind which perceives ideas, and which adopts what would now be called propositional attitudes (Salmon and Soames, 1989; Richard, 1990). It is instructive to follow this series of shifts, which can be construed as a progressive decentring of the site of cognition (Wilson, 2004).

First, there is classic Cartesianism, as traditionally understood (some authors have questioned whether this really corresponds to Descartes' own position: Baker and Morris, 1996; Sutton, 1998). On this view, there is an immaterial centre of thought, the Cartesian soul, in which all cognition takes place, linked to the body at the pineal gland. The first shift away from this picture gets rid of the insubstantial soul, but hangs on to everything else. This is 'Cartesian materialism', as it has been termed (Dennett, 1991). It retains the concept of a Cartesian 'theatre of consciousness' (only now it is in the brain, not the soul), where everything comes together at a central point, and where thoughts and experiences are processed. From here, a further shift takes us to *embodied cognition*, the claim that there may not be any centre of cognition at all, certainly not one which is conscious of every cognitive process (Clark, 1998; Hurley, 1998). The idea here is that the body is essentially implicated in the *processing* of information: it does not merely *supply* information through the senses. While this view is gaining ground philosophically, a lot of psychological work can be offered in support of it (e.g., Mackay, 1987; Edelman, 1989; Trevarthen, 1990); and it has been persuasively argued that it originates with, or was anticipated by, Merleau-Ponty (Kelly, 2000; Dreyfus, 2005).

So we move, in effect, from cognition located in the soul, to cognition located in the brain, to cognition located in the body. What all these views have in common, however, is location. Knowledge, thought and perception are ascribed, respectively, to the immaterial mind, the brain or the embodied person. With distributed cognition, we take a step beyond this need to attach cognition to *something*, or rather to some *one* thing. For certain cognitive tasks, the knowing, the perceiving and the believing can only be attributed to a network of things, to a cognitive system – if it can be attributed to anything. When I crimp the page, or insert a bookmark, the act of remembering cannot be attributed to me. It can only be attributed to the system consisting of myself, the book, the page and the bookmark. It is not located in any particular place. However simple the example, this is a more radical shift than the previous ones. And it is what justifies the claim that, even in embodied cognition, we are still approaching knowledge from a residually Cartesian perspective. For Cartesianism is the view that there is a knowing subject (whether it be mind, or brain or person); and with distributed cognition we no longer have one.

In view of the long history of Cartesian thought, most of us find it difficult to disengage from residually Cartesian assumptions, specific-ally the belief that an entire series of cognition-related concepts – belief, knowledge, perception, decision-making, expertise – are necessarily predicated of the individual. This is certainly true in the nursing literature, where epistemological discussion is almost wholly confined to questions about what the individual nurse can legitimately be said to know. Even Benner, probably the most philosophically sophisticated of nursing theorists, and influenced by the likes of Taylor, Merleau-Ponty, Heidegger and Gadamer, remains doggedly individualistic in her thinking. It is the expert nurse, the skilful practitioner, the moral agent, the embodied knower who is unequivocally the focus of her concerns (Benner and Wrubel, 1989; Benner *et al.*, 1996; Benner, 2000). She does, of course, emphasize the way in which the embodied person 'dwells in a culture' and 'belongs to a community'; and she says a great deal about the 'social embeddedness of knowledge'. However, these concepts are all part of her explanation of how the individual nurse becomes an expert, since cultural meanings are 'inscribed on the body', and learning to be a good practitioner involves 'developing moral imagination and skills' in a practice community, drawing on a wider practice tradition (Benner, 2000, pp. 8–9). There is never a sense that knowledge itself can be distributed; and, in fact, I suspect that this possibility is incompatible with her conception of nursing as a significant form of moral agency. Benner's account of expertise is, after all, a developmental one: nurses become expert by passing through a series of stages, acquiring a clinical grasp and skilful ethical comportment through experience, perceptual acuity and relationships (Benner, 2000, p. 13). There is scope for 'pooled expertise', learning from others, and the modelling of skills; but there is no space for distributed cognition, or the idea that knowledgeable agency might not be restricted to the embodied individual.

The fact that Benner is herself a forceful critic of Cartesianism is ironic, but not significant. She tends to associate Cartesian thinking with 'calculative rationality', and the concept of an 'embodied knower' is (for her) so completely antithetical to both rationality and calculation that it is sufficient to justify the claim to have transcended the Cartesian perspective. She has certainly transcended the classical form of Cartesianism, so perhaps this is ultimately a question of semantics; but it seems to me that we are in the middle of a long journey away from Cartesian epistemology, and that in hanging on to the idea of the individual 'expert knower', even an embodied one, Benner has retained too much of what needs to be relinquished (Paley, 2002).

The rest of the epistemological literature in nursing is largely devoted to a concept of 'knowledge' that is transparently one-dimensional, and its main concern is to argue that nurses have 'ways of knowing', or 'patterns of knowing', which are different from, but equal in status with, scientific knowledge (the *locus classicus* is Carper, 1999; but see also papers collected in Kenney, 1999; Polifroni and Welch, 1999; Higgs and Titchen, 2001, among other examples). This concept of knowledge is one-dimensional because it represents a mere sliver of the cognition spectrum, focusing on what nurses come to believe as the result of experience, intuition, moral sensibility, reflection and so on. All of these 'patterns of knowing' are mental states predicated of an individual Cartesian subject; and the obsession with such states of mind has limited enquiry into other cognitive tasks – perception, calculation, decision-making, analysis, assessment, risk evaluation, information processing, maintaining records, juggling needs and resources, devising standards, prioritizing and scheduling, to mention only the most obvious (Allen, 2004 is a persuasive account of nursing which recognizes the significance of cognitive activities like these). Systematic study of a wider range of cognitive tasks would make it more obvious, I think, that clinical cognition really is distributed; whereas a relentless pursuit of 'ways of knowing' will continue to blind nursing theorists to anything other than the contents of the individual nurse's mind.

■ Alternatives to the education reflex

A few pages ago, I asked why the education reflex, as a response to things-not-working-very-well, was so widespread, and I can now summarize my answer. Situations of the kind I described earlier are cognitive problems, and cognition is automatically associated with the (residually) Cartesian 'knowing' subject, an association which the nursing literature rarely, if ever, questions. So, when it is recognized that something isn't working very well, the natural assumption is that the knowledge and skills of some individual nurse, or group of nurses, require an upgrade. Someone needs educating.

The obvious question is what alternatives there are to the education reflex. The answer is surprisingly simple. If cognitive tasks are carried out by cognitive systems, networks of people and things, it may be possible to tinker with some other component of the system. Normally, we try to change the human element, by educating someone; but why not change something else instead? Design a new artefact, or reshape an old one; change a procedure, or modify the rules; reorganize the instruments, or revamp the instruction manual. Where cognition is distributed, we are not necessarily restricted to monkeying with people's minds.

Here is a simple example, taken from a US television show for children. Every year, a forest ranger has to measure the diameters of trees in order to estimate the amount of lumber in a particular plot of land. If she were to use an ordinary tape measure, she would have to measure the circumference of each tree, and perform an arithmetical calculation in order to work out its diameter. (The calculation is based on π, which is the ratio between the circumference and diameter of a circle ($c = \pi d$). If, then, the circumference of a certain tree is 6 feet, the diameter will be 1.91 feet.) In fact, however, a new kind of tape measure is used, one which is calibrated differently, and in such a way that it returns the diameter, not the circumference. The equation for converting circumference to diameter is, in other words, *built into* the tape. So, it is not necessary for the forest ranger to do any mental arithmetic; she simply holds the tape tightly round the circumference of the tree, as normal, and reads off the diameter directly (Pea, 1993). Of course, the tape cannot be used to produce ordinary measurements: it is naturally dedicated to this particular task. On the other hand, the possibility of an error in calculation has been eliminated, and the only other mistakes that can be made are procedural or perceptual (both of which were equally possible with an ordinary tape measure). The main cognitive burden has been shifted from the ranger's head to the instrument she uses.

☐ Calculating the dosage

This example suggests an effective method of reducing the Photofrin error rate. Instead of the nurse, or the junior house officer, calculating the dosage on the basis of weight, why not have a set of dedicated scales from which the dosage can be read off directly? This again shifts the cognitive burden to a piece of technology, and limits the scope for error to perception. In this case, however, the technology is not necessarily restricted to a single task, that of calculating Photofrin dosage. There are numerous drugs whose dosage is a function of weight, and the scales could be programmable. All the nurse would have to do, prior to weighing the patient, is select the relevant drug from a menu incorporated into the scales. The reading would be, not the patient's weight, but the correct dosage for the specified drug. This is a simple but innovative idea; and a patent for programmable scales has, in fact, been applied for. But, in the meanwhile, Axcan (manufacturers of Photofrin) have provided a ready-reckoning card, specifically for use with this drug; and a recent audit (Hodgson, 2004) shows that the error rate in the hospital trust concerned, over a six-month period, has been reduced from 47% to zero.

☐ Drug labels

In the Photofrin example, the cognitive problem is one of calculation; with Oxycodone, it turns out to be (partly) a matter of perception, because further investigation revealed that one important source of error was a

```
Ward 5 – Hospital Z                                        date
OXYCODONE (Oxynorm)                                        Qty: 10
Capsules
5 mg

exp Date                                                   D_____
Batch no:
Stock                                                      C_____

Store in a controlled drug cupboard
_____
KEEP OUT OF REACH OF CHILDREN                              Hospital Z
```

Figure 8.1   Oxynorm

```
Ward 5 – Hospital Z                                        date
OXYCODONE (Oxycontin)                                      Qty: 10
Modified-release tablets
5 mg

exp Date                                                   D_____
Batch no:
Stock                                                      C_____

Store in a controlled drug cupboard
_____
KEEP OUT OF REACH OF CHILDREN                              Hospital Z
```

Figure 8.2   Oxycontin

poorly designed label on the drug packaging. At the hospital concerned, medications are dispensed to the ward in plain white boxes, with a printed label which indicates the contents. The two Oxycodone labels are illustrated in Figures 8.1 and 8.2 (Kerr, 2004).

It is immediately apparent that discriminating between these labels will not be easy, unless the nurse is highly experienced and knows exactly what to look for. The only information that is highlighted (use of capitals) is the warning about children and the generic name for the drug. The critical data (OxyContin or OxyNorm) is in lower case and within parenthesis, and in the same font size as everything else; moreover, there is nothing on the OxyNorm label which makes it clear that this is the 'breakthrough' version of the drug. The two labels should be distinguishable at a glance, and they are not. This is all the more surprising in view of the fact that it has long been known that poorly designed labels are responsible for a significant proportion of drug administration errors (Hughes, 2001; Lyftingsmo, 2003;

American Society of Health-System Pharmacists, 2003), and some countries have introduced either legal standards for the labelling of certain drugs (Radhakrishna, 1999) or (as in Canada) voluntary standards incorporating minimum design requirements over and above legal obligations (Orser, 2000).

The design of labels, documents, computer screens, instruction manuals and other media intended to provide crucial information is a topic which has been increasingly studied in recent years (Winograd and Flores, 1986; Suchman, 1987; Norman, 1998). An interesting example in nursing is research by Effken, who has shown how monitors can be redesigned in order to help nurses recognize and understand the most significant information more quickly: 'making higher order variables visible in a haemodynamic monitoring unit improves the speed and accuracy of drug treatment for simple clinical problems for novices and experts alike, although novices improve more' (Effken, 2001, p. 250). She continues to study ways of modifying the intensive care environment in order to facilitate clinical decision-making; and it is worth noting that her work is explicitly based on the psychology of perception (Gibson, 1969; Gibson, 1986).

☐ Referral incentives

Now let me pick up the story of the cardiac rehabilitation referrals. A series of conversations with the ward nurses suggested that while the cardiology nurses were certainly inexperienced, they were fully aware of the function and significance of rehabilitation; so the training and induction programme that the CNS had been contemplating would have been pointless. Having abandoned this explanation, the CNS considered a number of other hypotheses, including the method for making referrals (phone calls rather than a form) and the distance separating the rehabilitation unit from the cardiology ward. But it appeared, on further investigation, that none of these alternatives could explain the referral pattern.

Here is a more plausible account. The most urgent incentive on the cardiology ward was to discharge patients as quickly as possible, in order to free up bed space. This is critical because the rehabilitation staff were willing to accept post-discharge referrals, and to see the patients at home. So the nurses on the ward had very little incentive to make a referral *pre*-discharge. If they needed the bed, they simply discharged the patient, assuming that they could refer to the cardiac rehabilitation unit later (although, not surprisingly, in some cases they forgot), and on the understanding that the unit would make a home visit. Ironically, then, rehabilitation unit staff were contributing to the problem themselves, in virtue of their willingness to accept referrals post-discharge. The solution to the problem is obvious: refuse to accept any more post-discharge referrals, but guarantee to see referred patients the same day, as long as the referral is made before 12:00 (McKay, 2003). This modifies the structure of incent-ives for staff on the ward: the interaction between the 'discharge' incentive and the 'referral' rule means that there is now pressure to refer patients promptly, in order to free up beds. As a result, behaviour on the ward changes, and a new pattern of outcomes emerges. In fact, this is how it turned out. The problem disappeared very quickly.

How is this situation analysed in terms of distributed cognition? First, the new system does not depend on whether the ward staff recognize the significance of rehabilitation. As it happens, they do recognize it, but that is not essential. The problem is not about knowledge and understanding, but about decision-making criteria, prioritization and memory, adding up to a different kind of cognitive task. The system introduced by the CNS distributes this task in a modified referral procedure, which makes no cognitive demands on ward staff. Nor does it require them to resist the 'discharge' incentive; instead, it exploits that incentive, working with the grain rather than against it. Just as, in the page-crimping example, the task of remembering is displaced by a series of motor procedures, so here the task of remembering and prioritizing is displaced by a simple administrative procedure.

☐ Self-referral

A rather different way of distributing the decision-making criteria in a cognitive system is illustrated by Husband's (1998) proposal, following his study of delays in the treatment of spinal cord compression: 'The finding that initial presentation directly to the oncology centre is associated with reduced delay to treatment... suggests that encouragement of increased self-referral by the patient to the oncology centre might be one solution to the problem, at least for those already under the care of the centre' (Husband, 1998, p. 21). In the Scottish example (Hutchison, 2003), a similar proposal involved issuing patients at risk of developing the condi-tion with a contact card, listing key signs and symptoms, and enabling them to present directly to the cancer centre. This reflects the fact that, in Husband's study, those patients who did self-refer direct to the centre were significantly more likely to be catheter-free and ambulant at time of treatment.

In this instance, the knowledge which the education reflex suggests should be planted, at considerable expense, inside a lot of professional heads is devolved to the contact card, with its weighted checklist of symp-toms and self-referral instructions. The function of the card is somewhere between a decision aid for patients (O'Connor *et al.*, 1999; Deyo, 2001) and an implementation-intention system, in which an intention to make a decision when certain circumstances arise is formulated beforehand (Goll-witzer and Bargh, 1996; Orbell *et al.*, 1997). This is a procedure which has been used to increase attendance for cervical cancer screening (Sheeran and Orbell, 2000). Its effect, like the other distributed systems I have considered, is to offload a certain cognitive task – here, making a decision about symptoms – on to an artefact-plus-procedure (in this case, specifically designed rather than improvised).

■ An equally brief conclusion

A quick summary may be in order. The education reflex is a pervasive response to things-not-working-very-well, at least partly because of a resid-ually Cartesian view of the knowing subject, and despite the fact that there is a good deal of evidence to suggest that 'educating somebody' is not effective without a substantial and expensive commitment from both teacher and learner. But abandoning Cartesianism makes it possible to understand many cognitive tasks in distributed terms, and to recog-nize the manner in which cognitive processes are routinely devolved to improvised or dedicated systems. This opens up the possibility of altern-ative responses to things-not-working-very-well, responses which are likely to be more effective (and which are certainly cheaper) than educa-tion. This is not, of course, to say that 'educating somebody' is never appropriate; that would be crazy. Neither is it to say that what I have described as the 'education reflex' applies to all forms of education. It is merely to observe that there are other ways of achieving certain object-ives, based on the idea that cognition is not exclusively located in the individual.

There are, no doubt, several matters arising. I do not have the space to deal with them here, obviously, but I will mention one. Distributed cogni-tion is one of a number of recent developments which seem to threaten conventional understandings of professional expertise. Another (related) example is evidence-based practice, which can also be construed as the devolution of clinical judgement to decision rules and procedures (Paley, 2006); and there is a growing literature, in nursing and medicine, which signals the panic induced by the claim that evidence-based, mechanical and actuarial methods are superseding the expert (Charlton, 1997; Mant, 1999; Barker, 2000; Fawcett *et al.*, 2001; Kitson, 2002; Upshur, 2002; Walker, 2003; Freshwater and Rolfe, 2004, and many others). My own view is that the notion of what it means to be an expert *is* changing, but this should be welcomed. Properly designed systems can do things more effectively than individual professionals, but it is important to emphasize that the professional still has a crucial role to play in those systems. What I think is implied is a shift in the relation been 'expert' and 'expertise'. Normally, we regard 'expertise' merely as an abstract term describing what experts have.

Semantically, 'expert' is the primary term. But we should now anticipate a reversal in polarity: 'expertise' becomes the central idea, and professionals participate in a series of networks, structures and systems which deliver expertise to clinical environments. So it is not just cognition that is distributed. Expertise is too.

Chapter 9

Particularizing the general: Challenges in teaching evidence-based nursing practice

Sally Thorne and Rick Sawatzky

■ Introduction

In modern times, a demand for formal accountability within health care service delivery systems has created a preference for practices that can be defended as 'evidence-based'. In this context, that which can be grounded in a particular kind and quality of evidence is privileged over that which is not, and public expenditure is shifting towards the activities and services for which there exists a credible body of evidence. Nursing has felt the pressure of the evidence-based imperative, and has responded by dramatically increasing the rate with which it frames its various knowledge claims as evidence of one form or another. Educators have taken up the challenge and developed an array of techniques and strategies by which nursing students are guided towards particular understandings of evidence and its applications within the practice context. Within this context, the gaze of the neophyte practitioner is increasingly directed towards the population, the system, and the epistemological underpinnings, and perhaps less often towards the patient as a unique and distinct individual. In recognition that much of what has been generated in the name of evidence has not achieved uptake within the clinical context, many practice settings are now dominated by an urgent mandate of knowledge transfer and research utilization. However, the precise role that evidence created on the basis of study of populations and systems ought to play in directing applications to particular instances in the practice context is rarely explicated.

In this paper, we argue that the conceptualization of evidence has become highly fluid within the discipline of nursing. In keeping with the complex nature of nursing, its epistemological diversity, and the methodological creativity inherent in its scholarship, various nursing authors position a wide range of definitional claims about what does and does not constitute evidence. They then tend to extrapolate arguments on the basis of those definitions, without due consideration for the degree to which they may misrepresent the common use of the notion outside of nursing's disciplinary context. In this manner they may then come to normalize ways of expressing nursing knowledge claims that are inherently problematic.

We attempt to illuminate and untangle some of the complex ways in which nurses have come to reference the notion of evidence within their theoretical discourse. Towards this end, we take a critical perspective towards some of the more problematic claims that have been made about evidence within our disciplinary literature, and examine the problems that inevitably arise from a failure to recognize the meaning and purpose of evidence within the larger discourse. Finally, we turn to the challenge confronting educators who seek to guide a new generation of nurses capable of discerning the nature and quality of evidence claims and of articulating the practice discipline's unique and distinct relationship to an evolving body of evidence. We see the conceptual slippage that has emerged in nursing as a phenomenon that is likely to emerge in other applied disciplines, especially those whose knowledge traditions straddle the social and the basic sciences, and those whose practice mandate ensures that the challenge of determining and defending 'right action' is taken up. Thus, our intention here is to challenge educators to wrestle with the idea of evidence as it manifests itself within our various disciplinary discourses. We do this so that they might guide the next generation out of the current conceptual wilderness and towards some epistemological clarity.

■ Structures and processes by which nurses think

As an applied practice science, nursing's thought and decision-making traditions have differed to some extent from those of other more circumscribed health and social service professions. Nursing's grounding is that of a human health and illness problem-solving orientation, inherently drawing upon a wide range of basic, applied and social scientific knowledge and conceptual structures within an individualized and relational context. Within this framework, academic nursing has attended to the theoretical and conceptual structure of its discipline with considerably more fervour than has been apparent in the other health and social service disciplines. This theoretical attention yields some insights into the challenges associated with understanding how nurses think.

In nursing, the role of theoretical models and conceptual frameworks that guide the clinical reasoning inherent in nursing practice has been the focus of several generations of scholarship. Such frameworks represent theoretically driven conceptual maps of the phenomena of concern to the discipline. They are understood to drive the *nursing process* by which nurses apply theoretical knowledge to their practice. The nursing process is the systematic mechanism with which individual nurses deal with multiple inputs in a dynamic living context and generate reasoned and defensible actions with regard to a valued outcome on behalf of those served (variously called clients or patients).

Because these frameworks and models explicitly orient nursing thought towards the application of general knowledge to the unique and particular instance, the precise role of nursing science within that theoretical reasoning process has always been somewhat difficult for the discipline to articulate. Nursing science has been understood as one element within the discipline's attempt to work out its complex relationship to both subjectively and objectively derived knowledge in matters pertaining to health and illness. Because nursing's emphasis is the very complexity of human health experience, its science draws our attention to the full range of experiential domains (from cell to soul, if you will). In this context, nurse scientists have traditionally engaged in competing strands of research development, capitalizing on both qualitative and quantitative investigative traditions.

These particular characteristics of nursing have powerfully influenced its trajectory with regard to the relationship between theory and science. In a very real sense, both theory and science serve the discipline's agenda of applying knowledge about the general to the context of the unique particular. Nursing practice, regardless of whether it is enacted at the individual, family, group, or societal level, has always held as a core value a unique kind of orientation to the holistically understood individual in context. Nursing has considered itself to have a unique relationship to the bodily, socially, psychically represented human experience of the person, and has considered this unique relationship to be fundamental to its disciplinary angle of vision on collective human health phenomena. The knowledge base upon which one refines how to accomplish nursing practice in all of its various dimensions therefore involves the generation and application of knowledge as a dialectic within which practice informs theory and theory informs practice in an iterative manner (also known as a *praxis* orientation). Thus, nursing's action imperative forces a degree of disciplinary comfort with diverse ways of knowing. This to say it assumes a knowledge development context that merges insights obtained through science with those gleaned from other forms of reason, pattern recognition, and experiential learning.

■ Problems in the understanding of evidence

In the context of the disciplinary theoretical tradition outlined above, nursing has encountered considerable difficulty in the uptake and interpretation of an evidence-based practice agenda. From our perspective, these problems arise in direct relation to our unique disciplinary *angle of vision* towards the challenge of health care and service delivery. They serve to illuminate the complex philosophical basis upon which the current agenda is mounted. We understand these challenges to reflect two distinct kinds of problems: those associated with distinctions between the various knowledge sources upon which nursing draws, and those associated with the fluidity with which the notion of evidence is defined within the discipline.

☐ Ways of knowing versus evidence

Since Carper's (1978) seminal work on 'patterns of knowing', nurses have referred to the different patterns of knowing to articulate the understanding that nursing knowledge extends beyond those questions for which empirical science has answers. The patterns of knowing represent diverse epistemological sources of ideas that, under certain circumstances, inform the development and application of nursing knowledge. Chinn and Kramer (2004) expanded Carper's work by referring to different ways of knowing that describe how nurses combine empirical knowledge with past experience and subjective understandings to inform their nursing practice. Examples discussed in nursing literature include the ways of knowing pertaining to skill, intuition, aesthetics, and therapeutic presence. Skill involves aesthetic expression in the form of skillful performance based on experience that is acquired by method of practice (Johnson, 1994; Chinn and Kramer, 2004). Aesthetic knowing can be seen as a reflective response to a nursing challenge from which a sense of meaning emerges. Intuition pertains to knowing that extends beyond the constraints of rational thought and that relies on an in-depth familiarity with the world of nursing (Rew, 1989). And personal knowing requires familiarity with physical, emotional, psychological, and social responses of the self and others as the basis for being therapeutically present with others in the world of nursing (Chinn and Kramer, 2004).

Although it is evident that various ways of knowing are and will be used in nursing practice, it is also important to recognize that not all ways of knowing result in knowledge that can be expressed as evidence. Conventionally, evidence draws on the philosophical premises of propositional knowledge to inform nursing practice in a reliable and consistent manner. Evidence is based on scientific and philosophical approaches to substantiate propositional knowledge claims.[1] Scientific approaches consist of systematic methods that combine logic with descriptions of directly and indirectly observable phenomena. Or, as argued by Kikuchi (2004), 'science inquires into the phenomenal aspects of reality' (p. 24). Philosophy, on the other hand, often relates to questions about metaphysical aspects of reality. These types of questions extend beyond the phenomenally oriented scope of science and are more appropriately addressed using philosophical approaches that rely on logic, argumentation, and common sense (Kikuchi, 2004). Examples include questions pertaining to the nature of reality (ontology), the way we come to understand or acquire knowledge (epistemology), and ethics or morality.

Although propositional knowledge is foundational to safe and competent nursing practice, nursing practice is inevitably influenced by other forms of knowledge that are not necessarily evidential in nature (Thompson, 2003). Examples in nursing literature include knowledge associated with personal knowing and various conceptions of aesthetic knowing (Carper, 1978; Chinn and Kramer, 2004) and intuition, which may also encompass knowing of a spiritual nature (Rew, 1989). These ways of knowing involve subjectivities that are, in their original form, not directly shareable beyond the immediate context of personal experiences. The resulting knowledge is of a fundamentally different nature than knowledge that conforms to the notion of evidence. Evidence pertains to knowledge that is shareable and applicable beyond the domain of personal perceptions, experiences, and beliefs. In this sense, evidence implies a degree of generalizability in terms of the patterns of phenomena to which a particular evidential claim applies. Subjective knowledge that is exclusively based on personal experience, intuition, or revelation does not constitute a shared form of knowledge that can be confirmed and argued as a basis for informing nursing practice (Johnson and Ratner, 1997).

In addition to the various ways of knowing commonly discussed in nursing literature, nursing practice is also inevitably influenced by ideologies. Ideology refers to beliefs about reality that have not been justified on scientific or philosophical grounds. These types of beliefs exist in three forms: (1) beliefs that have not yet been examined using scientific or philosophical approaches, (2) beliefs that have been examined but are not subjected to scientific or philosophical conclusions (for whatever reason), and (3) beliefs to which science or philosophy has not provided a conclusive answer. Such beliefs are held by people in a particular social context on the basis of them being shared as part of a larger belief system. It is quite apparent that people hold various ideological beliefs to be worthy with a great deal of certainty despite the lack of scientific or philosophical justification. Take for example the ideological belief that every person is innately good. In essence, this belief is an ideological position that cannot be justified scientifically or philosophically. Science cannot be used to determine the meta-physical properties of 'good', and philosophy is limited in justifying the universality of such a claim being true. Nevertheless, many nurses presumably hold some variant of this kind of ideological belief as foundational to their nursing practice.

Our discussion of various ways of knowing has several implications for how knowledge relates to nursing practice. Scientific and philosophical approaches provide the foundation for knowledge that is evidential (that is, reliable and verifiable) in nature based on the premises of empirical verification and philosophical argumentation. Evidential knowledge of this form provides the basis for informing nursing practice in a general and systematic sense. Though subjective knowledge and ideologies inevitably influence nursing practice, knowledge of this nature does not provide a foundation for evidential knowledge development, meaning that which can be used to provide general direction to nursing practice. For example, it is quite apparent that protocols for nursing practice cannot be solely based on a nurse's experiential knowledge. On the other hand, the application of protocols to unique situations requires a nursing judgement that is quite properly made in the context of a nurse's previous experience. It is widely agreed that safe and competent nursing practice extends beyond the mechanical application of protocols because it is contingent on the ability of nurses to recognize the particular instances in which protocols may or may not apply.

A brief reflection on the skill of providing an injection may help to more explicitly delineate the difference between evidential knowledge and other forms of knowledge. Almost anybody could follow the correct principles for administering an injection. These principles are based on scientific justification (e.g. using sterile technique) and philosophical justification (e.g. principles associated with respect or privacy). However, it has also been suggested that skill in this context involves ways of knowing that are aesthetic and personal in nature (Chinn and Kramer, 2004). In this sense, the actual skill of an injection is something that is developed through inner processes associated with practice and experience. As long as the principles are followed correctly, there is no scientific or philosophical basis for sharing or justifying these inner processes. As a result, nurses may have different perceptions and experiences pertaining to the performance of a skill, such as an injection; one nurse may feel particularly good about skillfully providing an injection, whereas another nurse observing may not share the same sense of appreciation for how adeptly the skill was performed. Assuming that all scientific and philosophical principles pertaining to injection administration were adhered to, it seems that the performing nurse and the observing nurse do not share the same frame of reference upon which their experiential understanding was based. This is because their perceptions and experiences are inherently subjective. Though evidence provides the foundational knowledge base for ensuring that all essential principles are systematically adhered to, the skillful enactment of a set of principles involves other ways of knowing (e.g. personal and aesthetic knowing) that are not readily subjected to scientific or philosophical scrutiny.

This example illuminates the kind of complexity inherent in how nursing thinks about its practice knowledge, and the legitimacy claims upon which it bases its understanding of clinical reasoning and practice action. Within nursing, there has always been a distinct sense that expert practice involves an increasingly fine-tuned capacity to know when and how to use, or possibly depart from, evidence-based practice protocols, by interpreting population-based knowledge in relation to the particular individualized contexts in which nursing care takes place. Thus, while it is unacceptable to ignore evidentiary claims in clinical reasoning, they inherently represent only a fraction of the advanced expert knowledge of nurses, whose practice domain is the unique holistic and complex client within a particular temporal, spatial, and relational context.

□   Shifting conceptualizations of evidence

A second set of problems arises from the various conceptualizations of evidence that have crept into the disciplinary literature as well as common discourse within nursing. The notion of *evidence*, as it has come to be applied within the medical and health care contexts, explicitly references a hierarchy of knowledge sources that are understood to be reliable and therefore credible foundations for clinical reasoning (Sackett *et al.*, 1996). In this context, the randomized controlled trial (RCT) has risen to become the gold standard for what constitutes evidence, often privileging those species of knowledge for which the RCT is a viable and practical option. This conceptualization contrasts with the legalistic definition of evidence, in which a wide range of forms of information may be understood as indicative of the truth or falsity of key facts, and may therefore be included within the human processes of reasoning conclusions. The commonly accepted medical definition of evidence has tended to explicitly set conditions for which certain forms of scientific proof are held to exist. These conditions are set against what is held to be the inherent unreliability of expert clinical knowledge or wisdom (Timmermans and Berg, 2003). While the law understands evidence as something that could potentially be misleading, medicine seems to have considered it something that almost always trumps all other competing claims (Rycroft-Malone *et al.*, 2004)[2]. Sometimes nursing has further complicated the scene by injecting a new twist on its definition of evidence[3]. Where conventional scientific facts are either absent from or irrelevant to a clinical reasoning context, some nurse authors have re-inscribed non-evidentiary sources of knowledge with terminological labels such as 'clinical evidence' in an attempt to justify their appropriate inclusion as a basis for clinical action (Clarke, 1999; French, 2002; Thompson, 2003). In the context of the raging agenda of evidence-based practice, this conceptual maneuver seems reminiscent of Lewis Carroll's Humpty Dumpty who argued that 'When I use a word . . . it means just what I choose it to mean' (1872, 1974, p. 179).

Despite these shifting conceptualizations, when empirical evidence is uniquely understood to be 'best' evidence, it is inherently assumed to supersede other forms of knowledge that differ in kind (such as physiologic principles or patient values) and that are not amenable to hierarchical ranking (Tonelli, 2001). Recognizing that much of what is carried out in the name of medicine and health care can never be subjected to RCTs by virtue of rationality, practicability, or ethics, we are left with a paradox in practice knowledge. As Grypdonck (2005) conceives of it, evidence-based health care has become 'an ideology that violates its own ideology' in that it cannot be subjected to the basic test that it sets for other knowledge claims. From her perspective, evidence-based health care assumes the relevance of confirmatory proof that one option will work above all others rather than seeking guidance as to the range of reasonable options from which a skilled clinician might appropriately draw. As such, it reflects a standardizing agenda, rather than one that involves individualization (Timmermans and Berg, 2003). The kind of science favoured by the evidence-based practice agenda becomes that which pays tremendous attention to subjects and little to representativeness of stimulus, thereby privileging those treatments and interventions for which confusing contextual contaminants (such as time, subjective awareness, etc.) can be controlled. And this, as we know, is almost never the case in the complex business of holistic nursing care delivered to diverse individuals in the context of their unique relational and sociocultural worlds.

It is undeniably the case that hierarchies of evidence are beneficial in evaluating knowledge pertaining to predictable relationships between well-defined phenomena. However, the degree to which evidence is justified in its application to practice is contingent upon the congruency between the form of evidence (e.g. as defined by the research design) and the nature of knowledge needed to inform a particular area of nursing practice. In other words, specific forms of evidence support specific kinds of conclusions associated with ways of knowing that answer specific types of questions to inform nursing practice. Though RCTs are highly effective in providing evidence pertaining to causal relationships (e.g. the effectiveness of specific interventions based on well-defined treatment outcomes), other forms of evidence are needed to understand the nature of phenomena and the various contexts in which particular phenomena take place (e.g. the secondary effects or meanings of such interventions within the larger personal or social context). For example, though RCTs provide compelling evidence about the efficacy of particular pain management strategies, other forms of evidence are needed to provide further insight into the experience of pain in the various contexts in which pain might occur. Nurses rely on highly reliable evidence based on RCTs to inform particular pain management strategies when the causal mechanism as well as the outcome is well understood in relation to the various situations in which the pain management strategy can be applied. However, nurses' understanding of pain and the nature of the desirable outcome requires a familiarity with the many and various ways in which pain may be experienced and expressed. The latter is best informed by knowledge that is more descriptive and inductive in nature.

Having identified the kind of evidence that is most compatible with the particular question arising from their practice, nurses also need to consider the degree of certainty that is needed before applying that evidence to practice. In applying knowledge to practice, nurses implicitly make a judgement about the degree to which an evidential claim applies to a situation encountered in nursing practice. The resulting degree of belief placed on an evidential claim represents a judgement of the certainty with which it holds true based on predefined premises that delineate the scope and context to which it applies. Statistical inference is foundational to deductive knowledge development where probability theory is used to objectively examine the truth or, from a Popperian perspective, falsity of propositional claims. The related assumptions of probability theory are well understood, and rest on the ability to measure and isolate or control all relevant phenomena. However, the complexity of factors associated with human experiences of health and illness precludes our ability to consistently consider all potentially relevant phenomena. It is therefore widely recognized that evidential knowledge based on statistical inference must be interpreted with a degree of tentativeness in terms of its application to particular situations. In essence, the nature of probabilistic relationships between phenomena implies that the causal mechanism is not fully understood. Because of this, nurses need to make a judgement about whether a particular situation is sufficiently congruent with the probabilistic patterns of relationships between phenomena upon with the evidential claim is based, before the evidential claim can be confidently applied.

The application of evidence to particular situations has been debated for a long time. The challenge is that the processes by which evidential knowledge is developed rely on inferential mechanisms by which particularities have to a large extent been averaged out. Obviously, particularities are inconsequential in relation to deterministic causal relationships which are generalizable in a strict sense. However, the nature of knowledge pertaining to human experience of health and illness is such that deterministic claims to generalizability of causal relationships can only seldom be made. For example, probabilistically defined causal relationships pertaining to a theory of stress and coping may be widely applicable to various contexts of nursing care. Nevertheless, there are numerous conceivable instances to which the theoretical notions underlying stress and coping theory do not apply (e.g. the notion of stress appraisal may not apply to a person who is cognitively impaired). The application of evidential knowledge of this nature, such as knowledge pertaining to stress and coping, requires an in-depth familiarity with the context in which this knowledge is used to inform nursing practice. Without this familiarity, nurses run the risk of unknowingly applying evidential knowledge to situations that do not conform to the general patterns of phenomena to which a particular evidential claim applies. To apply evidential knowledge, nurses need to be thoroughly familiar with the context to which such knowledge applies, while recognizing the unique idiosyncrasies that may occur in particular situations and that may lead to adverse outcomes if generalizable knowledge claims were blindly or uncritically relied upon.

The above arguments reveal that the application of evidence to practice is not merely a mechanical process, but involves a degree of judgement that relies on appropriate familiarity with the particular situation to which evidential claims may be applied (DiCenso, 2003; Rycroft-Malone *et al.*, 2004). Some evidential claims require only a small amount of individual judgement. For example, advanced life support (ALS) protocols can be readily and widely applied as a justified approach to responding to a cardiac arrest in most circumstances where resuscitation is considered a desirable outcome. Nurses do not need to rely on exhaustive judgemental processes to evaluate whether an ALS protocol applies to a particular situation in nursing practice because the premises for using ALS protocols are clearly delineated and understood. However, application of guidelines for pain management may, for example, not be as obvious. Pain by its very nature is uniquely experienced, interpreted, and managed. We hold distinct thresholds within which pain is tolerable and understandable, and value systems within which pain confers meaning. Although certain kinds of knowledge can be obtained about pain patterns across populations within highly controlled contexts, that information rarely provides us with any certainty as to the right answer with regard to this particular patient, at this particular time. Nurses use knowledge to offer the best options they know of within the context of the patient's experience, but recognize that pain management will always require sensitive ongoing assessment, careful intervention titration, and vigilant monitoring for unique response patterns.

■ Strategies for education

The value of an evidentiary basis in challenging persistent and problematic beliefs in health care delivery is somewhat obvious. The literature reflects numerous instances in which long-established protocols or widely accepted common sense interventions have been modified for the obvious betterment of patients on the basis of that which can be determined from a rigorous analysis of careful empirical testing (DiCenso, 2003; Barer, 2005). The value of empirical knowledge in shaping the standards of professional practice is undeniable. Skillfully navigating among empirical claims is therefore a vital competency within the fundamental disciplinary knowledge base of all professional health care providers, and must be a priority focus within educational programmes (Romyn *et al.*, 2003).

However, the ability to engage in critical analysis of the evidence-based agenda also seems requisite to the effective preparation of the neophyte professional entering today's health care ideological context (Mitchell, 1999). From the perspective of nursing, clinical reasoning must be based not only on a sound interpretation of what we know, but also on a thoughtful critical analysis of what we don't know and why we don't know it.

As Kitson explains, '. . . we need to recognize our theoretical and methodological blind spots and move from taking comfort in the certainties
derived from simplistic reductionistic approaches to acknowledging the
assumptions, biases, and weaknesses that characterize most of our scientific
investigations' (1999, p. 14). Further, we must beware of the tendency
within evidentiary knowledge to focus our attention on efficacy or effectiveness rather than understanding the processes and conceptual relationships underlying our evidential claims. Timmermans and Berg note that
'Proponents of evidence-based medicine are wary of reasoning from basic
principles or experience; they distrust claims based on expertise or patho-
physiological models. They prefer to remain agnostic as to the reason why
something should or should not work – rather, they objectively measure
whether or not it works in real-life settings' (2003, p. 3). It is also apparent
that the available evidence basis from which strong practice claims can be
derived is not built simply by harvesting scientific discoveries, but is inherently dependent upon programmes of research that may well have been
generated to serve certain social, ideological, and even economic interests
(Walker, 2003). That for which there is 'good evidence' is therefore not
necessarily inherently 'best practice' but rather represents a convention
within which the preponderance of scientific products is taken to represent
the most defensible decision.

It seems imperative, therefore, that, in their formative educational years,
neophyte nurses are taught to critically reflect upon the reasons underlying
the presence or absence of an evidence base within any particular context.
Further, they must also learn to distinguish knowledge claims that indeed
exist in the form of 'good' evidence from other forms of nursing knowledge
that essentially rely on ways of knowing that are subjective and possibly
ideological in nature (Winch *et al.*, 2002). Different aspects of nursing
practice are informed by different forms of knowledge. Some forms of
knowledge come with a degree of certainty and generalizability, whereas
other forms of knowledge may relate more specifically to the individual
case without having clearly understood generalizable implications. It is
therefore essential that we educate nursing students about the forms of
knowledge needed in relation to particular aspects of their nursing practice
(DiCenso and Cullum, 1998).

A related concern is that neophyte nurses may readily interpret the
prevailing notion of hierarchical evidence frameworks as implying that all
areas of nursing practice are best informed by the form of evidence that lies
at the top of the hierarchy while disregarding the basic scientific premise
that different forms of evidence serve different purposes in relation to
knowledge development. It is quite clear from our previous discussion
that the diversity of problems encountered in nursing practice necessitates diversity of epistemological approaches to knowledge development.
Neophyte nurses need to learn to associate appropriate epistemological
approaches to the type of knowledge needed to guide nursing practice by,

for example, distinguishing evidential knowledge pertaining to the various meanings of phenomena from evidential knowledge pertaining to efficacy of predefined interventions.

From our perspective, an appropriate educational mandate requires not only a reasonable sophistication with regard to systematic retrieval and critical appraisal of formal evidentiary claims pertaining to clinical practice situations, but also an appreciation for the philosophical underpinnings of the nature of knowledge within a socially mandated practice discipline. Students need guidance in locating protocols and clinical practice guidelines, and also in working out a defensible basis upon which variations and individualized applications can be justified. Thus, we believe the continual grounding of nursing scientific knowledge within our disciplinary theoretical tradition is of vital importance. The models and frameworks that are so often discarded nowadays as inconvenient remnants of an immature disciplinary science may well serve as the ideal foundation for a philosophical understanding of the complexity and context within which nursing exists. Although the original authors may have understood the value of their conceptual models to be more theoretical in the conventional sense, we understand them as entirely philosophical in nature, reflecting ideas about problem-solving, reasoning, individualizing, and weighing options that remain contemporary and fresh in the world of practice knowledge application. We conceive of that body of conceptual work as a powerful orienting structure for making explicit the values underlying professional nursing, articulating the intellectual challenges inherent in applying general knowledge in particular contexts, and interpreting the social mandate governing the actions nursing takes on behalf of those it serves. Thus the emergence of an evidence base for good practice and the refinement of a conceptual orientation towards the unique individual should not be seen as mutually exclusive intellectual directions for an applied health discipline.

Students will need to be aware of competing discourses between, on the one hand, expanding the definition of evidence to the point at which it includes all knowledge forms that might be brought to bear on a particular clinical decision and, on the other hand, arguing for increasing refinement of the exclusive domain of a certain species of knowledge that we ought to refer to as 'evidence'. The issue here is not what each of us personally prefers to consider 'worthy' knowledge applicable to good practice decisions, but rather how we collectively come to an understanding of the conventions and processes by which we will eliminate poor practices and support the uptake of practices with established benefit. By attempting to be overly generous in our collective definitions of what constitutes evidence, we inherently complicate our capacity to strive towards the values for which the evidence-based agenda was created.

Within this context, students will need to develop competencies with a sophisticated form of analysis and of articulating the reasoning underlying their clinical decisions. Their task will not simply be one of discriminating strong from weak evidence, but rather one of discerning the nature and substance of evidentiary claims and interpreting the meaning of the presence or absence of such claims. For example, they will need to know when and how to defend certain kinds of clinical practices for which a conventional evidence base such as RCT may be unavailable or inherently impossible. They may also need to know how to recognize the presence of confusing or ambiguous findings from empirical studies to sharpen their critical analysis in relation to a phenomenon until such time as the weight of the available evidence makes the interpretation more persuasive. And they will also seek to understand how to advocate for appropriate variances within a health care climate in which certain compelling evidentiary claims take on ideological dimensions. In order to engage in the world of increasingly sophisticated and compelling evidence claims, their relationship to evidence will have to be intimate and dynamic. If we aspire to educate our students towards clarity in thinking and morality in purpose, the manner in which we collectively approach the complex universe of evidence-based practice claims will be inherently complex and philosophical. By teaching them to understand the structure and function of a scientific claim, and to understand the complex and problematic world into which that claim is set forth, we may be able to better prepare them for the kind of thinking that will facilitate the underlying values for which the evidence-based movement was advanced without falling prey to an uncritical acceptance of its dominant rhetoric.

◼ Conclusion

Through this examination of the challenge confronting educators within the discipline of nursing who attempt to wrestle with the complexities of applying an evidence-based agenda to a particularized practice discipline, we hope we have illuminated problems confronting those educators across various disciplines who seek to enlighten the next generation towards a meaningful engagement with a world of competing knowledge claims. We have illustrated the manner in which nursing's indelicate straddling of science and philosophy may have created a somewhat confusing notion of what constitutes a theory, the remnants of which remain embedded in our disciplinary thinking. From our perspective, this same slippage around whether theoretical claims are or are not meant in the scientific sense haunts much of the writing within the social sciences today. We have also demonstrated how a commitment to explicating and valuing diverse ways of knowing have inadvertently privileged the incontestability of subjective knowledge as a viable source of sound clinical decisions.

In the current academic context, many disciplines are similarly confronting the schisms in scholarly discourse that can arise from an uncritical adherence to ideas. We have also recognized that the ideas that are shared within a discipline, in this case nursing, represent a deeply felt conviction for many of its members. Our relationship to a health professional discipline typically extends well beyond a vocational option and into the domain of a calling or moral imperative. In this context, we may be prone to an unsophisticated conflation between probability and 'truth'. This same notion creeps into the educational challenge in other disciplines when our rhetoric attributes ideology to the 'other' but not to ourselves. We therefore see the educational implications that may be drawn from this analysis as applicable beyond the confines of our own discipline.

In a world in which nurses will face increasingly complex clinical challenges and confront an expanding array of administrative and consumer pressures with regard to evidence claims, it is imperative that the discipline adopts a clear and unambiguous mechanism by which to consider what does and does not constitute evidence. In order to do this, we must come to agreement on the reasoned basis by which we would distinguish between the various forms of knowledge upon which our clinical mandate relies and the terminology with which we reference our epistemological underpinnings. The urgency of public accountability for health care expenditures and resource allocation decisions will only extend the demand for justifications on the basis of that which is evidence-based. Our credibility as a discipline, in an increasingly vigilant accountability context and with an increasingly informed health consuming public, will depend on our collective capacity to interpret and explain the sources of knowledge upon which we rely and the manner in which we use and apply those sources. Nurses of the future must find solid grounding upon which to base evidence claims that can be understood beyond the syntax of the discipline and can stand the test of public scrutiny while also being sensitive to and creative within the development of the discipline. Towards this end, educators must tackle the complex challenge of navigating the discipline's epistemological complexity, and translating its various elements into a credible relationship with the notion of what constitutes evidence.

■ Notes

1 Conventional understandings of evidence are based on the epistemological premises of propositional knowledge, where knowledge is defined in terms of justified true beliefs. Scientific and philosophical approaches are used as the foundation for justifying, or substantiating, beliefs with the purpose of developing a body knowledge that is 'evidential' in nature. A belief essentially refers to a proposition that can be articulated, and justification refers to a systematic process by which we argue or substantiate a particular belief to be true or warranted. Justification is therefore not seen as universally conclusive; there exist differences of opinion about the degree to which particular beliefs are justified. The notion of 'true' has an ontological implication in that reality exists in a form that is independent of human consciousness.

2   While it is often argued that the enactment of evidence-based medicine inherently reflects application of inscrutable scientific facts to the individual context (Sackett *et al.*, 2000), the emphasis within the movement is always on factual information that withstands a highly rigorous systematic review (Cochrane, 1999), the spirit of which has been described as 'purity and exclusion' (Traynor, 2002, p. 164).

3   Note that the phenomenon of redefinition of evidence to include clinical expertise is not unique to nursing and has also has also been reported within medicine (Buetow, 2002).

Part 4

Politics of Education, Knowledge and Society

Chapter 10

Little narratives of nursing: Education in the Postmodern University

Gary Rolfe

■ Introduction: After Auschwitz

Some of us are beginning to suspect that the post-Enlightenment project of modernity; of liberal education; of the elimination of illness and disease; of truth and justice for all, is going wrong. For some, the promise of modernity became perverted early in the twentieth century, culminating in *Auschwitz*, 'which can be taken as a paradigmatic name for the tragic "incompletion" of modernity' (Lyotard, 1992, p. 30). For Lyotard, the breakdown is irretrievable: 'the project of modernity [. . .] has not been forsaken or forgotten, but destroyed, "liquidated" ' (Lyotard, 1992, p. 30). For others, Auschwitz marked a nadir and a turning point in the restoration of the 'uncompleted project of modernity' (Habermas, 1981). For Habermas, modernity is not *in*complete (partial) but *un*completed (*as yet* unfinished).

In any case, what remains 'after Auschwitz' (Adorno, 1973) is not the original Enlightenment dream, if for no other reason that, following the holocaust, the human race realized that it could no longer trust itself. Auschwitz pushed reason and rationality to their limits, perhaps to their logical conclusion: 'the summit of reason, order, administration, is also the summit of terror' (Readings, 1991, p. 22). After Auschwitz, we have handed over the governance of the major institutions which have hitherto driven the Enlightenment dream to the impersonal 'free market' forces of democratic liberal capitalism. For some, the triumph of capitalism represents a confirmation of the Enlightenment values of truth and justice; for others, it signals a step towards the post-Enlightenment 'new dark ages' (MacIntyre, 1985, p. 263).

In this chapter, I intend to explore the effects of the ethos of free market capitalism in the 'new dark ages' on the institution of the University in general, and on nursing education within the University in particular, and suggest an alternative based on the writing of Bill Readings and Jean

François Lyotard. I will begin by examining the traditional role of the University and its relationship with knowledge generation and dissemination.

■ Knowledge, grand narratives and the University

In his well-known work *The Postmodern Condition: A Report on Knowledge*, Lyotard (1984) identifies the narrative as the organizing principle of knowledge. Pre-modern or 'traditional' narratives offer more or less straightforward storied accounts of knowledge, and can be couched in a great variety of different language games (following Wittgenstein, 1958) such as the prescriptive (instructing), the performative (enacting), and the interrogative (enquiring). Traditional narratives 'allow the society in which they are told, on the one hand, to define its criteria of competence and, on the other, to evaluate according to those criteria what is performed or can be performed within it' (Lyotard, 1984, p. 20). The validating criteria of pre-modern narratives thus rest with the society in which, and on whose behalf, they are told.

In contrast, modern or 'scientific' narratives employ a single language game: denotation. Science has the single aim of describing, and thus a single criterion for acceptance: truth[1]. Furthermore, the scientific narrative does not present itself as a simple and straightforward story. Whereas traditional narratives are validated through the act of telling and by the status accorded by society to the narrator and the audience, scientific narratives are self-validating, insofar as the criteria for the validation of the truth-content of the narrative forms part of the narrative itself. Whereas traditional narratives simply tell the story, scientific narratives are metanarratives, since they also tell the story of why the story has to be true. So, for example, a scientist's narration of her research project includes not only an account of the findings, but also the story of how those findings were achieved and why they are valid and accurate (that is, an account of the methodology and method).

When a metanarrative extends its boundaries of validation beyond itself, it becomes a grand narrative: 'a story that claims the status of a *universal* metanarrative, capable of accounting for all other stories in order to reveal their true meanings' (Readings, 1991, p. xxxiii, my emphasis). For example, Christianity tells the story of Christ as the son of God (narrative), the story of why it is true that Christ is the son of God (metanarrative), and the story of why this story is more true than all other competing stories about God (grand narrative). For Lyotard (1984), the Enlightenment project produced two grand narratives which structured and organized our knowledge up to and beyond Auschwitz. The first, which he termed the 'speculative grand narrative', regarded knowledge as an end in itself with truth as its goal. As Lyotard notes, the speculative grand narrative derives from the work of Schleiermacher and Humboldt, is oriented towards a training for citizenship that has a spiritual and moral dimension (Lyotard, 1984), and is most often encountered in arts and humanities departments of the University. Lyotard's second grand narrative is the grand narrative of emancipation, which regards knowledge as a means to the end of freedom and justice. For Lyotard, this grand narrative has its origins in the French Revolution with the ideals of universal education and the power of science to reduce suffering and transform society. The grand narrative of emancipation, of knowledge as a means of improving quality of life, takes a pragmatic approach to truth and is encountered most often in the University in departments of natural, biological, social and political sciences.

For Lyotard (1984), the task of uniting these two grand narratives of science and the arts fell to the discipline of philosophy, which 'must restore unity to learning, which has been scattered into separate sciences in laboratories and in pre-university education' (p. 33). Clearly, however, the unifying grand narrative of philosophy never achieved its goal: university disciplines are becoming ever more fragmented and specialized; philosophy departments (at least in the UK) have diminished substantially in number since the 1980s, and many philosophers now reject the very idea of a universal grand narrative. Lyotard traces this 'deligitimation' of knowledge (p. 37) to the post-war boom in technology and 'the redeployment of advanced liberal capitalism [...] a renewal that has eliminated the communist alternative and valorized the individual enjoyment of goods and services' (p. 38).[2] Under 'advanced liberal capitalism', knowledge is no longer legitimized by an appeal to either truth or justice; rather, 'in matters of social justice and scientific truth alike, the legitimation of that power is based on its optimizing the system's performance – efficiency' (p. xxiv). After Auschwitz, knowledge is valued in terms of its efficiency[3] and profitability in a market-driven economy rather than for its potential to fulfil human goals of truth and justice. *Liberal-Capitalism* has become the new grand narrative of the University, the validating principle for knowledge and the driving force of research and development in contemporary society. As a result, knowledge is a commodity to be bought and sold in the marketplace, and as Readings (1996) tells us, the commoditization of knowledge has succeeded in reducing it to the status of information.

This shift from a focus on knowledge and the pursuit of truth and justice to a focus on information and the pursuit of efficiency has, in Readings' words, left the University in ruins. For Readings (1996), a central and very telling example of the ruined University is the rise of the discipline of cultural studies. First, he points out, culture becomes a legitimate field of study only when the University *as a whole* is no longer concerned with it:

> Thus, Cultural Studies must be understood to arise when culture ceases to be the animating principle of the University and ... becomes instead an object of study among others, a discipline rather than a metadisciplinary idea (Readings, 1996, p. 92).

The suggestion is that the University is no longer operating in the service of society in general and culture in particular, but for the efficient running of the nation state and multinational corporations.

Secondly, and in a similar vein, the word 'studies' should alert us to the fact that there are other things we can do with culture apart from studying it, and that culture is neither a traditional nor a natural focus for our studies. Thus, the rise of disciplines such as cultural studies, sport studies, business studies and indeed, nursing studies only becomes possible when studying becomes merely one activity among many in the University, and where it is not self-evident that study is the most appropriate approach to certain subjects. Thus, the fact that it is possible to make the statement 'I am doing cultural studies at university' without it being taken for a tautology should alert us to the changing role of the University away from its central role in determining the *cultural* norms of truth and justice and away from a focus on disciplines that are self-evidently foci of *study*. The word 'studies' thus signals a categorical difference between the disciplines in which it forms part of their title (either explicitly or implicitly), and those such as mathematics, chemistry and philosophy, where the addition of the word 'studies' is neither necessary nor meaningful.

In fact, we could argue that the *study* of business, sport or nursing (to take just three fairly arbitrary examples) is not the primary aim in any of these disciplines, but is merely the means to some other end. In other words, business, sport and nursing are neither arts, sciences nor even humanities disciplines, but *technologies*.[4] Of course, the individuals who are studying these subjects might argue that they are following the speculative grand narrative in their pursuit of business, sporting or nursing knowledge for its own sake or for some aesthetic end, or else are following the emancipatory grand narrative by making a contribution to justice, freedom and better business, sport or nursing care through science. Indeed, the move of nursing into the University in the UK during the 1990s was undertaken with a great deal of emancipatory zeal and with high expectations for nurse education. However, from the perspective of the grand narrative of Liberal-Capitalism, academics in these disciplines are engaged primarily, albeit unwittingly, in the generation and application of *information* about business, sport or nursing with the aim of maximizing efficiency and the potential for profit.

■ Nursing studies and the new technologies

I am suggesting that nursing studies can be seen as part of the rise of the 'new technologies' within the University, which include cultural studies, film studies, sport and leisure studies, educational studies, business studies and a host of other applied subjects (see also Bearn, 2000). I am making a distinction here between the old and new technologies. The 'old technologies' such as engineering and fine art were already located within the University prior to the grand narrative of Liberal-Capitalism and can, with some justification, be said to contribute towards the Enlightenment project of knowledge, truth and justice. The 'new technologies' such as sport and leisure studies and nursing studies could be said to owe their existence within the University solely to the new Liberal-Capitalist grand narrative, and would appear to be far more oriented towards the goals of efficiency, profitability and the free market than the ideals of the Enlightenment. Whilst nurse education, and even nursing as an academic discipline (along with similar disciplines such as teacher training and social work), perhaps pre-dated the grand narrative of Liberal-Capitalism and might with some justification be said to contribute towards the Enlightenment project of a better life through the application of science, its integration into the University and its subsequent transformation into nursing *studies* in the 1970s in the USA, the 1980s in Australia, and the 1990s in the UK was at least partly driven by capitalist considerations of economy, efficiency and the modernization of the health service. In the more humanistic of the new technologies such as nursing, a tension has therefore arisen between the post-Enlightenment values of many academics and the emerging grand narrative of Liberal-Capitalism.

Under the grand narrative of Liberal-Capitalism, these new technologies are beginning to replace the humanities, arts and sciences as the most popular disciplines in terms of student numbers, with the subsequent closure of traditional University departments such as chemistry, history and even sociology. In fact, it could be argued that without the grand narrative of Liberal-Capitalism, nursing studies and the other new technologies would find it difficult even to establish a foothold in the University. Certainly, these new technologies do not sit well within the traditional grand narratives of the University, since they share the ethos of neither the sciences nor the arts and humanities. Indeed, we need only examine the long-standing and as yet unresolved debate about whether nursing should be regarded as an art or a science to suspect that perhaps it is neither. Whilst some writers have argued for nursing as a 'craft' (Barker and Buchanan-Barker, 2004), I believe that the term 'new technology' offers a more accurate description.

I shall now examine several problems posed by the new technologies in general, and nursing studies in particular, and attempt to show why neither the traditional grand narratives of the Enlightenment University nor the new grand narrative of Liberal-Capitalism fully resolves them.

■ The problem of professional practice

All of the new technologies are concerned with some form of professional activity outside of the University, and most academics in these disciplines are themselves former practitioners who continue to value practice for its own sake; as something *intrinsically* as well as extrinsically worthwhile which they wish to carry on doing. On a more pragmatic level, many academics would argue that practice provides them with credibility in the classroom, whilst others push the argument further and maintain that regular practice is necessary in order to maintain their status as experts. Finally, practice is also seen as a means of informing teaching with up-to-date examples and cases, and a few academics would claim that it also contributes to their knowledge base through reflection-on-action, case studies and small-scale action research.

However, the important position accorded to professional practice by many nurse academics is neither acknowledged nor valued within the traditional grand narratives of the University. In fact, we have already seen that in most of the traditional sciences, arts and humanities disciplines, this split between academic work within the University and practice outside of it is meaningless, since for these academics, theorizing and research *is* their practice. Thus, one of the ways (perhaps the primary way) of practising sociology, mathematics, geography and so on is to work in a university department in what Lyotard (1992, p. 76) refers to as the 'cognitive profession'. The same cannot be said for many of the new technologies; it is not strictly accurate for an academic working in a university department of nursing to claim that she is doing nursing, nor for an academic working in a department of business studies to claim that she is running a business. Nursing and business are not 'cognitive professions' and are not usually practised from within university departments. With a few notable exceptions such as medicine and architecture, the Enlightenment University not only refuses to value professional practice by academics, it fails even to recognize it as an issue.

We might imagine that the problem would be resolved as the post-Enlightenment grand narrative of Liberal-Capitalism begins to emerge from the ruins of the traditional University, since under Liberal-Capitalism, knowledge is no longer valued solely as a means to the end of truth and justice, but rather as a route towards greater efficiency and profitability. Thus, in the UK during the 1960s and 1970s, the new Liberal-Capitalist University appeared to be shifting its focus from knowledge generation to knowledge application. This shift in focus was reflected in the proliferation of 'sandwich courses' in the newly chartered universities which included a substantial practical component, along with the emerging practice-based agenda of the polytechnics, which generally valued the practical application of knowledge over pure research.

However, by the time that nursing studies in the UK entered the academy in the 1990s, the agenda had shifted once again from knowledge *application* to knowledge as a *commodity* to be bought and sold in the marketplace, thereby reinforcing the traditional University focus on the production of knowledge through research. This renewed and intensified concern with research activity has (perhaps ironically) strengthened the hand of academics in the traditional cognitive professions, for whom (as we have seen) practice *is* research. However, for those academics in the new technology disciplines, the theory–practice dilemma has simply been replaced with a new teaching-research dialectic.

■ The problem of research

It is clear, however, that this return to research is somewhat different under the grand narrative of Liberal-Capitalism. Whereas the Enlightenment project regarded research alongside theorizing as part of a general strategy for producing knowledge and thereby arriving at truth, the Liberal-Capitalist University promotes it as a machine for generating information. For example, C. Wright Mills, a social theorist firmly attached to the values of the Enlightenment University, gave the following advice to his students:

> Avoid the fetishism of method and technique. Urge the rehabilitation of the unpretentious intellectual craftsman, and try to become such a craftsman yourself. Let every man be his own methodologist; let every man be his own theorist; let theory and method again become part of the practice of a craft. Stand for the primacy of the individual scholar; stand opposed to the ascendancy of research teams and technicians. Be one mind that is on its own confronting the problems of man and society (Mills, 1970, p. 246).

Clearly, Mills regarded researching and theorizing as simply two similar and largely interchangeable species of scholarly activity from which the academic could pick and choose to suit her own preferences, claiming elsewhere that 'I do not like to do empirical work if I can possibly avoid it' (p. 225). However, it would be difficult to imagine an academic getting away with such a sentiment today in the Liberal-Capitalist University, where the ascendancy of the research team is complete, the fetishism of methodological rigour is beyond reproach, and the information generated by doing empirical research has significantly higher value than the knowledge generated by theorizing. Thus, whilst the Enlightenment University might have conducted nursing research in order (at least ostensibly) to further the Enlightenment quest for truth, justice and a better life for all, the Liberal-Capitalist University does so in order to generate information to be sold in the marketplace, or in the case of nursing, kudos and funding in the UK's Research Assessment Exercise (RAE).[5]

Importantly, one of the consequences of this commoditization of knowledge as information is a move away from the rigours of the academy towards those of the manufacturing industry and the production line. Efficiency is the new criterion of quality, research is now assessed in terms of throughput rather than process, and university departments are judged according to the amount of research funding that comes in, and the number of peer-reviewed papers in 'high quality' journals that go out.[6] Even the assessment of the quality of the journals is the outcome of a simple mathematical computation based on the number of citations that the journal receives. It is hardly surprising, then, that the edict 'publish or perish' (or, in its current form, 'research or perish') is fast becoming a reality for all academics in the Liberal-Capitalist University. Lyotard puts it rather more starkly: 'the application [of efficiency] . . . necessarily entails a certain level of terror, whether soft or hard: *be operational or disappear*' (Lyotard, 1984, p. xxiv, my emphasis).[7]

Whilst we might imagine that the research culture of the new technologies such as nursing studies might flourish under the Liberal-Capitalist criterion of efficiency, it is once again the 'cognitive profession' of traditional academics which has adapted best. Part of the explanation undoubtedly lies in the fact that, despite changes in validity criteria, the new goal for research of producing marketable information relies on very similar production processes to the old Enlightenment goal of knowledge generation. This can be seen by the way in which the aims of experimental nursing research have shifted seamlessly from the generation of knowledge to the new task of judging the effectiveness and efficiency of treatment interventions.

However, the problem for nurse academics and other new technologists is perhaps more deep-seated than simply a shift in focus from generating theoretical knowledge to evaluating the effectiveness and efficiency of treatment interventions. First, we have seen that a number of nurse academics continue to struggle with balancing their roles of teacher and practitioner, so that the emphasis on a third role of researcher is often the final straw. Secondly, and linked to this, is the point that many academics from the new technologies regard the *transmission* of knowledge to other practitioners through teaching as a more important aspect of their role than the *generation* of knowledge through research. Producing new nurses is, understandably, seen as being of greater value than producing new knowledge or information.

Thirdly, and perhaps most importantly, there is a mismatch between the knowledge requirements of the new technologies such as nursing and output of the Liberal-Capitalist research machine. The grand narrative of Liberal-Capitalism has championed large-scale generalizable quantitative research and, specifically, the randomized controlled trial (RCT) as the government-sponsored 'gold standard' research method for nursing. These methods are perfectly attuned to the Liberal-Capitalist aims of rationalizing services and nursing care, since they produce decontextualized statistical information that can be used as a rational basis for making large-scale decisions, and which is easily packaged for sale. However, the new technologies such as business studies, hotel and catering and nursing are concerned largely with inter-personal relationships and with meeting the needs of individuals, and these concerns value contextualized and individualized knowledge from small-scale qualitative studies as perhaps more important than the production of marketable information from RCTs. However, the gold standard quantitative methodologies have somewhat marginalized the small-scale qualitative 'little narratives' of research, and whilst some nurse academics have followed the path of least resistance by chasing six-figure grants for large-scale quantitative research projects, others have refused to become part of the new research machine.

There is an added irony that whilst researchers have undoubtedly seen their status greatly increased under the grand narrative of Liberal-Capitalism, the degree of 'intellectual craftsmanship' (Mills, 1970) involved in working for the research machine has almost certainly diminished. Many academic departments, particularly in the new technologies, appear to be developing offices full of high-status, well-paid 'research clones' (to use the terminology of one of my colleagues) whose sole job is to write research bids, manage the work of research assistants and produce research papers.

■ The problem of teaching and learning

Perhaps unsurprisingly, academics in the new technologies such as nursing studies tend to place a greater emphasis on teaching and learning than their colleagues in more traditional disciplines. However, whilst we might have expected the production of professional practitioners to be more highly regarded in the Liberal-Capitalist University than the production of knowledge, we have seen that it is research that continues to dominate over teaching. Thus, whilst nursing and the other new technologies attract large numbers of undergraduate students along with the accompanying per capita funding, the criterion for academic excellence continues to be performance in the RAE. Because of the significantly higher demand for teaching in the new technologies, many nurse academics find it impractical to devote sufficient time and energy to both research *and* teaching, and are being forced to choose between the two. A number of nursing departments are therefore dividing (whether overtly or covertly) into separate teaching and research institutes, with a disproportionate amount of the income of the department going to fund the latter.

If we shift our focus from pre- to post-qualifying education, we can see that the most significant impact of the Liberal-Capitalist grand narrative on teaching is not its effect on nurse academics, but on students. First, the commoditization of knowledge has had a profound influence on the way that students are coming to regard post-qualifying education programmes. The fact that much post-graduate nurse education is no longer free at the point of delivery has emphasized to students that when they enrol on courses and pay their fees, they are purchasing a commodity. Furthermore, as academic qualifications become more important for promotion within the nursing profession, students become less interested in the educational experience and more focussed on the outcome. For all the good intentions behind the modularization of courses, one of the unintended effects is that some students do not wish to buy the educational process, nor even the knowledge and information identified in the learning outcomes of the modules, but the CATS points awarded on successful completion of the module.[8]

The more cynical reader might suspect that some of the new technology departments of the University are beginning to resemble *Bureaux des Changes*, where students are able to shop around to obtain the best exchange rate of pounds sterling for CATS points, which they are then able to convert back into hard cash in the form of promotion and salary increase. Whist this is perhaps a rather extreme scenario, we should bear in mind that such a situation would have certain benefits for both parties, since most University departments have almost unlimited CATS points at their disposal but very little disposable cash.

Secondly, the commoditization of knowledge has also influenced the way that the University is organizing itself and its students. Readings (1996) has observed that the recent preoccupation with issues of 'quality' and 'excellence' is a strong indicator that the University has become a 'bureaucratic corporation' that is being run exactly like any other large business. Readings argues that the term 'excellence' is now synonymous with the *administration* of process rather than with the process itself, and that 'quality' of output now usually refers, rather ironically, to an increase in *quantity*. Until very recently, the UK 'Teaching Quality Assessment' (TQA) in the UK was concerned predominantly with the smooth passage of students through the educational system in the most efficient way and the shortest time possible, and the *quality* of teaching being assessed by the TQA was based largely on the *quantity* of students (in terms of hitting recruitment targets), degrees awarded (amount, time taken and classification), attrition rates, library funding and stock, and of course, paperwork. The obvious implication is that an excellent lecturer is one who efficiently administers the students through the system in such a way as to facilitate the quality targets of the University rather than for any intrinsic (or even extrinsic) benefits to the student, and the student ultimately becomes a means to the end of accumulating a high score on the TQA and the conversion of student fees into CATS points.[9]

Readings suggests that there are a number of questions to be asked of such a value system:

> Are grades the only measure of student achievement? Why is efficiency privileged, so that it is automatically assumed that graduating 'on time' is a good thing? How long does it take to become 'educated'? [. . .] Is the best University necessarily the richest one? What is the relation to knowledge implied by focusing on the library as the place where it is stocked? Is quantity the best measure of the significance of library holdings? Is knowledge simply to be reproduced from the warehouse, or is it something to be produced in teaching? (Readings, 1996, pp. 25–26)

It could be argued, then, that the post-Enlightenment grand narrative of Liberal-Capitalism has enabled the emergence of the new technologies such as nursing studies, but that the free-market value system of efficiency, effectiveness and the production of information has, in fact, proved to be an inhospitable climate for the development of these practice-oriented disciplines.

■ Towards a Postmodern University

If nursing studies and the other new technologies are to survive and compete in the post-Enlightenment University, an alternative to the grand narrative of Liberal-Capitalism must be sought. We have seen that, for some writers, the solution is the restoration of the 'uncompleted project of modernity' (Habermas, 1981) and the post-Enlightenment grand narratives of truth and justice. Others, however, believe that modernity is dead (or, at least, that it is very unwell) and that the grand narratives of the Enlightenment should no longer impose their values on the University. The more radical of these voices argue not for a new grand narrative to replace truth and justice, but rather a postmodern[10] attitude of 'incredulity towards all grand narratives' (Lyotard, 1984). That is not to say that we should reject truth and justice as irrelevant or unsuitable values for the University, but that we should be incredulous towards their claims to be universal taken-for-granted narratives applicable to all disciplines in all situations. Such an attitude of incredulity has a number of profound and far-reaching implications for the University as a whole, but particularly for the new technologies such as nursing studies where the pursuit and development of theory and practice remain separate enterprises.

If we adopt an attitude of incredulity or disbelief towards the *very idea* of a grand narrative, then how are we to legitimate nursing knowledge and theory? If there is no grand narrative, no overarching criterion for making judgements about truth claims, then how are we to recognize good research and valid knowledge? The answer favoured by certain postmodern writers is that we should look *not* to the *origins* of knowledge and theory but to its *goal*. Lyotard (1984) pointed out that, for the modernist researcher, the validity of the knowledge generated by a research project rests with the credibility of the researcher and the validity of the methods used. Thus, 'within the bounds of the game of research, the competence required concerns the post of sender [of the research findings] alone' (p. 25, parenthesis added). For the postmodern researcher, however, knowledge is not validated by an appeal to the rigours of the method or methodology employed in the study, but by an appeal to the utility of the knowledge *in practice*. Thus, whilst the validity of modernist scientific knowledge is the responsibility of the researcher or 'sender' of the knowledge, including her status within the scientific community, postmodern narratives[11] 'are legitimated by the simple fact that they do what they do' (p. 23). This, of course, is a pragmatist view of truth, and to echo Rorty (1991), pragmatism views truth as what it is useful for us to believe. The emphasis for Rorty is not only on truth as being what is good or useful to believe, but more importantly, that it should be believed by *us*. It is not the researcher who decides what counts as knowledge, but the recipients of that knowledge, the community for whom the knowledge is intended, and in the case of knowledge about practice, that means practitioners. The aim of the researcher is not to impose her authority on the study, but to enter into a dialogue with her readers in order to attempt to convince them of its worth. The postmodern turn therefore implies a shift in the responsibility for validating the text from the writer to the readers, and thus from a single 'authorized' version of knowledge to a plurality of competing versions according to the needs, requirements and judgements of each individual reader (Barthes, 1977).

We can, perhaps, see why the Liberal-Capitalist University might reject such a position, since it eschews the idea of a quality benchmark or seal of approval endorsed by academic experts. If the quality (or truth, or whatever else we might wish to call it) of the knowledge is assessed by the individual user of that knowledge according to her individual needs, then knowledge can never be decontextualized and packaged as universal, value-free information.

The shift from the Liberal-Capitalist University to the Postmodern University is thus *literally* a matter of judgement. For Readings, the challenge was 'to think what it may mean to have a *University that has no idea*, that does not derive its name from an etymological confusion of unity and universality' (Readings, 1996, p. 122, my emphasis). The ideas of unity and universality are both counter to the idea of the Postmodern University that has no idea (or, we might say, no 'big idea', no grand narrative). The question therefore becomes one of how judgement might be possible in the University that subscribes to no grand narrative, in which the task of making judgements about the validity of knowledge is dispersed amongst a wide community of practitioners and other interested parties who value difference over consensus or unity of thought. We cannot simply return to the modernist notion of critique, since critique depends on the assumption that the University is still concerned with issues of truth and falsehood rather than with successful or unsuccessful performance. Neither can we refuse to judge, since 'those in the University are called upon to judge, and the administration will do it for them if they do not respond to the call' (Readings, 1996, p. 130). As academics, we are in the judgement business: we have to make judgements about what to include in curricula, to evaluate the work of our students, and to choose between competing knowledge claims. As Readings states, we have to respond to the call. Fortunately, 'responding does not, however, mean proposing new criteria, but finding ways *to keep the question of evaluation open*, a matter for dispute – what Lyotard would call the locus of the differend' (p. 130, his emphasis).

The notion of the *differend* is central to Lyotard's resolution of the postmodern problem of the delegitimation of knowledge. A *differend* is a site of dispute between two competing claims from different knowledge communities 'which cannot be equitably resolved for lack of a rule applicable to both arguments' (Lyotard, 1988, p. xi). Such situations rarely arose in the Enlightenment University, which strove for unity/universality (universitality?) and a single knowledge community, and where disputes could be settled by recourse to the dominant grand narrative, that is, by the application of critique. Neither do they arise in the Liberal-Capitalist University, where disputes are resolved according to the criteria of efficiency and funding[12]. Lyotard refers to such disputes as litigations, which can be settled by the application of a single rule of judgement recognized by both parties, whether it be the accepted research validity criteria, RAE scores or hard cash. *Differends*, disputes between parties who cannot agree on which criteria to abide by, are more problematic, since *any* rule of judgement 'would wrong (at least) one of them (and both of them if neither side admits this rule)' (Lyotard, 1988, p. xi).

The role of the postmodern academic is not, as it is in the Enlightenment University, that of an intellectual 'who helps forget *differends*, by advocating a given genre [...] for the sake of political hegemony' (Lyotard, 1988, p. 142). It is not, as it is in the Liberal-Capitalist University, that of an administrator, striving for the illusion of excellence, where excellence itself is merely 'a non-referential [or, perhaps, a self-referential] principle that allows the maximum of uninterrupted internal administration' (Readings, 1996). The postmodern academic is concerned neither with intellectual critique nor with administrative excellence, but rather with postmodern *judgement*, which is to say, 'in detecting *differends* and in finding the (impossible) idiom for phrasing them' (Lyotard, 1988, p. 142). For Lyotard, this fundamental requirement of the Postmodern University falls to philosophy. The philosopher makes 'enigmatic' judgements, judgements without rules: 'This is, after all, what Aristotle calls prudence. It consists in dispersing justice without models' (Lyotard and Thébaud, 1985, p. 26). Lyotard's philosopher does not usually reside in a department of philosophy. Postmodern philosophy, as Derrida (1982) taught us, is not a discipline but a way of thinking, a way of *being* in the University. Postmodern philosophers are at home in any department, any discipline. The philosopher should be regarded as being in the same category as the intellectual she is coming to replace.

■ Conclusion: A re-Enlightenment

The Enlightenment University, driven by the grand narratives of knowledge and justice and united by the discipline of philosophy, lies in ruins. It has been replaced by a commercial enterprise whose primary aims are the generation and sale of information and academic credits, united by bureaucrats and the self-referential illusion of quality.

This shift in the function of the University from the generation and dissemination of culture to the generation and sale of information has enabled the entry of the 'new technologies' such as nursing studies into the sphere of higher education, but it has not created the conditions for them to flourish, since the source and destination of nursing knowledge is primarily situated in a realm of practice that lies outside of the University. If nursing is to survive as an academic discipline, a new 'Posthistorical' (Readings) or Postmodern (Lyotard) University is required, in which the academic functions as a 'philosopher', as an arbitrator between the many competing little narratives arising not only from academic theorizing and research, but also from practitioners in the 'new technologies' and, importantly, the recipients of these practices.

This chapter has explored a blueprint for rebuilding the University outlined by Bill Readings just before his death in 1994, based on Lyotard's themes of knowledge, justice and philosophy for a postmodern world (see also Blake *et al.*, 1998, ch. 7). We have, in a way, come full-circle back to the concerns of the Enlightenment University. Of course, Lyotard's notions of knowledge and justice are rather different from those of the age of the Enlightenment. As he points out, he is interested in a model of knowledge legitimation 'that has nothing to do with maximized performance, but has as its basis, difference' (Lyotard, 1984, p. 60). Similarly, he is searching for 'an idea and practice of justice that is not linked to that of consensus' (Lyotard, 1984, p. 66), but rather to the idea of difference.

And yet, significantly, it remains the job of the philosopher to unite them in an attempt to move the Postmodern University and the 'new technologies' forward. Lyotard's postmodern philosopher is not concerned with unifying thought or resolving disputes 'for the sake of political hegemony', but is concerned rather with 'finding the (impossible) idiom for phrasing them', with the opening-up of discussions that have no resolution and encouraging what Derrida (1982) referred to as *différance*, the perpetual deferral of a final resolution of intellectual dispute. Ultimately, however, the postmodern philosopher is engaged in the very same activity as her predecessors since the time of the Ancient Greeks: 'to find, if not what can legitimate judgement, then at least how to save the honor of thinking' (Lyotard, 1988, p. xii).

■ Notes

1 More specifically, a correspondence theory of truth in which a denotative statement is true if and only if the statement is an accurate description of an event or thing existing 'in the world'.
2 This was written in 1979, and foreshadows the rise of 'Thatcherism' in the UK, 'Reaganomics' in the USA, and the disintegration of the Soviet Union.

3 Indeed, we might view Auschwitz as the prototype for efficiency, as representing the 'administrative murder of millions' (Adorno, 1973), in which the trains to the death camps always ran on time.

4 Or, put another way, whilst a sociologist might be defined as someone who studies and researches in the field of sociology, and a historian is someone who studies and researches in the field of history, a nurse is not usually defined as someone who studies and researches in the field of nursing. Consequently, whilst the term 'nurse academic' is necessary to distinguish between nurses working inside and outside of the University, the corresponding terms 'sociologist academic' and 'historian academic' are more or less tautological.

5 The RAE is a form of assessment of each university, and its departments, in the UK, upon which it is judged how much money should be given for research funding to a particular department, dependent upon the judged quality of its research output. Published scores and grading are involved. The system is nationally organized, time-consuming, expensive and not without controversy.

6 Based on the UK Research Assessment Exercise (RAE) criteria.

7 Whilst the meaning of being operational is, in this case, fairly straightforward, the act of disappearing can be interpreted in a variety of ways. A recent draft paper from a UK university (which will remain anonymous for obvious reasons) entitled 'Research Inactive Members of Staff' discussed a number of soft and hard levels of terror for dealing with 'difficult cases' of staff who would not or could not 'achieve research performance of an international quality' in time for a forthcoming RAE. These included 're-designating members of staff to administrative or other related grades by mutual agreement', voluntary early retirement/severance, redundancy and disciplinary procedures.

8 The Credit Accumulation and Transfer Scheme (CATS) is a points system recognized by all UK Higher Education institutions as a method of quantifying credit for a particular module or programme. CATS points can be accumulated towards an academic award or can be 'cashed in' as exemption from certain modules.

9 This process has recently been modified, and the Quality Assurance Agency (QAA) now conducts 'Institutional Audits' which include an element of self-assessment by the educational institution. Whilst the focus of quality assurance has begun to shift towards a more qualitative evaluation, it is as yet too early to assess the full impact of this initiative. In any case, quantitative measures such as progression, retention, completion and employment data continue to figure prominently in the assessment process (QAAHE, 2002, p. 25). Furthermore, the seemingly liberal practice of self-audit is itself subject to an overall institutional audit and a number of specifically targeted discipline audits by members of the QAA, prompting comparisons with Foucault's notions of the 'normalizing gaze' and the 'panopticon' (Foucault, 1977), as disciplinary technologies of self-regulation.

10 Compare Lyotard's view of postmodernism as a reaction against liberal capitalism with that of Betts (2005), for whom 'in the economic conditions of the Western, postmodern world, everything is for sale' (p. 176).

11 For Lyotard (1984), the 'postmodern condition' marked a return to the pre-modern narrative form as the pre-eminent means for legitimating knowledge.

12 For example, TQA decisions are based on the smooth administration of the student through the system and RAE submissions are judged in part on the amount of research funding obtained by the department.

Chapter 11

Care of the self in a knowledge economy: Higher education, vocation and the ethics of Michel Foucault

John S. Drummond

■ Introduction

> Knowledge and information today is being produced
> like cars and steel were produced a hundred years ago
> (Stiglitz, 1999, p. 2).[1]

This remark by Joseph Stiglitz, as well as the title of his paper, refers to what is now commonly referred to as a 'knowledge economy'. Perhaps it is time to place recent policy developments in the education of nurses and health care professionals in this wider context. Such a discourse now permeates UK government policy at all levels.[2] The term 'knowledge economy' is, as one would expect and as Stiglitz emphasizes (see further below), primarily a signal for strategists and policy-makers that it is time to take note of a fundamental shift in the role and treatment of knowledge in both the manufacturing and service sectors. The latter includes health and education. It is important, therefore, that we begin to grasp the concept in the terms and purposes of these policy-makers, and are able to reflect on its implications for the treatment of knowledge and educational practice. That is essentially the purpose of this chapter. It begins with an outline of what different commentators have intended by the term 'knowledge economy' and how that is held to differ in emphasis from its predecessor, an 'industrial economy'. The chapter then examines the presence of 'knowledge-economics' in the discourse-practices of education. To inform the analysis from a philosophical perspective, the chapter introduces Michel Foucault's concept of ethics as a relationship that one has with one's self (*rapport à soi*). In filtering the implications of a knowledge economy through Foucault's notion of *rapport à soi*, I develop the idea that educators are now being asked to carry out a work on themselves that is presented as a prescriptive

194

moral code. Two questions are asked. First, in the changing context of a knowledge economy, what might it mean to carry out a work on one's self? Second, what are the potential relations between such a work and what it means to engage in what now appears to be the ever-changing business of education? Introducing the dimension of Foucauldian ethics will allow us to consider the knowledge economy in a manner that introduces the self into a relation with knowledge, and yet which also calls us to work on our selves in manner that is a permanent provocation with respect to its incitements. In the final part of the chapter, I argue that a knowledge economy requires a new kind of critical awareness in which both an ethics and aesthetics of education may play a central part. I do this by introducing the ancient Greek concept of the 'care of the self' (*epimeleia heautou*)[3]. In various places throughout the chapter I will use nursing and nurse education as particular illustrations of the general points I seek to make. There are two reasons for this. First, the notion of caring is obviously pertinent to nursing in ways that would be seen as uncontroversial, but also in ways which I will argue apply in principle across the health care education sector as a whole. Second, nurse education, as a recent newcomer to the higher education sector and because of its largely practical orientation, is particularly vulnerable to the incitements of a knowledge economy in ways that may compromise the notion of the care of the self by the transformation of 'care' into an increasingly technicist concept that is penetrated by economic rationality. But again, and as with the first reason, the points I make about caring in the context of nursing is to use nursing as symptomatic of a more general trend. But first, an overview of significant features of a knowledge economy.

■ What is a knowledge economy?

The term 'knowledge economy' is often used these days to distinguish it from its nominal predecessor, 'industrial economy'. A main feature of what is often referred to as post-industrial society is a shift in emphasis from manufacturing to service industries (Bell, 1973). Such a trend has manifested steadily since the post-war economic optimism of the 1960s, and more noticeably during the 1980s as much of heavy manufacturing industry experienced intermittent recession and decline. However, although the knowledge economy in which we increasingly find ourselves may be predominantly post-industrial, the relation between the two is not one of identity. As Bell recognizes, 'knowledge economy' is not simply an alternative term for a predominance of service industries over manufacturing. It relates rather to the technological infrastructure of knowledge and an increasing shift in the treatment of knowledge itself. This is what we go on to examine by outlining four significant features of this shift.

First then, a knowledge economy is one that moves from an economy of scarcity to an economy of abundance (Stiglitz, 1999). This is to say that knowledge is not like other resources. A useful way of reflecting upon this is to recognize that knowledge, as a resource, is not ecology-dependent in the sense of 'raw material'. It doesn't become depleted like rain forests or fossil fuels; rather, it grows and cross-fertilizes. A resource that continues to expand rather than diminish is perhaps a curious phenomenon when conceived of in economic terms. Normally, a resource that is abundant would, at least in the pure case, decrease in financial value. But with knowledge it is different, due principally to its increasing commodification in a fiercely competitive global economy (Stehr, 1994). Over the past few decades, this difference has impacted on the culture of the academy in particular ways, a point to which I return below.

Second, and significantly, knowledge by its very nature does not fit into the traditional distinction between use value and economic value. What is meant by this is that knowledge begins to be treated not simply as something that is acquired to be *used* or *applied* in the making of a product or provision of a service, but also begins to be treated *as* a product, a commodity in its own right. It thus accrues an economic value that is not exchanged in the traditional sense of goods and services. This is to say that the same knowledge can be sold again and again; thus it begins to circulate as a product in the economy. This applies especially to the generation (and appropriation) of knowledge that creates competitive advantage in new markets, or, just as importantly, identifies more efficient ways of doing things that either generate profit or save time (and therefore capital). In this respect, the economic value lies not in the knowledge itself but in the bearers of the knowledge in the markets of employment. It is 'human capital' that is exchanged, a point of obvious significance for the 'business' of education. This is because knowledge becomes something that must be invested in, either by new entrants into the arena of human capital (students and job-seekers), or by the constant training and re-training of workforces as new configurations of knowledge come on stream (Deleuze, 1995; Rose, 1999). Moreover, if consumers are to be incited, or indeed obligated towards such investment of their selves as 'human capital', then knowledge itself (the product) must be rendered 'commercially' viable in relation to marketing, branding, packaging, purchasing and consummability. In this respect, knowledge in the educational sector begins to be 'treated' as something that can be 'sent out', 'handed over', 'transmitted' or 'downloaded' (Lyotard, 1984). The emphasis upon perpetual training and re-training stems from a fear of falling behind, of becoming cognitively (and thus economically) disadvantaged (Department of Trade and Industry, 1998; Stiglitz, 1999).

Third, and importantly for our purposes, in the academy there is a concomitant shift in the function of human capital, which is to say a shift in the relation between knowledge and the knower. In a knowledge economy, there has been a tendency for educational systems to become culturally grounded less in people (lecturers and students) and more in the *regulated transparency* of competencies, outcomes, and standards of proficiency. Educational institutions may say that they are student-centred, when actually they are becoming more knowledge-centred in the quest for transparency and innovation where programmes and modules are increasingly treated as products.[4] Human capital must be made to fit into predetermined regimes and processes. It is in this manner that knowledge, as a commodity, becomes, as it were, exteriorized from the knower; 'treated' separately from the knower. Knowledge becomes the benchmark or the system-serving outcome to which the learner/worker must step forward, and not without a degree of respect, or even unquestioning reverence. The benchmarking of academic levels and standards of various university degrees in the UK is a case in point (Quality Assurance Agency for Higher Education [QAAHE], 2001, 2004). This also resonates with the culture of accountability, transparency and standard(ization) as knowledge begins to be treated as a commercial product in the 'business' of education, a trend that Marshall (1996) refers to as 'busnorationality'. The exteriorization of knowledge from the knower stems from the increasingly overt tendency to use knowledge solely or at least predominantly for the cultivation of human capital. This shift in the way that knowledge is treated minimizes the nature of knowledge as an aspect of personhood and the enrichment of personhood, a point to which I return later.

Fourth, and finally, there is a shift from a weighty economy to a 'weightless economy' (Stiglitz, 1999, p. 2). What this means is that the technologies that generate, store, transmit or conduct knowledge are becoming increasingly invisible to the naked eye and therefore the public eye. They recede into the electronic enclaves of miniaturization, or indeed back into mystery as a new techno-epistemic priesthood emerges with its micro-waves and lenses, its pulses and bytes. Perhaps the point to be made here concerns the increasing tendency for education to be treated as the mere *transfer* of knowledge from a source to a recipient (Standish, 1999). There is a danger therefore that the important distinction between knowledge and information may become increasingly blurred in the sense that knowledge may be increasingly presented and packaged in forms that can be transmitted through various electronic media. Of course, it depends on how such media are used in the construction of knowledge, and here I have merely pointed to a danger with respect to the treatment of knowledge as that which cultivates *and* informs human capital. Castells puts this point well when he notes that

> To be sure, knowledge and information are critical elements in all modes of development, since the process of production is always based on some level of knowledge and in the processing of information. However, what is specific to the informational mode of development is

the action of knowledge upon knowledge itself as the main source of productivity. (Castells, 1996, p. 17)

Moreover, it is worth adding to Stiglitz's insight that there is perhaps a certain irony here in that, as certain forms of information technology recede into invisibility there is, at the same moment, an expansion of the technologies of transparency and accountability imposed upon the education sector by the *qualitariat*, a point that I develop further below.[5]

The four trends outlined above do not constitute a sudden rupture. Arguably, knowledge, especially technical or professional knowledge, has always had an implicit economic value as well as an explicit use-value, an element of competitiveness and jealously-guarded ownership in relation to markets and livelihoods. It makes sense, however, to speak of a knowledge-economy when this trend crosses a notional threshold such that the very volume and exponential increase in the sophistication of knowledge puts the economic value on a par with its continuing use-value and, indeed, often precedes it.[6] This latter fact is one of which governments have become increasingly aware as evidenced by calls to produce workforces (human capital) who will engage in more flexible, enterprising and competitive ways of thinking (Department of Trade and Industry, 1998; World Bank, 1998). It is in this respect that, in line with such economic policy, a certain type of culture in the education sector requires to be established, hence the increasing role of governments in the standards and content of higher education, along with the funding of research and development. The aim is obviously to seek to establish and further reinforce a structural isomorphism between economy and academy (Hartley, 2000) in which the academy is increasingly re-organized and positioned to *serve* the economy (Burbules and Torres, 2000). This is well-summarized in Stiglitz's (1999, p. 3) claim that a certain 'techno-scientific way of thinking' requires to be 'more pervasive in every corner of life.' The point to be developed in the next section is that the increasing penetration of a knowledge economy into the ethos of both the academy and practice incites us not simply to embrace this change in the treatment of knowledge, but also to carry out a work on our selves with respect to it.

■ The knowledge economy and *Rapport à Soi*

It is in the context of the above that we now take what may appear to be a sudden change of direction by turning to the work of the French philosopher-historian Michel Foucault. This, perhaps surprisingly, will not focus directly on Foucault's work concerning power/knowledge for which he is probably best known, but on his last two major published works (1984b,c), in which Foucault conducted a genealogy of how the ancient Greeks sought to constitute themselves as moral subjects.[7]

What is of interest here is not the central theme of sexuality that Foucault researched for this purpose, but rather the template that he used to extrapolate and discuss his findings. I briefly summarize this before returning to its relevance for our discussion on a knowledge economy.

Foucault's analytical template starts from the given position that people conduct themselves against a cultural background, part of which is constituted by a network of moral codes. Such moral codes are socially situated discourses that emerge historically and contingently in ways that, in a given culture, relate the individual to a series of abstract concepts and collectives – such as pleasure, business, marriage, the law, the market place, duty and so forth. These moral codes need not be exhaustive or even explicit but they are always there in the background as an indeterminate network of prescriptions and expectations regarding conduct. These 'codes of conduct', however, do not, in and of themselves, constitute the ethical dimension in Foucault's intended sense. Rather Foucault (1986, p. 352) uses the word 'ethics' to refer to the implications of these moral codes for 'the kind of relationship you ought to have with yourself (*rapport à soi*)'. *Rapport à soi* refers therefore to 'how the individual is supposed to constitute himself as a moral subject of his own actions' (ibid.). Foucault identifies four interrelated dimensions to *rapport à soi*. The chapter now turns to a consideration of these dimensions against what are arguably the background 'codes of conduct' implicit in the expectations and incitements of a knowledge economy as it impacts on education and practice. Note here that I am not referring explicitly to professional codes of conduct such as that of the UK Nursing and Midwifery Council (2004a) which are designed to protect the public.

☐   Mode of subjection *(mode d'assujettissement)*

The mode of subjection refers, as Foucault (1986, p. 353) says, to 'the way people are invited or incited to recognize their moral obligations' in a given context. Familiar examples would be the discourses that constitute a religion, a work ethic, or perhaps patriotism and duty in times of national crisis. Against the background of a knowledge economy, the mode of subjection operates in various ways, all coming under the twin citadels of lifelong learning (Scottish Office, 1998; Scottish Executive, 1999) and quality assurance. This is to say that a knowledge economy requires the enculturation of a learning society in the former respect and a transparency of performance in the latter. It is in this context that we have become familiar with such well-worn phrases as purchasers and providers (of knowledge); practice-development; evidence-based practice; the audit-trail; credit-points and their accumulation; accreditation of prior learning

(APL); reflective diaries; learning contracts, learning outcomes, and, of course, the ever ubiquitous continuing professional development (CPD) portfolio, presented as a kind of regulatory bank account of the performing *ego* – evidence that, as a unit of human capital, one has been carrying out a work on one's self (United Kingdom Central Council [UKCC], 1999; Nursing and Midwifery Council [NMC], 2006a,b). As noted above, this relates also to perpetual training and re-training. To stand still and wonder is somehow to move backwards. All of the above elements contribute to a kind of 'knowledge-economics' and have more or less been interiorized into the cultures of the academy and practice. Note, however, that such an infrastructure has little to do with education in a substantive sense. The elements of 'knowledge economics' are dedicated largely to the administration of transparency such that they may act as a constraint on the enrichment of the self through an engagement with knowledge in ways that are not predetermined or measurable.

☐   Ethical substance *(substance éthique)*

Substance éthique refers to that aspect of the self that is to be worked upon in relation to moral conduct; or put differently, that which is targeted by the 'modes of subjection'. It may be feelings, intention, desire or indeed physical states that instantiate an excess of habit. The question for us, therefore, is what is it about our selves that requires to be worked upon in a knowledge economy such that to fail to do so may be seen to fail professionally and hence morally? It seems all too obvious to state that it is our standard of performance and our creative output that we are incited to attend to, a certain epistemic work ethic that exercises its power in obligatory courts of judgement such as the UK Research Assessment Exercise (RAE), Enhancement-led Institutional Review (QAAHE, 2003), and the capturing of new markets with 'innovative' degree programmes. Note how, even if it is unintentional, all of this has the ring of 'could be guilty unless proved innocent'. It is as if there is always a lack that stains us, as if our worth must be consistently reaffirmed. The self becomes always an economic work-in-progress. It is in this respect that Masschelein (2001) talks of living always on the edge of exclusion; working permanently to preserve inclusion in the academy. If, as suggested above, to stand still is to move backwards, then running is often merely to survive – to stand still with the seal of approval, until the next time. We call this continuing professional development; lifelong learning; when actually it would not be unreasonable to refer to it as the commodification of the self. The relation between the self and knowledge becomes increasingly positioned into one of conjoint commodification – the unit of human capital and the economic worth of the knowledge that is possessed and disseminated, including research outputs in the form of publications.

☐   Technologies of the self *(practiques des soi)*

Foucault (1986, p. 354) describes this as answering the question, 'What are the means by which we can change ourselves in order to become ethical subjects?'. How are we to work on the ethical substance? The notion of technologies of the self is, of course, nothing new. We are familiar with such things as regimes of training, diet, meditation, prayer, fasting, exercise, abstinence, penance and so forth. In this cultural sense, such activities are seen as means-to-an-end with regard to the self, or perhaps in some cases as ends-in-themselves. With a knowledge economy, however, things appear slightly different in that the work we must perform on our selves is not *primarily* for the self as an end-in-itself, its moral progress or ethical sagacity, but rather for the solvency of an economic enterprise. What then is this work? It is precisely that. Labour! But it is a labour that takes a peculiar form in that we are incited to manage ourselves in such a way that the enterprisation of the self may increasingly form the sediment of one's interiority. This is to say that an ethos of economic enterprisation becomes an interiorized quality of the way that academic life and work is motivationally framed and perceived to the detriment of more substantive educational pursuits – a self that is incited to focus on nothing more than ongoing survival as it performs its tasks from one episode of judgement to the next, the pressure and the upshot of which is 'be operational (that is, be commensurable) or disappear' (Lyotard, 1984, p. xxiv, parenthesis in the original).

☐   *Telos*

Finally then, we have *telos* into which the modes of subjection, ethical substance and *practiques de soi* can all be subsumed. By *telos*, Foucault is referring to the kind of being we aspire to become, or are incited to become. In other teleologies, this may be a being who is virtuous; self-masterful; virile; compassionate, athletic. In terms of a knowledge economy, we are openly incited to become *Homo economicus*, to keep the dollars flowing and the cash-tills ringing. But we are also incited to become *Homo qualitarianus* where the standard is that dictated by how the knowledge 'out there' has been organized and packaged – the benchmark, the outcome, the competency – the act of technicist knowledge upon the relation between knowledge and the self. There is, of course, a certain irony in all of this insofar as the incitement to innovation of performance in teaching and research must be accompanied by an obligatory infrastructure of compliance to standardization. The point made here is that when the infrastructure dominates that which it is intended to serve, innovation may be stifled rather than enhanced. Moreover, the very notion of 'innovation' becomes a measure of its economic value, which seems to ignore the fact that innovation is by its very nature indeterminate.

If we take the original points made on the knowledge economy at the beginning of this chapter, and combine them with their summarized filtration through Foucault's four dimensions of *rapport à soi* outlined above, then it becomes possible to stop and wonder what may be happening to us. It is the apparent inevitability of the way that knowledge is treated in a knowledge economy that heralds a need to reflect on its purpose and implications in a time of perpetual change. It is to this notion of the 'treatment' of 'knowledge by knowledge' in education that I now wish to turn, for it is in the treatment of knowledge in this manner that the educator is incited to form what must also, of necessity, amount to a certain relationship with her self. It is at this point that I use nursing as a particularly apt example to draw out features that, although perhaps less obvious in non professional programmes, are nevertheless increasingly emerging.

■ Atomization and transversality

In vocationally-orientated programmes, when knowledge is commodified it tends first of all to be atomized, which is to say broken down into its performative components. Chosen elements of that atomization can then be re-packaged into new configurations of competencies, or proficiency standards and outcomes that bring into being new forms of human capital as a function of performativity. An example in the UK is the rise and rise of the healthcare assistant; another is the rather ambitious project of the generic 'healthcare worker' as a precursor and low-level hybrid of doctor/nurse/paramedic. It is in this manner that atomization serves to augment transversality of outcomes across what were traditionally the domains of different professions. By transversality of outcomes is meant those vocational learning outcomes that can apply across different professions. Atomization and transversality are, of course, the implicit processes involved in the practice of 'skill-mix'.[8] For example, we have, in the UK in healthcare system, already witnessed the atomization of care into that which is 'personal' and that which is 'nursing', into that which is described as basic and that which is technologically enhanced, or extended, and into that which is universal for a given case and that which is particular deviation from it. That is also why nursing programmes have often been incited to have exit qualifications in years one and two of what is nominally a three-year programme (UKCC, 1999). Knowledge, in this sense, becomes more malleable to economies of scale and efficiency. It is centrifuged to its performative essence, before being re-spun as part of the quest of capital to colonize this resource and bring it into circulation on its own terms. Such knowledge is not therefore politically neutral. Neither, notwithstanding widening access and social inclusiveness, is it a product of the enterprise of human development. It is worth remembering that in the Enlightenment of the eighteenth century, the cry of post-Enlightenment rationality was the emergence of reason over faith, and the knowledge this would produce for the benefit of all – part of what became the grand narrative of modernity. But now, with the increasing shift from use-value to economic value, this armoury of the *ego* has itself begun to be colonized by the very epistemic ethos it sought to undermine in terms of private self-interest, the irony being that, over two hundred years later, it is done in the name of modernization.

A further and indeed greater danger than atomization and transversality is a marginalization of those epistemic dimensions that are difficult to render transparent in the process of enterprisation. As professional knowledge becomes increasingly exteriorized from the knower, the more reflexive aspects of cognitive activity, *and the disciplines associated with them,* tend to be squeezed out as more and more focus is given, not to what might constitute education, but to *learning* as a purely commercial enterprise. Yet it is these more intangible, perhaps even playful aspects of cognitive engagement that actually *constitute* an important part of education, as opposed to mere training, even higher-order training. This has implications for educators, particularly when such vocational programmes of preparation are increasingly held up as the ideal model. For example, Bearn (2000, p. 231) identifies nursing as part of the new 'professional intelligentsia' in the universities in that they learn 'skills immediately necessary for the efficient functioning of the current system [ ]'. And nothing more! In such a system-dominated world, knowledge and people (human capital) are not so much cared for as managed. In this respect, when education becomes system-dominated, there is a real danger that teaching becomes an outcome-orientated transaction in an epistemic marketplace, an increasingly pressurized transmission, and possibly an unwitting marginalization of the ethical and aesthetic richness that educational encounters can bring.

As a response to the dangers of this marginalization, I want, in the final section of the chapter, to introduce the basic elements of a more positive account of *rapport à soi*, one that invites the self into a different form of relationship with itself; one that is not simply functional for knowledge-economics dressed up as education. As stated above, the idea that I am entertaining here can be encapsulated in the ancient Greek concept identified in Foucault (1984c, 1986) as *epimeleia heautou*. It is this that I now go on to explain.

■ Education and the *epimeleia heautou*

Education is not a neutral activity. It carries with it responsibilities and choices that entail both ethical and aesthetic dimensions that are, *ipso facto,* part of the *telos* – that which we seek to become. It is in this respect that *epimeleia heautou* can be broadly translated as 'taking care of one's self', and, in the context of this chapter, is intended to capture what it means to be an educator in these dimensions. It is important to realize, however, that *epimeleia heautou* represents not just an ideology or an attitude.

> The term *epimeleia* designates not just a preoccupation, but a whole set of occupations; it is *epimeleia* that is employed in speaking of the activities of the master of a household, the task of the ruler who looks after his subjects, the care that must be given to a sick or wounded patient [...]. With regard to oneself as well, *epimeleia* implies a labour (Foucault, 1984c, p. 50).

We noted above that a knowledge economy incites us to carry out a work on our selves (*practique de soi*) – to *labour* in the name of the solvency of an economic enterprise. When this labour is applied, not to the cultivation of the economy, but rather to the cultivation of the self, this is *epimeleia heautou*, even if, in vocational programmes such as nursing, the economic aspects of healthcare delivery cannot be completely jettisoned. However, the difference between 'cultivation of the economy' and 'cultivation of the self' remains an important one in that it relates not only to the dominant purpose of the labour but also to the element of choice involved. The *epimeleia heautou* is not imposed on one by means of a policy or statutory obligation. Rather,

> [ ] it is a choice about *existence* made by the individual. People decide for themselves whether or not to care for themselves [...]. It was a question of making one's life into an object for a sort of knowledge, for a techne, for an art [...] the main area to which one must apply aesthetic values is oneself, one's life, one's existence (Foucault, 1986, pp. 361–362, emphasis in the original).

An immediate clarification is required here. By 'aesthetic values' in the above quote, Foucault is referring to an *askesis* (an inner striving to develop oneself ethically and reflexively) rather than to forms of egotism or self-indulgence.[9] Moreover, and as Pierre Hadot (1992) recognizes, for the ancient Greeks, the cultivation of the self *qua* self was only one aspect of *epimeleia heautou*.[10] The concept also entailed an important relation between the self and the collective. In the context of our discussion, this relation centres on knowledge and the role it plays in education. To be an educator who engages in *epimeleia heautou* is to have a certain relationship with one's self (*rapport à soi*) that is also a sign of the nature of one's attachment to the collective through the treatment of knowledge as it relates to *educere*. This is to say that the notion that, for a teacher, the three elements, *rapport à soi*, knowledge and *educere*, could somehow operate separately is inconceivable. Yet as indicated in the opening section of the chapter, it is the very separation of these elements that constitutes a striking feature of how they appear to be 'treated' in a knowledge economy:

use-value to economic value (commodification of knowledge); exteriorization of knowledge from the knower (commodification of the other), and the positioning of the would-be educator as *Homo economicus* and *Homo qualitarianus* (commodification of the self). This is in stark contrast to the ethical dimension of the *epimeleia heautou* in which care of the self, care of knowledge and care of the other are inextricably related in the pursuit of an *askesis*. In vocationally orientated programmes such as nursing, it is particularly important that the care of knowledge can be a medium through which the self and the other are treated as ends-in-themselves and not simply as functional for the efficiency of a system. Nursing is a particular case in point in that the engagement with nursing knowledge reflects the concept of a 'self' in need of care, this arguably being the central element of nursing's raison d'etre. But at the same time, nursing, as part of healthcare, is also by pragmatic necessity system-orientated where the self can easily become marginalized by system requirements. Thus the treatment of the self as an end-in-itself is important in nursing programmes and should be reflected in the way in which the nursing student herself is educated if she is to carry this principle into practice. This point is also highlighted in different ways in the opening chapter by Anne Scott in the present volume. Of course, it is important that these two ends, care of the self and system efficiency, are not treated as being mutually exclusive, but to embrace the *epimeleia heautou* is to keep the relation between these ends in a state not of absolute opposition, but certainly that of an enigmatic ambivalence of a perhaps longed-for harmony, on the one hand, and a permanent provocation, on the other. This is important to emphasize because the incitements of a knowledge economy often seem to reinforce the impression that the species known as 'Man' might live by bread alone.

It is for this reason that it is important to argue for the preservation of these educational pursuits that have little obvious economic value. Professional integrity requires this sustaining ambiguity or else political and ethical arguments all too easily become instruments on the altar of transparency and efficiency. Moreover, it is important for nursing that the notion of care, although not without controversy and productive debate, does not become analysed down into the conceptual bones of the performative and the expressive. Such an analytical move, while certainly possible, is a rather flat and hollow victory. The professional act of caring is not only about what can be verified. It is also about the attachment of the carer to the human condition, to a philosophy of both the individual and the collective that, while it may prove difficult (or even impossible) to comprehensively define, may nevertheless withstand the vagaries of economic rationalism. This point can be put more forcefully when we consider that for some, in educational programmes such as nursing, espousing the virtues of perhaps high-blown critique and obscure aesthetic pondering doesn't seem to make any economic sense. If we follow this through, then what happens is that economic rationality and system-competence can declare open season on what it increasingly defines as 'pointlessness'. What's the point in having philosophical discussions and theories about 'care' or 'play' or 'beauty' as part of everyday professional life? What's the point in even entertaining the possibility of an aesthetic dimension to care or education?[11] To assert that there *is* no point is only to assert that there is no *economic* point, or that which may contribute to system-efficiency. Note, therefore, that it is in more than subtle ways that economic rationality can so easily present itself as knowledge-economics by, more subtly still, donning the mask of specious philosophical analysis. So what's the point of the *epimeleia heautou*?

What I am thinking of here is not an education *in* ethics or values (which is already possible), but rather the ethics *of* education where *educere* (as drawing out) manifests as part of an ethos that underpins the relation of the educator to the student, a relation that also imbues the *treatment* of the knowledge that is being considered; its precious value, but also its limits, its ambiguity, even its transience, and yes, sometimes its beauty. This also signals (without seeking to define) an aesthetic dimension to *epimeleia heautou* by which is intended a certain attention to judgement in relation to the best way to go about things. Thus the aesthetic dimension of *epimeleia heautou* is not primarily where one might expect it to be. It does not, for example, lie in mere expressiveness of skill, although I see no intrinsic reason why it may not be found there without pretending to some pastiche of the fine arts (with regard to nursing, see Wainright, 2000; Edwards, 2001 on this point). Neither does it lie in a cool discernment of what might count as 'quality' across a range of transparent indicators identified by the *qualitariat* (although, again, there is no intrinsic reason why it may not also be found there). But it does not come from there. It arises, as Bearn (2000) states, from a passion, an aesthetic engagement, a feeling that *there is something happening here*, a cultivation of the self that goes beyond mere competence as defined in a list of skills. *Educere* is an act of passion that, while it is currently obliged to struggle in an infrastructure that is sometimes alien to it, and while it may to good effect utilize learning and teaching technologies, has no need ultimately to rely upon them. As Gordon Bearn puts this latter point,

> Good teachers are passionate about something and that passion will keep them and their lectures, seminars and classes off-balance, because the rhythm of passion is unpredictable. If it were not it would not be a passion. With passion, a teacher can excite students using any pedagogical technology; without passion even the most sophisticated technology is just wires (Bearn, 2000, p. 254).[12]

The *epimeleia heautou* then has two interdependent dimensions, the ethical and the aesthetic. The ethical has three aspects: care of the self, care of knowledge, and care of the other. The aspects of the aesthetic dimension are a perhaps curious combination of a cultivation of judgement of what is best to do regarding the ethical dimension (care of the self, care of knowledge and care of the other) and a passion for engaging in it. This is not indoctrination, but enculturation. With the increasing domination of the academy by economic requirements, the site of ethico-aesthetic diversity lies in a cultural pluralism that the economy can never wholly capture.[13] Education as a practice (not a set of policies) will always be more of a cultural than an economic or even scientific phenomenon. While there is certainly satisfaction to be gained and congratulations to be given in the fact that a particular group of students have passed their exams, have qualified as nurses or specialist nurses, and are now competent to function in the system at whatever level, perhaps, as educators, we should also ask the question, 'did we manage to engage them in the *epimeleia heautou*, or will the system take them somewhere along the line?' One of the purposes of the educator who embraces the *epimeleia heautou* is to nurture those who will one day replace her.

■ Conclusion

The purpose of this chapter has been to introduce into the work of thought the fact that many changes occurring in education today (nurse education being a particularly clear example) can be identified as stemming from features that correspond to the incitements and obligations of a knowledge economy. There is, of course, a sense in which it may be difficult to see anything intrinsically wrong with this, and it has not been the intention of this chapter to be epistemologically luddite with regard to change that brings demonstrable improvements in the *provision* of education, particularly wider access and social inclusiveness. But such good intention does not detract from an obligation to recognize the dangers that ensue when, through the process of atomization and transversality, education, and in particular vocationally orientated education, is melted down into lists of competencies, and strings of modules each with its numerical value, or abstract and often banal statements that are held to represent a totality, and by which yet another brand of human capital may be produced and reproduced for scales of economic efficiency. Although education may be possible within such a system, such is not sufficient to be *identified* with education. Of course, this is a modest point, and while understanding the obligatory requirements of universities to be economically efficient, my argument is based on the broader underlying premise that the incitements of a knowledge economy lead to a treatment of knowledge in which, as units of human capital, people are treated as a means to an end – that of the solvency of an enterprise. Moreover, the *modes of adjustment* to such a change seek to interiorize this economic principle as a *telos* in the minds of educators, where the infrastructure of knowledge-economics dominates the educational process, constrains it, seeks to assume its identity, and, ironically, perhaps even destroys it.

It is thus that the obsessive search for transparency on behalf of the *qualitariat* may be taking us not into light but into a kind of muddy technicism that actually detracts from the quality of education that is putatively sought. As a counter to this trend, I have sought merely to introduce the foundations of the *epimeleia heautou* as an important, and I would argue necessary, dimension of the *educational* enterprise, this being as much an evocation as a proceduralization. This is obviously not to denigrate the notion of competence or proficiency in terms of knowledge and skills that professions such as nursing require to learn to practise safely (NMC, 2004b). It is rather to go beyond competence in a manner that promotes an ethical and aesthetic reflexivity in relation to the application of that knowledge and the practice of these skills in a highly system-orientated environment that is healthcare. Such a reflexivity therefore must also form part of the culture and way in which nurses and other health care professionals are educated.

We may say of the *epimeleia heautou* that, for the educator, it is that which brings to knowledge a different form of value: that which gives abundance and buoyancy to the work of thought and affect; which exteriorizes not knowledge from the knower, but rather economics from knowledge, and interiorizes a set of values grounded in a passion, not only of expression, but for the *epimeleia heautou* itself so that it may be passed on from one generation to another. In a knowledge economy, it is the challenge of the *epimeleia heautou* that the educator faces today. This has always been difficult, but we must ask if it is now more difficult than it was before.

■ Notes

1 This statement was made when Joseph Stiglitz was Chief Economist at the World Bank.

2 For example, at the time of writing, the Scottish Executive currently has over 200 papers on its WEB site that make specific reference to the knowledge economy. See http://www.scotland.gov.org.

3 *Epimeleia heautou* can be translated as 'care of one's self'. '*Epimeleia*' (επιμέλεια) from both ancient and modern Greek means assiduity, attention to, care of a person or thing. '*Heautou*', from ancient Greek in the third person neuter, means one's self. *Heautou* also carries masculine and feminine alternatives that I will not use here.

4 How often have we heard the question of how this or that degree is to find its 'niche' in the market?

5 I owe the term '*qualitariat*' to David Hartley (see Hartley, 1997).

6 The arms and space races of the cold war are cases in point, not to mention well-publicized competition in the computer software industry. To this we might also add the 'race' to own different strands of the human genome. The threshold referred to above seems to be crossed in the middle decades of

the twentieth century, and is associated with technology and the increasing globalization of competitive markets (Stehr, 1994).

7 These two books were part of a larger genealogical project on sexuality that remained unfinished at the time of Foucault's death in 1984.

8 Note how in the concept of skill-mix there is rarely any mention of people as ends-in-themselves. This is another example of exteriorization of knowledge from the knower. In nursing, skill-mix used to be an *intra*-professional practice of atomization. In healthcare, it is now an *inter*-professional practice of transversality.

9 This is arguably in contrast with Foucault's 'aesthetics' in his article 'What is Enlightenment?' where he posits 'the dandy' as living his life 'as a work of art' (see Foucault, 1984a).

10 See also Davidson (1994).

11 For a brilliant exposition of 'pointlessness' in education, see Bearn (2000).

12 With the word 'passion', Bearn is referring not to emotive excitement, and certainly not loss of control, but to an intensity of engagement that is also a caring for something.

13 See Hartley (2000) on this point.

Chapter 12

Gadamer's *The Enigma of Health*: Can health be produced?

Michael A. Peters, Keith Hammond and John S. Drummond

◼ Introduction

There are very few philosophers of health who have emerged from the mainstream Western tradition which is perhaps not surprising given the deep cultural preference of early modern thought for the separation and hierarchization of the mind/body, and rationalism and philosophy of the theoretical over practical knowledge. Indeed until very recently philosophy of health *per se* was not a topic that registered in any well-defined area like political philosophy, philosophy of education or philosophy of science for example. At first, the closest we get to it is as an offshoot of applied ethics in relation to medicine, which has received an impetus with bioethics[1] or a concern with Eastern philosophy which focuses on self-knowledge. These deep cultural biases may also explain why the contemporary philosophy of the body, which developed out of the phenomenology of Merleau-Ponty and has origins going back to Nietzsche, was slow to develop (see Peters and Burbules, 2004).

Of course the situation has changed significantly in recent decades, in which a more philosophical and critical approach to both the concept and pursuit of health has emerged. Various journals devoted to philosophical enquiry into medicine, nursing and health education are now engaging with the concept of health and its variables in more general terms that go beyond the traditional boundaries of what began as medical ethics. Added to this, there are those who have approached the topic through the field of health education and promotion. The work of David Seedhouse (1997, 2005) serves as an exemplar here (see also Chapter 2 in this present volume), and from a different direction through philosophy of science, aspects of the work of Bruno Latour (1993, 2004). Also notable through a critical social theory approach is the work of Graham Scambler (2001, 2002), and Scambler and Higgs (1998).

There are also examples of interest in the political economy of health, approached from different angles in relation to inequalities in the third world as a result of neoliberalism and globalization (see, e.g. Gough, 1979; Teeple, 1995; Navarro, 1999; Pollock and Price, 2000).

There is little doubt then that health as a concept worthy of critical and philosophical enquiry is now very much at large in a rich and growing literature. However, rather than engage directly with this literature, with which many readers will already be familiar, we wish to conclude this introduction by taking a different route. In summarized form this will begin with Hippocrates and take us to modern health care and the institutionalization of modern science. We do this not as a historical undertaking but to set a certain context that will inform the rest of the chapter.

In one sense it could be argued that before the institutionalization of modern science, a Hippocratic approach to medicine resided in a kind of practical wisdom – a philosophy of *phronesis*. Hippocrates or rather the *Hippocratic Corpus* – which comprises some 60 medical treatises written in the late-fifth-century or early-fourth-century BCE – was inspired by the Pre-Socratics and referred to the body, based around appropriate diet, treatments, and a code now famous as the Hippocratic Oath, which established a covenant by the physician or healer in favour of the sick, to keep them from harm and injustice and to share the art of healing with others without fee. The Oath, which is still the basis for present-day medicine, states, 'I will follow that system of regimen which, according to my ability and judgement, I consider for the benefit of my patients, and abstain from whatever is deleterious and mischievous'. It also states that the physician will refrain from taking advantage of the sick, while preserving their privacy.[2] Whilst still binding, it is clear that the fundamental message of the Oath does not have the force it once had for medical practice, or indeed health care in more general terms, a point which we come to further below.

It is similarly clear that conceptualizations of health and disease have changed greatly since the time of Hippocrates. In his time and after, the symptoms produced by an illness were viewed as the natural response of the body to an affliction. But in the mid-eighteenth and nineteenth centuries, the conceptualization of disease began to change. In the classical medicine of the eighteenth century, it was held that the symptoms of a disease were a manifestation of the sickness itself, implying that treatment of the symptoms was treatment of the disease (Foucault, 1974; Risse, 1986). In this way, different diseases were classified as distinct ontological entities, in terms of genera and species. While this shifted the understanding of the body away from the Renaissance 'medicine of the library' and the enigma of the Galenic Humours, it also laid the foundations for a further and more profound epistemic shift that would lead to the gradual emergence of modern biomedicine. In other words, a shift from treating the relation between symptoms and disease as one of identity to one where symptoms were a manifestation of pathophysiologies that often bore no obvious relation to the symptoms themselves. The move towards the medicalization of health and the body thus began with this profound shift that stretched over a hundred years – a period not insignificant for other gradual epistemic shifts in science, technology, and the economics and geography of industrial production, shaping this new approach to the body in what arguably saw the beginnings of a political economy of health. This epistemic shift has brought great benefits to health care, particularly in the economically rich countries of the West, benefits and advances that previously were literally inconceivable. It has also brought with it certain consequences on a political register.

Today commentators talk of the medicalization of health and the body to analyze the way in which health care services have become more inequitably distributed in relation to need and the way they are increasingly inappropriate in emphasis and organization, with the result that health care often continues to be an instrument of commercial interest and social control (Sanders, 1985, n.d.; Scambler, 2002). The term 'medicalization' is often used in relation to women's health and control over their bodies, old age and mental health.[3] It can refer to the way in which commodification distorts health needs, especially in the areas of pharmaceutical products, and increasingly also medical equipment. In these related cases it is sometimes claimed that the health care industry functions to create or 'produce' needs, to limit low-cost and convenient solutions, and to control the market in ways that are inimical to equity in health care. Of equal concern is the 'production' of the image of the beautiful body and its conflation with the appearance of health.

In many respects, these cultural and political concerns reflect an emerging philosophical literature that questions whether health can be produced at all, or, put differently, what such production actually entails and what it can be taken to mean. Foremost in the mainstream philosophical literature pushing this enquiry, and in many respects presaging the contemporary literature, is the work of Hans-Georg Gadamer (1900–2002). Gadamer's (1996) *The Enigma of Health* gives us a series of essays written as meditations on health over the period 1963–1991. What emerges in Gadamer's analysis is that health, although it can be restored, is not something that can be made or produced beyond its natural state. Health is simply a feature of our 'being' in the world. Health is a condition of our natural existence, which for the most part functions outside of conscious thought until we fall ill or are injured. We think about health, mostly when we are ill or not well for some reason or another, or in terms of maintenance (which we are coming to further below). Once the equilibrium of health is regained, it moves back to being forgotten as we get on with life. This is the central antinomy informing Gadamer's concept of health that stands at the heart of the discourse and practice of health. This chapter examines Gadamer's enigma and uses it to explore dimensions of the economy and institutionalization of health and health care, before considering the implications of this for educators of health care professionals. To do this, we now begin with Gadamer's central ideas. We then seek to associate their implications with a consideration of aspects of the work of Ivan Illich on iatrogenesis before returning once again to Gadamer and the enigma of the very concept of health itself. Our central argument at this point is one that identifies a conceptual space between the concept of health and the pragmatics of its restoration. It is in this enigmatic space that attempts are made to invest in the concept in various ways that, while attempting to 'produce' health, are not necessarily productive. In particular, and against the received convention, we contest the view that health is somehow 'more' than the absence of illness or disease. It is the attempt to produce this enigmatic 'more' that leads to the distortion of both health maintenance, and the relation between health and a good life in a political economy of health.

■ Gadamer's *The Enigma of Health*

Gadamer's thesis is that health cannot be produced and that health is fundamentally in a state of 'being' which we do not think about until it leaves us as in periods of illness, disease or injury. As soon as health returns or is restored, it moves back into a state of being forgotten until such times as it is threatened once again and comes to the front of our consciousness. What unfolds in the *Enigma of Health* is a philosophical exploration of this puzzle, which Gadamer calls the 'miracle' of health. For Gadamer, as we might expect, reflecting upon health is yet another occasion for hermeneutics and in some 13 papers, written on very different occasions between the early 1960s and the late 1980s, Gadamer pursues the notion of 'balance' found in health. And whilst this collection does not give a systematic philosophy of health, the essays are remarkably consistent with one another, as each points to confusions about the enigmatic character of health – confusions that are then exploited in the health industry but not in older traditions of the 'art of healing' that Gadamer claims from the ancient Greeks. The point of showing the hidden aspects of health is to challenge the idea of it being derivable from modern technology. Whilst we value science's capacity for objectification which is fundamental to the acquisition of knowledge, there is no similar process involved in understanding health. 'Health' simply 'does not present itself to us' in a similar manner according to Gadamer (1996: 107). Health is always positioned between our having 'too much' of what is good in life and having 'too little'. Health, he warns, 'is not something that can simply be made or produced' and handed over as any other commodity. Gadamer's approach thus implies a whole new critique of the health 'business'.

Gadamer states the reality of health becomes all too clear 'when it is a question of applying scientific knowledge to our own health' from the 'perspective of science'. When we are ill, it is as if we are separating the illness off from ourselves, as the subject or person involved. The illness is treated as if it possessed an independent existence which we seek to destroy. In so doing we see that health always stands within a broader horizon of nature. 'Every therapy stands in the service of nature' claims Gadamer, meaning even those therapies which we administer to ourselves (1996: 111). Health, he says, is ultimately 'care for our own health' as 'an original manifestation of human existence' (1996: vii). Thus, health is not produced but is created in the choices of how we steer our lives. Within this exposition there is of course a critique of other ideas about health that are promoted in the scientific culture of modernity which we take up later.

Gadamer makes the point that 'it is part of our nature as living beings that our conscious self-awareness remains largely in the background so that our enjoyment of good health is constantly concealed from us'. Even so 'its hidden character' still 'manifests itself in general feeling of well-being' (1996: 111). This well-being Gadamer locates in between artful 'construction' and letting things be 'as they are' that makes us 'open to new things, ready to embark on new enterprises and, forgetful of ourselves, we scarcely notice the demands and strains' which our 'bureaucratized life form puts on us' (ibid.). In this way health is always about granting us freedoms. It can never just be about learning the right health regime. Health is about finding our own way in life. Health is thus about the deep recognition of our own health needs that begin with our own judgements. This works in contrast to the world of modern health care, education and social policy that seeks universal standards of 'objectivity'. There is a natural form of 'measure' which things bear within themselves. If health is difficult to really measure, it is because it is 'a condition of inner accord, of harmony with oneself that cannot be overridden by other, external forms of control', writes Gadamer (1996: 108).

Gadamer's enigma thus highlights the value of ordinary experience where 'everyone's private and personal existence' develops out of an 'encounter with themselves and their fellow human beings' (1996: 104). Everyday experiences are different to those of the natural sciences in that ordinary experiences 'have a common quality: what we learn from them becomes experience only when actually integrated into the practical consciousness of acting human beings'. When so integrated, this experience grounds daily life in balanced processes that evolve in the blood and guts of 'subjective' existence. It is not through a specialist or professional sort of knowledge of the doctor, lawyer or teacher that the good life is lived. Ordinary 'experiential' knowledge is 'largely unverifiable and unstable' and yet Gadamer places this sort of knowledge at the irreducible heart of the concept of health. He claims this encounter with the ordinary experience is one that 'science cannot ignore' as he pulls the concept back from standardization, claiming the fundamental fact remains, that 'it is illness and not health' that confronts us as though it is 'opposed to us' (1996: 107). It is illness that forces itself on our subjectivity and never health in the promissory form of technology or health products, which result in a kind of 'healthism', health for its own sake.

The *Enigma of Health* reclaims the value of ordinary practical truths – truths that cannot be about controlled conditions or methodological procedures. The aim is to show that scientific knowledge cannot be taken as the only activity creating legitimate knowledge. We agree with the Gadamerian claim that the restriction of truth to purely scientific know-ledge devalues ordinary or practical wisdom (*phronesis*). It restricts all questions of truth to questions of scientific competence, conforming mani-festly to philosophical 'positivism in all its varieties, which rejects concep-tual construction and pure speculation as it claims that nothing which is capable of being experienced can remain withdrawn from the compet-ence of science' (Gadamer, 1996: 2). With this approach, scientific method overrules anything unpredictable, accidental, contrary to expectations so that the claim of the universal establishes itself without variance. Gadamer considers this approach a prejudice of the Enlightenment. He claims our 'forgetful' encounter with ourselves is the 'enigma' that is always health. The commercial innocence of this position, we argue, is pursued in clear opposition to the technical outlook, in education as well as health, later in this chapter – taking the thrust of Gadamer's case in a direction that is against an instrumental perspective on professional thought and the broader civilizing patterns of western modernity. The technocratic outlook, according to Gadamer, flattens and gives a rather one-sided view of health issues. So the general theme of his *Enigma of Health* follows that of *Truth and Method* (Gadamer, 1976) where the approach derived from the natural sciences is said to be 'altogether unsuitable' for the conceptualizing of health. Like art or history, Gadamer's notion of health embraces the world of another sort of enquiry, a world of hermeneutical enquiry – involving a reading of ourselves against the 'whole' that is in the world of nature. So Gadamer argues for a re-positioning of health in the balanced conditions of forgetful subjectivity. We later claim that this has enormous consequences for those like Illich who have a similar approach in educational and third-world issues.

Gadamer asserts throughout these talks and essays that medicine involves the restoration and not the production of health. To make this point clear, he re-examines the Greek term *techne*. He states, 'the discovery of the concept of techne and its application to medicine marked a first decisive commitment towards everything that essentially characterizes western civil-ization' (1996: 31). But Gadamer counsels caution with the term saying it 'does not signify the practical application of theoretical knowing' but rather 'a special form of practical knowing' in 'the free-thinking investiga-tion of things' that is in 'the spirit of *logos*' or 'the explanatory grounds of everything we hold as true' (ibid.). Here there is a return to the ground of

Heidegger where *techne* is rendered as 'a special modification of what art means' which is unique to health work. The point of Gadamer's spelling out this meaning is that it clearly repositions the notion of health – moving it away from something that is produced by science and more towards the art of emulating nature, or indeed in the recognition that we are part of nature (Latour, 2004). The concept of health is thus embedded in an artful practice. It is put back into the subjective conditions of living a good life, engrained in a culture that values living life well. Gadamer thus realigns health, moving the concept away from *epistemai* (pure or abstract knowledge for its own sake) because *epistemai* is 'precisely what practice is not'. Practice, as in heath practice, is more of a *phronesis*, a kind of practical knowledge which 'as steadily increasing experience, is gathered from life and the circumstances of human actions' (1996: 5). Contemporary professional health practice, while often manifesting these qualities at the level of individual care, also incline towards the terms of specialisms, seeing itself as 'science' or 'technique' that captures 'experience in a wholly new sense' as formulated by Descartes' where 'the ideal of certainty became the standard for all understanding' (ibid.). The shift occurs with the rise of modern science, moving the relationship of theory and practice away from experience and towards the division we know now in the theory and practice of science. Here experience 'ceased to be a source or starting point of knowledge and became, in the sense of "experiment", a tribunal of verification before which the validity of math-ematically projected laws could be confirmed or refuted' (1996: 5). So contemporary science becomes a mode of enquiry that moves towards a 'novel relationship to practice, namely that of constructive projection and application' (1996: 6). Thoughtful experience that informs the good life is relegated to a lower division of knowledge. Practice, as in wise 'authentic' life choices, falls from the frame and with it the subjective focus on 'being' in the world.

Gadamer's approach to human health is thus more concerned with the thoughtful deliberations of a good life practice than it is with technical interventions. Indeed, for Gadamer, the more scientific we become in our life the less we are able to make thoughtful decisions about our own life practices. For Gadamer it is the general faculty of wise judgement that determines health. Summarizing his approach, he states, 'the more strongly the sphere of application becomes rationalized, the more does proper exercise of judgement along with practical experience in the proper sense tend to atrophy' (Gadamer, 1976: 101). However, it is important to note that Gadamer is never against science as such but he does consider human health to be a problem located as much in the subjective experiential concerns of the humanities as in the often-forced technical applications of science in a political economy of health.[4] Misplacing the problem, he thinks, weakens the modern human if taken as a pursuit in itself beyond the artful pragmatics of maintenance. Gadamer tries to anchor the puzzle of health in a more appropriate, ontological mode of understanding human life as a whole in all its mysteries and richness. The *enigma* that is health then for Gadamer is concealed or hidden, and misunderstood in the dominant ethos of Western modernity.

■ Gadamer and the political economy of health

Gadamer makes the case clearly that although health professionals can often do much to restore health, they cannot produce it any more than they can produce happiness or material wealth, and that to think in such productive terms misconstrues the relationship between theory and practice and especially misunderstands the nature of *techne*. This position is in part commensurate with that taken up by Ivan Illich who highlights the problem of *iatrogenesis* to describe reactions caused by drugs, operations and invasive procedures, or indeed an insidious and often institutionalized neglect, increasingly reported, for example, in caring for the elderly (Scottish Commission for the Regulation of Care, 2006). In short, these days *iatrogenesis* is a concept used to refer to illnesses, errors or misadventures caused by the caring professions. It is estimated that 80,000 people in the US alone die from *iatrogenesis* in any one year, though this figure, whether correct or not, does not take into account a more pervasive ethos which is disabling in one form or other to 'patients' of Western-style medical health.[5]

In both *Medical Nemesis* (1974) and *The Limits to Medicine* (1978), Ivan Illich encapsulates and develops his central thesis concerning the disabling effects of institutionalization in a scientific and technological age that he first raised in *Deschooling Society* and later developed in *The Disabling Professions*.[6] In the early 1970s Illich pursued a central argument famously worked out in *Deschooling Society* that he refined and applied in *Tools for Conviviality* and other works. Illich argued that in schools and other industrial institutions process and substance become confused so that the pupil is "schooled" to confuse teaching with learning and grade advancement with education, and the patient comes to mistake the bureaucratization of medical treatment for health care. Analogously, social work is mistaken for the improvement of community life, police protection for safety, military poise for national security, the rat race for productive work. As he goes on to write, 'Not only education but social reality itself has become "schooled"' (Illich, 1970).[7] Illich's critique, then, is a critique of institutionalization, commodification and experts in a political economy. He argues that 'Universal education through schooling is not feasible' and he uses deschooling as the paradigm of deinstitutionalization, leading to deschooling society. He argues that schools are 'manipulative institutions' and that 'the institutionalization of values leads inevitably to physical pollution, social polarization, and psychological impotence'. Schools like welfare bureaucracies in general claim a monopoly of the social imagination and set up a table of what is valuable and feasible. He writes: 'This monopoly is at the root of the modernization of poverty'. And this is why we must disestablish schooling and set up 'convivial institutions' or 'learning webs'. Illich elaborates:

> A good educational system should have three purposes: it should provide all who want to learn with access to available resources at any time in their lives; empower all who want to share what they know to find those who want to learn it from them; and, finally, furnish all who want to present an issue to the public with the opportunity to make their challenge known (ibid.).

In days well before the invention of the Internet he was the first to use the terms 'opportunity web' and 'network' to designate specific ways of providing access to resources and emphasized those networks such as the telephone and the postal service that are primarily accessible to individuals who want to send messages to one another, without other pre-selecting channels or materials. Illich, who died in 2002, proposes a critique of modernity, of modern institutions that performed the opposite of their intended function and he found the roots of this process in the institutionalization of charity in the thirteenth-century Church.

Illich's arguments were taken up strongly in the field of mental health where new drugs such as chlorpromazine and the antidepressants, imipramine and iproniazid, developed during the 1950s, permitted community care approaches in the 1960s and 1970s. Deinstitutionalization policies also coincided with the growth of civil rights and a new dawning awareness of patients' rights. In the 1980s, right-wing groups who argued that welfare created a 'culture of dependency' appropriated the same deinstitutionalization arguments. These arguments reinforced traditional political arguments concerning the romantic origins of individualism, the economic vitality of capitalism, and the belief that the market was a morally better form of political economy than any form of state intervention.

The basis for his argument in *Medical Nemesis* (Illich, 1976) is the view that the medical establishment has become a major threat to health, and hospitals have become monuments of narcissistic scientism. The medicalization of life that developed with the advance of capitalism and medical technology has encouraged people to give up the autonomy and control over their own bodies. He talks of both clinical *iatrogenesis* and social, cultural and structural *iatrogenesis*, and wants to limit the institutionalization of medicine as a form of governmentality. In a more recent piece Illich (1994) proposes a manifesto for 'hygienic autonomy' where he claims certain liberties for those who would celebrate living rather than preserve 'life'. These liberties can be paraphrased as follows:

- the liberty to declare myself sick;
- the liberty to refuse any and all medical treatment at any time;
- the liberty to take any drug or treatment of my own choosing;
- the liberty to be treated by the person of my choice – that is, by anyone in the community who feels called to the practice of healing, whether that person be an acupuncturist, a homeopathic physician, a neurosurgeon, an astrologer, a witch doctor or someone else;
- the liberty to die without diagnosis.

Illich's arguments are often seen as bold, challenging, and not without virtue in the questioning of health care establishments and their often impositional regimes of knowledge and practice, particularly in the field of mental health with its Cartesian residues subsumed into pharmacological adventures. There is also virtue in the notion that disorders or illnesses will keep appearing, or new ones will be identified as such. And certainly choice is important in an increasingly informed society on health care matters, as health is now on the consumerist agenda through various forms of media and different forms of investment in the concept. That said, although Illich's arguments are important in that they invite thought as to what we are about, they may also appear as somewhat wayward if taken always to their literal extremes. Certainly many people in ill health (and their carers) who are suffering would not agree with all of his proclamations. For example, to the parent or parents of a child who develops a life-threatening form of meningitis, or an acute asthmatic attack, Illich's arguments will come across as profoundly irrelevant. To many they will appear as an invitation to adopt a certain passive stoicism reminiscent of some kind of premodern (or indeed postmodern) fundamentalist bio-theocracy. Disease kills more people every minute of every day than *iatrogenesis* (including witch-doctors and astrologists) ever did. But Illich has a point when he makes a distinction between the sciences or empirical pursuits of healing, on the one hand, and their institutionalization on the other, and particularly so with respect to the education of practitioners who then reproduce such institutionalized regimes. It is perhaps ironic that Illich's notion of 'learning webs' has indeed become more prolific through the Internet, but as an adjunct to, or often integrated into mainstream education, and not as a pure alternative to it. Add to this that, with respect to 'citizens', health as a concept and its pursuit through various means is now, in some respects, approaching what Illich wished, but not necessarily in the way he wished. Let us expand on this.

The concept of health and its pursuit as a life-choice, or for improvement of ailments or diseases, is now very much in the public domain. It has broken through the barriers of the professions and their citadels. Much health information now comes through call centres, the media (especially the Internet) and not from the health care professions, although health care researchers and practitioners are often the source of it. However, and as noted above, this has also tended to incorporate health and healing into a consumerist agenda which lends a certain irony to Illich's idea of choice or 'liberty' as noted above. By this we mean that a capitalist ethos is now very much investing in health pursuits through the media – magazines, TV, Internet, radio, alternative therapies, dietary programmes, regimes of abstinence, fitness videos and DVDs. The point we are making here is that not only is the epistemic gap between health care professionals and patients becoming narrower, but also that the idea of the production of health (in Western societies) is becoming increasingly conflated with the philosophical idea of 'the good life', where a conflation wrongly treats two concepts as if they were one and the same. We develop this point below by returning now to Gadamer.

■ Health and the good life

Our highlighting of aspects of Illich's work serves to take us back to Gadamer and the relation between the concept of health, on the one hand, and the more philosophical idea of 'the good life' on the other. The idea of 'the good life' is obviously not a scientific one. While health care and other sciences and technologies may be utilized in the pursuit of the good life, it would appear odd if they were dominant over other dimensions such as the moral, the aesthetic, the political, the ecological, the interpersonal and so forth. Thus while, for any individual, an absence of any illness or disease, or ailment or infliction must be pleasing in the pursuit of the good life, it is not always a necessary condition, just as it is not a sufficient one. This should not be construed as a passive or negative statement, for it is also often the case that if one is not treated for certain illnesses or pathologies (which are treatable), then one will most likely die, in which case the idea of the good life becomes redundant. However, it still remains the case that the pursuit of health and the pursuit of the good life are not the same, which is not to say that there is never any relation between them. Put like this, the statement seems rather modest if not downright obvious. But it also serves as an entrée to a related set of issues of which health care educators and practitioners are becoming increasingly aware. This takes us to the next section of the chapter that examines the relation between health and the good life from a different direction, which will include an examination of the concept of health itself. This will then lead to the concluding section of the chapter in which we consider the implications for educators of health care professionals.

An important and evident issue that we have not yet discussed in this chapter is that the *idea* of a relation between health and the good life has moral overtones which have always been present to a degree in health care discourse. This can be described as a tension between victim-rescuing and victim-blaming. We are familiar with the current emergence of 'lifestyle' where certain participants appear to invite various pathologies upon themselves, both to their own cost and to the cost of the nation in a political economy of health. We refer to such things as smoking, drug taking, alcohol, obesity, dietary habits and a sedentary disposition. This has now reached the stage where certain voices are calling into question whether such individuals actually deserve health care intervention if they do not change their ways. This is not simply a scientific proclamation; it is also moral in that it is held that such pathologies arise because such individuals have been pursuing not a 'good life', but a 'bad life'. It is in this respect that the concept of health (for various reasons that we attend to below) begins to infiltrate the philosophical idea of the good life. It would, however, be a mistake to think that the emergence of a victim-blaming ethos is a contemporary phenomenon. For example, in premodern times the visitation of disease was often held to be divine retribution for a life badly led. In the eighteenth and nineteenth centuries, the illnesses of the poor were often proclaimed as a consequence of their own lack of moral fibre or hygiene. This served to reinforce the idea that moral rectitude and health came to go together in the idea of the good life.

What has changed, however, is that the distinction between victim-rescuing and an increasing ethos of victim-blaming now has various health care sciences to back it up – not only to enable the distinction, but also to legitimate it in ways that were not necessarily available before. A further development is that health is now as much a consumerist 'product' and slogan as it is an actual state of affairs. This takes us to our next point, which is that the very concept of health and its pursuit (whether through treatment or prevention) is undergoing a profound change, at least in post-industrial societies with sustainable economies, disposable incomes and a large and liberal media industry. It is worth examining this further as it sets a context that will take us to the concluding section of the chapter.

There is a very real sense in which health as a concept does not have any 'outside'. By this we mean that it is increasingly composed of multiple elements that render it difficult to detail in any definitive sense, hence Gadamer's notion of the 'enigma' of health. Indeed the very concept of health usually only makes an appearance because of its emerging absence, whether insidious or sudden and dramatic, which is to say in states of illness or disease. It is interesting therefore that the World Health Organization, and various other accounts of health, state that it is somehow more than the 'mere' absence of illness or disease. It is this 'more' that fractures the concept into multiple elements that render the concept itself as virtual as it is actual. This is to say that the concept begins to be invested in through various means by different groups for different reasons. These reasons embrace the whole spectrum of liberal capitalist societies, ranging across the application of biomedical science, pharmacology, health care technologies, political economy, aesthetics, consumerism and commodification, spirituality, fitness products including media, personal growth, physical appearance, dietary regimes and supplements, regimes of caution, self-help and abstinence. All have something called 'health' or 'improved health' as their putative goal, or at least claim to contribute to its pursuit. We are not arguing here that there is anything *intrinsically* wrong with these developments – doubtless all or most have their virtues in given contexts of what is now blatantly a 'health industry'. Again, following Gadamer, our point is rather that the concept of health keeps slipping away into the enigma that it has always been. A different way of putting this would be to say that the concept of health is not for defining or delineating, or even analysing as in necessary and sufficient conditions. Rather it is a virtual and mobile concept that is used to justify various pursuits. It is for *using* in the construction of ourselves, or indeed in the would-be construction of our interiority by others. In this respect the concept of health is similar in principle to other concepts such as happiness, justice and human rights to name a few, although of course the detail of the multiplicity of elements is not the same in each case.

This is obviously not to say that the concept of health is vacuous, without diversities of meaning or purpose, or indeed reality. But the purpose of the concept, and the ways in which it is used, takes precedence over some ultimate meaning. It is this that leads us to say, if somewhat flatly, that the main purpose for which the concept of health is used with reference to people is indeed the treatment of, or elimination of, or reduction of, or prevention of disease by whatever means. As Gadamer indicates, such pursuits have always been part of the human condition. This therefore calls into question the idea that the concept of health alludes to something 'more' than the 'mere' absence of illness or disease when the absence of any illness or disease would be a good place to start and, indeed, finish. What could this 'more' possibly mean beyond the pursuit of some ideal state? We are of course aware that the concept of health is used metaphorically in a multitude of ways as in 'healthy cities', 'healthy climate', 'spiritual health', 'healthy relationships' and so forth, but these can all be reduced to the pursuit of the absence of their negative elements, including that of the 'healthy lifestyle'. It is the idea of the 'healthy lifestyle' that once again relates such pursuits to the idea of the 'good life' with its moral, political, economic, aesthetic and epistemic dimensions. But the philosophical idea of the 'good life' is itself a concept and while (as in the case of health) it is certainly possible to describe the fluctuation and changing of its elements, it is ultimately a concept that is *used* to justify and give meaning to certain pursuits and judgements. In short, then, the concept of health and the good life are in a way of being, a point emphasized time and time again by both Illich and Gadamer.

There is virtue in the fact that concepts such as health, the good life, human rights and so forth are for using in various contexts rather than for delineating in some fixed epistemic and pre-packaged moral programme. This means that such concepts are open to contestation, creative changes in their elements in the work of thought and practice. This 'work of thought and practice' is as hermeneutic as it is scientific in the bio-medical sense, which is to say that interpretive understanding and objective explanation are inextricably linked in the consideration of illness or disease that has manifested in a human life. Every decision made by health professionals with regard to patient care is a judgement that occurs in a situated context where the subjective and the objective are engaged in a perpetual dialectic when considering the question 'what is the best thing to do here?' It is interesting that, in the nursing literature, the hermeneutic dimension has largely been ascribed to the patient (*this is what it means to me*), while the scientific dimension has largely been ascribed to the clinical sciences (*here is the objective data we have gathered for evidence-based practice*). This dichotomous reasoning misses Gadamer's point that both dimensions are contextually situated in a manner that perpetually interact for better or worse. They fibrillate as elements of the concept of health and of the idea of the good life, respectively. This has implications for the educators of health care professionals and it is this with which we now conclude.

■ Conclusion

It would be easy to reduce the argument thus far to the cliché that we must take the 'patient's' view of things into account. While we would certainly agree, this has to mean more than drawing the patient into a purely scientific dimension (as in informed consent and information-giving for example, important though these are). It also has to mean drawing the hermeneutic dimension out into a more integrated perspective. For educators of health professionals this means developing a curricular approach that embraces not only the sciences of life, but also the perspective of the quality of a human life that is led in multiple dimensions, and of which the enigmatic issue of health is only a part. As noted above, while this argument may appear somewhat attenuated in cases of acute medical emergencies, or dramatic and sudden crises requiring life-saving interventions, we also have to remember that many pathologies are prodromal and rumble on through a life led. Add to this that many manifestations of pathology are evidenced in a chronicity that never quite goes away, and in which medical sciences are subsumed into the larger hermeneutic of the idea of the good life in all of its dimensions (Thorne, 1993). Thus bringing the hermeneutic dimension back into curricula and educative practice means more than taking account of the phenomenology of the patient-experience. Let us explain what we mean by this.

We noted above that the concept of health, and the pursuits it gives rise to in its name, is undergoing a profound change, particularly in Western liberal capitalist societies. We also took the view that the concept of health is virtual, a concept composed of many changing elements; that it is therefore *used* in a multitude of ways by different groups for various reasons. We also argued that there is a certain virtue in 'thinking' of the concept of health in this way. While, on the one hand, it will lead inevitably to a clamour of voices that seek to 'capture' certain elements of the concept at the expense of others, on the other hand it keeps the concept (and its pursuits) open to debate as we engage with its ever-shifting scientific and hermeneutic horizon. This puts into a wider context the rather facile distinction between victim-rescuing and victim-blaming. Rather, what we seek is an interactive ethics, aesthetics and epistemology of exploration and not a scientist morality of accusation or benign domination. Thus we would argue that health care curricula require increasingly to take all of these factors into account. We now explore this.

We say 'explore' advisedly because, as educators ourselves, we do realize that programme content and curricular design are always challenging matters at both undergraduate and postgraduate levels of academic and professional preparation. Add to this that how health care students or trainees are educated is increasingly under political, media and governmental scrutiny (particularly in the case of nursing), then we seem to have something of a 'hot potato' on our hands. Regarding programme content, we are also aware of the old adage *we can't cover everything*, but we are not arguing for 'everything'. We are arguing for 'something' that takes the education of practitioners beyond scientifically informed and skill-based competence and safety; not something that denies the importance of such competence but something that enhances and takes it beyond the boundaries of its own limits and introspection. It is important that practitioners have a grasp of the bigger picture in which they are engaged. There is an entrée into this through courses on health care ethics that may take us back to the parent discipline of philosophy, and relate to political economies of health, and to examine ways in which the concept of health justifies various pursuits. We would argue that health care ethics be subsumed into the parent discipline and to have courses or modules on the philosophy of medicine, nursing or the philosophy of health and health care. Such programme content could embrace many issues that we have covered here but we would suggest doing this in such a way that is focused and coherent and not disparate.

We need to do this in such a way that concepts and debates thereof are introduced at undergraduate level, then followed up at postgraduate level when health care practitioners have more practice-experience to relate to. We end with an old adage from Plato: 'The unexamined life is not worth living.' With respect to the idea of the good life, this applies not only to the recipients of health care interventions, advice and proclamations – it applies also to health care practitioners and, in the context of this book, those who seek to contribute to their educational and formative experiences as they meet and are forced to ponder on the hermeneutic horizons that are now with us, and those that are yet to come.[8]

■ Notes

1 A good example of this bias is revealed in the APA Newsletter on Philosophy and Medicine at http://www.apa.udel.edu/apa/publications/newsletters/medicine. html (accessed 14/05/06) where most articles focus on medical ethics. There are some promising exceptions. See Timothy Murphy's 'Gay and Lesbian Health Care as Politics/Ethics' (vol. 98, no. 2, Spring 1999). On the philosophy of medicine, see also Pellegrino (1986), Caplan (1992), Velanovich (1994). For philosophy of nursing, see Edwards (1998, 2001).

2 For the full statement, see the translation by Francis Adams at http://classics.mit.edu/Hippocrates/hippooath.html.

3 On medicalization, see Foucault (1974) and Conrad (1992); and on the medicalization of women's bodies, see Morgan (2003).

4 The recent debate about the scrutiny of children's school packed lunches in the UK being a case in point. In particular, and quite sublimely, there was the incident when a young girl the contents of whose packed lunch box was judged to be perfectly 'healthy', apart that is from a jaffa cake as a 'treat'. The girl was not allowed the jaffa cake. It was taken from her. We are speechless here and can only ascribe such an act of deprivation to both ignorance and stupidity (see the archives of BBC news at http://www.bbc.co.uk).

5 For reports and relevant statistics, see the American Iatrogenic Association at http://www.iatrogenic.org/index.html.

6 For many of Illich's book as full texts accessible on the Internet, see http://www.preservenet.com/theory/Illich.html.

7 See http://www.ecotopia.com/webpress/deschooling.htm for the full text of *Deschooling Society.*

8 We should perhaps end by noting that Gadamer lived to over 102 years of age. While, on the one hand, this may give his meditations on health a certain authenticity, it is, on the other hand, not without a certain irony, or indeed 'enigma' (see Dalmayr, 2000).

Suggestions for further reading

This book has been compiled in the knowledge that its readers are likely to come to it with varying degrees of familiarity with philosophy in general and philosophy of education in particular. Some of its chapters perhaps stand as helpful ways into enquiry of this kind, especially where they draw upon a literature and write in idioms that are more generally familiar in the academic study of nursing; others do not hold back from addressing complex philosophical problems related to nursing practice and from engaging with the demands of the texts these problems have generated on their own terms. What we propose in the following brief suggestions for further reading is relevant especially to those who are comparatively new to philosophical enquiry, particularly as this relates to education, though our proposals are intended also as indicators of the state of the art.

Those seeking further understanding of the scope and possibilities of philosophical enquiry into education are well served by three recent books that purport to offer not only a broad overview of the field but also examples of work at its cutting edge. *The Blackwell Guide to the Philosophy of Education*, edited by Nigel Blake, Paul Smeyers, Richard Smith and Paul Standish (Blackwell, 2003), presents 20 major topics, each of which is covered by a pair of leading authors in the field. Chapters begin by providing an outline survey of the way the topic in question has been addressed, before proceeding to a more searching critical elaboration of particular issues. A complementary volume, *The Blackwell Companion to the Philosophy of Education*, edited by Randall Curren (Blackwell, 2003), brings together original essays on a wide range of subjects, once again by accomplished authors. *The RoutledgeFalmer Reader in Philosophy of Education*, edited by Wilfred Carr (RoutledgeFalmer, 2005), is a shorter collection of previously published papers, selected on the basis of their quality, influence and representativeness, and preceded by a substantial and provocative introduction. We recommend the above works as showing what it is *to do* philosophy and what it is to do this in relation to education. Philosophy does a disservice to itself if it is a mere rehearsal of the ideas of the great thinkers. Nevertheless, we recognize that some readers will be interested in reference works that identify succinctly key thinkers and ideas that are in play. A useful and accessible collection of short philosophical introductions to central topics in education is offered by William Hare and John Portelli's *Key Questions For Educators* (Caddo Gap Press, 2007). A synoptic guide to leading thinkers who have influenced education in philosophical ways is provided by two volumes in the Routledge Key Guides series: *Fifty Modern Thinkers on Education: From Piaget to the Present Day*, edited by Joy Palmer and David E. Cooper (Routledge, 2001), and *Fifty Major Thinkers on*

Education: From Confucius to Dewey, with the same editors working in collaboration with Liora Bresler (Routledge, 2001). *Philosophers on Education: New Historical Perspectives*, edited by Amelie Oksenberg Rorty (Routledge, 1998), provides a history of the views of philosophers on the impact and directions of education.

A number of journals are dedicated to the philosophy of education, some the product of illustrious traditions. Of particular note are *Educational Theory*, *Educational Philosophy and Theory*, *The Journal of Philosophy of Education* and *Studies in Philosophy and Education*. The vibrancy of the field is reflected by the introduction of two new journals in recent years: *Theory and Research in Education* and *Ethics and Education*. All these journals are, of course, also available online, and other resources are available in this way. The *Encyclopaedia of Philosophy of Education* is an expanding repository of articles on key figures influencing philosophy of education and on its central topics. The newly established and innovative Blackwell Portal for philosophy of education also offers a rich range of resources: it provides opportunities to post comments on articles recently published, with quick links and cross-referencing to leading journals in the field, advanced search features, occasional discussion groups and other special features, as well as resources for teaching.

For those interested in pursuing the more specific topics that have emerged in the preceding chapters, the works highlighted for consideration by our contributors are obvious examples of relevant further reading, and we encourage their pursuit. A number of chapters draw on questions concerning practical reason. In this respect, Aristotle's account of *phronesis* in the *Nicomachean Ethics* is particularly to be recommended. For an elaboration of this notion in relation to the education of teachers, Joseph Dunne's influential book *Back to the Rough Ground: Phronesis and Techne in Modern Philosophy and in Aristotle* (University of Notre Dame Press, 1993) repays careful study. Questions concerning practical reason and competence are also to the fore in the work of Hubert Dreyfus, a helpful and accessible introduction to which is provided by his *On the Internet* (Routledge, 2001). A more Kantian approach to practical reason is pursued in the writings of Onora O'Neill, of which *Autonomy and Trust in Bioethics* (Cambridge, 2002) and *A Question of Trust*, the BBC Reith Lectures of 2002 (Cambridge, 2002), may be of particular interest. Mary Midgley's writings introduce complex philosophical ideas in ways that make them admirably accessible and clear, and *The Myths We Live By* (Routledge, 2003), which dispels the modern myth that science is the only way to understand the world, is particularly recommended. Two useful collections whose relevance the titles make apparent are *Bioethics: An Anthology* (Blackwell, 2006) and *A Companion to Bioethics* (Blackwell, 2001), both edited by Helge Kuehse and Peter Singer.

Some may wish to pursue in more detail the work of particular post-structuralist philosophers as they have been applied to a broad range of educational issues. The following texts are perhaps of a more specialist nature, but are still accessible to the interested reader. The collection edited by Michael Peters, *Education and the Postmodern Condition* (Bergin and Garvey, 1995) relates mainly to aspects of the work of Jean-François Lyotard, with a short foreword written by Lyotard himself. A searching study of the resonance of this author's work for education is also provided by the collection edited by Pradeep A. Dhillon and Paul Standish, *Lyotard: Just Education* (Routledge, 2000), while Bill Readings elaborates a strongly Lyotardian line of thought in his *The University in Ruins* (Harvard University Press, 1996). Lyotard also figures alongside other poststructuralist thinkers in Nigel Blake, Paul Smeyers, Richard Smith and Paul Standish's *Thinking Again: Education after Postmodernism* (Bergin and Garvey, 1998), while the Nietzschean ideas upon which much poststructuralist thinking draws are thematized in their *Education in an Age of Nihilism* (RoutledgeFalmer, 2000). *The Therapy of Education* (Palgrave Macmillan, 2006), by Smeyers, Smith and Standish connects similar lines of thought with questions of practice more obviously related to health care. For those attracted to Foucault there is James Marshall's *Michael Foucault: Personal Autonomy and Education* (Kluwer Academic Publishers, 1996), but we also especially recommended the many published articles by Jan Masschelein and his collaborators. Educational issues informed by the work of Jacques Derrida are addressed in a very creditable collection edited by Gert Biesta and Denise Egéa-Kuehne entitled *Derrida & Education* (Routledge, 2001). John Caputo's outstanding, artfully titled *Deconstruction in a Nutshell: A Conversation with Jacques Derrida* (Fordham University Press, 1996) is recommended as an entry into this author's work, while James Williams' *Understanding Poststructuralism* (Acumen, 2005) provides a lucid, general guide to the thought of Foucault, Derrida, Kristeva, Lyotard and Deleuze.

Finally, for anyone seeking clarification of philosophical terminology, we recommend the use of a philosophical dictionary, of which there are several good examples. We suggest *The Oxford Dictionary of Philosophy*, edited by Simon Blackburn (2005), *The Cambridge Dictionary of Philosophy*, edited by Robert Audi (1999), and *The Penguin Dictionary of Philosophy*, edited by Thomas Mautner (2005).

References

T.W. Adorno, *Negative Dialectics*, trans. E.B. Ashton (London: Routledge, 1973).

D. Allen, 'Re-reading nursing and re-writing practice: towards an empirically based reformulation of the nursing mandate', *Nursing Inquiry*, 11.4 (2004) 271–283.

P. Allmark, 'Health, happiness and health promotion', *Journal of Applied Philosophy*, 22.1 (2005) 1–15.

P. Allmark, 'Choosing health and the inner citadel', *Journal of Medical Ethics*, 32 (2006) 3–6.

P. Allmark and A. Tod, 'How should public health professionals engage with lay epidemiology?', *Journal of Medical Ethics*, 32 (2006) 460–463.

American Society of Health-System Pharmacists, ASHP presents comments at Food and Drug Administration (FDA) Public Workshop on Risk Management. ASHP Government Affairs Regulatory Summary, 10.5 (2003). Online at: http://www.ashp. org/gad/monthlyupdates/regulatory/May_2003.cfm. Accessed 31/10/05.

An Bórd Altranais, *Scope of Nursing and Midwifery Practice Framework* (Dublin: An Bórd Altranais, 2000).

H. Arendt, *The Human Condition* (Chicago: Chicago University Press, 1998).

Aristotle, *The Nicomachean Ethics*, trans. Sir David Ross (1953) Revised by J.L. Ackrill and J.O. Urmson (Oxford: Oxford University Press, 1980).

G. Armitage and H. Knapman, 'Adverse events in drug administration: a literature review', *Journal of Nursing Management*, 11 (2003) 130–140.

A.D. Baddeley, *Human Memory: Theory and Practice* (London: Psychology Press, 1997).

G. Baker and K.J. Morris, *Descartes' Dualism* (London: Routledge, 1996).

M. Barer, 'Evidence, interests and knowledge translation: reflections of an unrepentant zombie chaser', *Healthcare Quarterly*, 8.1 (2005) 46–53.

P. Barker, 'Reflections on caring as a virtue ethic within an evidence-based culture', *International Journal of Nursing Studies*, 37 (2000) 329–336.

P. Barker and P. Buchanan-Barker, 'Caring as a craft', *Nursing Standard*, 19.9 (2004) 17–18.

C.A. Barry, 'The role of evidence in alternative medicine: contrasting biomedical and anthropological approaches', *Social Science & Medicine*, 62 (2006) 2646–2657.

R. Barthes, The death of the author. In: R. Barthes, *Image Music Text*, trans. S. Heath (London: Fontana, 1977).

BBC 1. Scotland Panorama Programme (London: BBC, September, 30th, 1999).

G.C.F. Bearn, Pointlessness and the university of beauty. In: P.A. Dhillon and P. Standish (eds), *Lyotard: Just Education* (London: Routledge, 2000).

W. Bechtel and A. Abrahamsen, *Connectionism and the Mind: Parallel Processing, Dynamics, and Evolution in Networks, 2nd Edition* (Oxford: Blackwell, 2002).

C.M. Begley, A.M. Brady, G. Byrne, P. Griffiths and P. Horan, *A Study of the Role and Workload of the Public Health Nurse in the Galway Community Care Area* (Dublin: Trinity College, School of Nursing and Midwifery Studies, 2004).

D. Bell, *The Coming of Post-Industrial Society: A Venture in Social Forecasting* (New York: Basic Books, 1973).

P. Benner, *From Novice to Expert: Excellence and Power in Clinical Nursing Practice.* (Menlo Park, CA: Addison-Wesley, 1984).

P. Benner (ed.), *Interpretive Phenomenology* (London: Sage, 1994).

P. Benner, 'The roles of embodiment, emotion and lifeworld for rationality and agency in nursing practice', *Nursing Philosophy*, 1.1 (2000) 5–19.

P. Benner and J. Wrubel, *The Primacy of Caring: Stress and Coping in Health and Illness* (Menlo Park, CA: Addison-Wesley, 1989).

P. Benner, C.A. Tanner and C.A. Chesla, *Expertise in Nursing Practice: Caring, Clinical Judgment and Ethics* (New York: Springer, 1996).

P. Benner, P.L. Hooper-Kyriakidis and D. Stannard, *Clinical Wisdom and Interventions in Critical Care: A Thinking-in-action Approach* (Philadelphia: WB Saunders Company, 1999).

J.L. Bermúdez, *Philosophy of Psychology: A Contemporary Introduction* (London: Routledge, 2005).

L.A. Bero, R. Grilli, J.M. Grimshaw, E. Harvey, A.D. Oxman and M.A. Thomson, 'Closing the gap between research and practice: an overview of systematic reviews of interventions to promote the implementation of research findings. The Cochrane Effective Practice and Organization of Care Review Group', *British Medical Journal*, 317.7156 (1998) 465–468.

D.M. Berwick and T.W. Nolan, 'Physicians as leaders in improving health care', *Annals of Internal Medicine*, 128.4 (1998) 289–292.

A.C. Tina Besley, 'Foucault and the turn to narrative therapy', *British Journal of Guidance & Counselling*, 30.2 (2002a) 125–143.

T. Besley, *Counselling Youth: Foucault, Power and the Ethics of Subjectivity* (Westport, CT: Praeger, 2002b).

T. Besley, 'The body and the self in the New Zealand health & physical education curriculum', *New Zealand Journal of Educational Studies*, 38.1 (2003a) 59–72.

T. Besley, 'Heidegger and Foucault: truth-telling and technologies of the self', *Technology, Culture & Value: Themes from Heidegger, ACCESS Critical Perspectives on Communication, Cultural & Policy Studies, Special Issue*, 22.1 (2003b).

T. Besley, 'Self denial or self mastery: Foucault's genealogy of the confessional self', *Poststructuralism and the Impact of the Work of Michel Foucault in Counselling and Guidance, British Journal of Guidance & Counselling, Special Issue Symposium*, 33.3 (2005).

A.C. Tina Besley and R.G. Edwards, 'Symposium', *Poststructuralism and the Impact of the Work of Michel Foucault in Counselling and Guidance',British Journal of Guidance & Counselling, Special Issue Symposium*, 33.3 (2005).

C.E. Betts, 'Progress, epistemology and human health and welfare: what nurses need to know and why', *Nursing Philosophy*, 6 (2005) 174–188.

J. Bird, *The Heart's Narrative: Therapy and Navigating Life's Contradictions* (Auckland: Edge Press, 2000).

N. Blake, P. Smeyers, R. Smith and P. Standish, *Thinking Again: Education after Postmodernism* (Westport, CN: Bergin and Garvey, 1998).

N. Blake, P. Smeyers, R. Smith and P. Standish, *Education in an Age of Nihilism* (London: Routledge Falmer, 2000).

N. Blake, P. Smeyers, R. Smith and P. Standish (eds), *The Blackwell Guide to Philosophy of Education* (Oxford: Blackwell, 2003).

J. Blustein, *Care and Commitment* (Oxford: Oxford University Press, 1991).

G. Blunden, H. Langton and G. Hek, 'Professional education for the cancer care nurse in England and Wales: a review of the evidence base', *European Journal of Cancer Care*, 10.3 (2001) 179–182.

S.N. Bolsin, 'Education and debate: the Bristol cardiac disaster', *British Medical Journal*, 317: (1998) 1579–1580.

M. Bowman, *The Professional Nurse. Coping with Change, now and the Future* (London: Chapman & Hall, 1995).

A.L. Brown, D. Ash, M. Rutherford, K. Nakagawa, A. Gordon and J.C. Campione, Distributed expertise in the classroom. In: G. Salomon (ed.) *Distributed Cognitions:*

Psychological and Educational Considerations (Cambridge, UK: Cambridge University Press, 1993).

A. Bryans, The nature and application of professional knowledge in community nursing assessment. Unpublished PhD Thesis (Glasgow: Glasgow Caledonnian University, 1998).

R. Bubner, *Modern German Philosophy* (Cambridge: Cambridge University Press, 1981).

S. Buetow, 'Beyond evidence-based medicine: bridge-building a medicine of meaning', *Journal of Evaluation in Clinical Practice*, 8.2 (2002) 103–108.

S. Buetow, Opportunities to elaborate on casuistry in clinical decision making. commentary on Tonelli. Integrating evidence into clinical practice: an alternative to evidence-based approaches. *Journal of Evaluation in Clinical Practice*, 12, 248–256, *Journal of Evaluation in Clinical Practice*, 12 (2006) 427–432.

S. Buller and T. Butterworth, 'Skilled nursing practice – a qualitative study of the elements of nursing', *International Journal of Nursing Studies*, 38.4 (2001) 405–417.

N. Burbules and C. Torres (eds) *Globalization and Education: Critical Perspectives* (New York & London: Routledge, 2000).

C.C. Butler, R. Pill and N.C.H. Stott, 'Qualitative study of patients' perceptions of doctors' advice to quit smoking: implications for opportunistic health promotion', *British Medical Journal*, 316 (1998) 1878–1881.

T.N. Byrne and S.G. Waxman, *Spinal Cord Compression* (Philadelphia: F.A. Davis, 1990).

A. Campbell, Education or Indoctrination? The issue of autonomy in health education. In: S. Doxiadis (ed.), *Ethics in Health Education* (Chichester: Wiley, 1991).

J. Campbell, *Reference and Consciousness* (Boston: MIT Press, 2003).

A.L. Caplan, 'Does the philosophy of medicine exist?', *Theoretical Medicine*, 13 (1992) 67–77.

B. Carper, 'Fundamental patterns of knowing in nursing', *Advances in Nursing Science*, 1.1 (1978) 13–23.

B.A. Carper, Fundamental patterns of knowing in nursing. In: E.C. Polifroni and M. Welch (eds), *Perspectives on Philosophy of Science in Nursing: An Historical and Contemporary Anthology* (Philadelphia: Lippincott, 1999)

L. Carroll, *Through the Looking Glass* (London: The Bodley Head, 1872–1974).

M. Castells, *The Rise of the Network Society* (Oxford: Blackwell, 1996).

S. Cavell, *Must We Mean What We Say?* (Cambridge: Cambridge University Press, 1976).

S. Cavell, *The Claim of Reason* (Oxford: Oxford University Press, 1979).

S. Cavell, *Philosophical Passages: Wittgenstein, Emerson, Austin, Derrida* (Oxford: Blackwell, 1995).

S. Cavell, Performative and passionate utterance. In: *Philosophy the Day after Tomorrow* (Cambridge, MA: Harvard University Press, 2005).

B.G. Charlton, 'Restoring the balance: evidence-based medicine put in its place', *Journal of Evaluation in Clinical Practice*, 3.2 (1997) 87–98.

P.L. Chinn and M.K. Kramer, *Integrated Knowledge Development in Nursing*, 6th edn (St. Louis: Mosby, 2004).

A. Clark, *Being There: Putting Brain, Body, and World Together Again* (Cambridge, MA: The MIT Press, 1997).

A. Clark, Embodied, situated and distributed cognition. In: W. Bechtel and G. Graham (eds), *A Companion to Cognitive Science* (Oxford: Blackwell, 1998).

J.B. Clarke, 'Evidence-based practice: a retrograde step? The importance of pluralism in evidence generation for the practice of health care', *Journal of Clinical Nursing*, 8.1 (1999) 89–94.

Clinical resource and Audit Group, *A Prospective Audit of the Diagnosis, Management and Outcome of Malignant Cord Compression* (Edinburgh: Scottish Executive, 2001).

A.L. Cochrane, *Effectiveness and Efficiency: Random Reflections on Health Services* (London: Royal Society of Medicine Press, 1999).

P. Conrad, 'Medicalization and social control', *Annual Review of Sociology*, 18 (1992) 209–232.

A. Cribbs and A. Dines, What is health promotion? In: A. Dines and A. Cribb (eds) *Health Promotion: Concepts and Practice* (Oxford: Blackwell, 1993).

J. Cromwell, W.J. Bartosch, M.C. Fiore, V. Hasselblad and T. Baker, 'Cost-effectiveness of the clinical practice recommendations in the AHCPR guideline for smoking cessation'. *Journal of the American Medical Association*, 278 (1997) 1759–1766.

F. Dalmayr, 'The enigma of health: Hans-Georg Gadamer at 100', *The Review of Politics*, 62.2 (2000) 327.

A.I. Davidson, Ethics as aesthetics: Foucault, the history of ethics and ancient thought. In: J. Goldstein (ed.), *Foucault and the Writing of History* (Oxford: Blackwell, 1994).

D. Davis and A. Taylor-Vaisey, 'Translating guidelines into practice', *Canadian Journal of Nursing Research*, 157 (1997) 408–416.

D. Davis, M.A. O'Brien, N. Freemantle, F.M. Wolf, P. Mazmanian and A. Taylor-Vaisey, 'Impact of formal continuing medical education: do conferences, workshops, rounds, and other traditional continuing education activities change physician behaviour or health care outcomes', *Journal of the American Medical Association*, 282.9 (1999) 867–874.

L. de Raeve, *Nursing with Integrity*. Unpublished PhD Thesis (Swansea: University of Wales, 1998).

G. Deleuze, *Negotiations, 1972–1990*, trans. M. Joughin (New York: Columbia University Press, 1995).

D. Dennett, *Consciousness Explained* (Boston: Little, Brown & Co, 1991).

Department of Trade and Industry, UK, *Our Competitive Future: Building the Knowledge-driven Economy: Analytical Background* (London, Cm4167, 1998). Available at: http://www.dti.gov.uk/comp/competitive/an_reprt.htm (accessed 30/01/06).

Department of Health, *Making a Difference. Strengthening the Nursing, Midwifery and Health Visiting Contribution to Health and Health Care* (London: Department of Health, 1999).

Department of Health *Choosing Health: Making Health Choices Easier* (London: Department of Health, 2004).

J. Derrida, *Margins of Philosophy*, trans. A. Bass (Hemel Hempstead: Harvester Press, 1982).

J. Derrida, *Limited Inc.*, trans. S. Weber and J. Mehlman (Evanston, IL: Northwestern University Press, 1988).

J. Derrida, 'The future of the profession or the unconditional University (Thanks to the 'Humanities', What *Could Take Place* Tomorrow). In: H. Worth and L. Simmons (eds), *Deconstructing New Zealand: Re-writing Godzone at the Millennium* (Palmerston North: Dunmore Press, 2000).

J. Derrida, *Paper Machine*, trans. R Bowlby (Stanford: Stanford University Press, 2005).

R. Descartes, *Discourse on Method*, trans. F.E. Sutcliffe (London: Penguin, 2001).

J. Dewey, *Experience and Education* (New York: Touchstone, 1977).

J. Dewey, *Art as Experience* (New York: Perigree, 2005).

R.A. Deyo, 'A key medical decision maker: the patient', *British Medical Journal*, 323 (2001) 466–467.

P. Dhillon and P. Standish (eds), *Lyotard: Just Education* (London: Routledge, 2000).

A. DiCenso, 'Evidence-based nursing practice: how to get there from here', *Nursing Leadership*, 16.4 (2003) 20–26.

A. DiCenso and N. Cullum, 'Implementing evidence-based nursing: some misconceptions', *Evidence-Based Nursing*, 1.2 (1998) 38–40.

P.M. Dodek and J.M. Ottoson, 'Implementation link between clinical practice guidelines and continuing medical education', *Journal of Continuing Education in the Health Professions*, 16 (1996) 82–93.

P. Dourish, *Where The Action Is: The Foundations of Embodied Interaction* (Cambridge, MA: The MIT Press, 2004).

D. Dowding, P.A. Scott, K Niven, A. Taylor and A. Morrison, Examining the interventions of nurses in acute medical and surgical units in Scotland. In: N. Oud (ed.), *ACENDIO: Proceedings of the third European Conference of the Association of Common European Nursing Diagnoses, Interventions and Outcomes in Berlin 2001* (Bern: Verlag Hans Huber, 2001), pp. 136–137.

R.S. Downie, *Government, Action and Morality* (London: Macmillan, 1964).

R.S. Downie, *Roles and Values: An Introduction to Social Ethics* (London: Methuen, 1971).

R. Downie, C. Fyfe and A. Tannahill, *Health Promotion Models and Values* (Oxford: Oxford University Press, 1990).

W. Drewery and J. Winslade, The theoretical story of narrative therapy. In: G. Monk, J. Winslade, K. Crocket and D. Epston (eds), *Narrative Therapy in Practice: The Archaeology of Hope* (San Francisco: Jossey-Bass, 1997).

H. Dreyfus, *Being-in-the-World: A Commentary on Heidegger's Being and Time, Division I* (Cambridge: MIT Press, 1991).

H. Dreyfus, Responses. In: M. Wrathall and J. Malpass (eds), *Heidegger, Authenticity, and Modernity: Essays in Honor of Hubert L. Dreyfus, Volume I* (Cambridge, MA and London: MIT Press, 2000) pp. 305–341.

H. Dreyfus, *On the Internet* (London and New York: Routledge, 2001).

H.L. Dreyfus, Merleau-Ponty and recent cognitive science. In: T. Carman and M.B.N. Hansen (eds) *The Cambridge Companion to Merleau-Ponty* (Cambridge, UK: Cambridge University Press, 2005)

H.L. Dreyfus and S. Dreyfus, *Mind over Machine: The Power of Human Intuition and Expertise in the Era of the Computer* (Oxford: Blackwell, 1986).

H. Dreyfus and C. Spinosa, 'Highway bridges and feasts: Heidegger and Borgmann on how to affirm technology', *Man and World*, 30.2 (1997) 159–178.

J.S. Drummond, 'Nietzsche for nurses: caring for the Übermensch', *Nursing Philosophy*, 1.2 (2000) 147–157.

J.S. Drummond, '*Petit Différends*: A reflection on aspects of Lyotard's philosophy for quality of care', *Nursing Philosophy*, 2.3 (2001) 224–233.

J.S. Drummond, 'Freedom to roam: a Deleuzian overture for the concept of care in nursing', *Nursing Philosophy*, 3.3 (2002) 222–233.

J.S. Drummond, 'Nursing and the avant-garde', *International Journal of Nursing Studies*, 41 (2004) 525–533.

J. Dunne, *Back to the Rough Ground: Practical Judgement and the Lure of Technique* (Notre Dame: University of Notre Dame Press, 1997).

J. Dunne, Arguing for teaching as a practice: a reply to Alasdair MacIntyre. In: J. Dunne and P. Hogan (eds), *Education and Practice: Upholding the Integrity of Teaching and Learning* (Oxford: Blackwell, 2004).

J. Dunne, What's the Good of Education? In: W. Carr (ed.), *The Routledge Falmer Reader in Philosophy of Education* (London: Routledge Falmer, 2005).

G. Edelman, *The Remembered Present: A Biological Theory of Consciousness* (New York: Basic Books, 1989).

S.D. Edwards, 'What is philosophy of nursing?' *Journal of Advanced Nursing*, 25 (1997) 1089–1093.

S.D. Edwards (ed.), *Philosophical Issues in Nursing* (Basingstoke: Macmillan, 1998).

S.D. Edwards, *Philosophy of Nursing: An Introduction* (Basingstoke: Palgrave Macmillan, 2001).

J.A. Effken, 'Informational basis for expert intuition', *Journal of Advanced Nursing,* 34.2 (2001) 246–255.

M. Ekebergh, M. Lepp and K. Dahlberg, 'Reflective learning with drama in nursing education – a Swedish attempt to overcome the theory praxis gap', *Nurse Education Today,* 24 (2004) 622–628.

L. Ewles and I. Simnett, *Promoting Health: A Practical Guide to Health Education,* 1st edn (Chichester: Wiley, 1985).

T.A. Faunce and S.N. Bolsin, 'Three Australian whistle sagas: lessons for internal and external regulation', *Medical Journal of Australia,* 181.1 (2004a) 44.

T.A. Faunce and S.N. Bolsin, 'Supporting whistleblowers in academic medicine: training and respecting the courage of professional conscience', *Journal of Medical Ethics,* 30.1 (2004b) 40.

J. Fawcett, J. Watson, B. Neuman, P.H. Walker and J.J. Fitzpatrick, 'On nursing theories and evidence', *Journal of Nursing Scholarship,* 33.2 (2001) 115–119.

M. Fitzpatrick, *The Tyranny of Health: Doctors and the Regulation of Lifestyle* (London: Routledge, 2001).

M. Foucault, *The Order of Things* (New York: Random House, 1970).

M. Foucault, *The Birth of the Clinic: An Archeology of Medical Perception,* trans. A.M. Sheridan Smith (New York: Vintage Books, 1974).

M. Foucault, *Discipline and Punish: The Birth of the Prison* (London: Penguin, 1977).

M. Foucault, Two lectures. In: C. Gordon (ed.), *Power/Knowledge: Selected Interviews and Other Writings 1972–1977 by Michel Foucault.* (Hemel Hempstead: Harvester Wheatsheaf, 1980c).

M. Foucault, What is Enlightenment? In: P. Rabinow (ed.), *The Foucault Reader* (London: Penguin, 1984a).

M. Foucault, *The Use of Pleasure: History of Sexuality, Vol. 2* (Harmondsworth: Penguin, 1984b).

M. Foucault, *The Care of The Self: History of Sexuality, Vol. 3* (Harmondsworth: Penguin, 1984c).

M. Foucault, On the genealogy of ethics: an overview of a work in progress. In: P. Rabinow (ed.), *The Foucault Reader* (London: Penguin, 1986).

M. Foucault, Technologies of the self. In: L.H. Martin, H. Gutman and P.H. Hutton (eds), *Technologies of the Self: A Seminar with Michel Foucault* (Amherst: University of Massachusetts Press, 1988).

M. Foucault, Governmentality. In: G. Burchell, C. Gordon and P. Miller (eds), *The Foucault Effect: Studies in Governmentality* (Hemel Hempstead: Harvester Wheatsheaf, 1991).

M. Foucault, The ethics of the concern for self as a practice of freedom. In: P. Rabinow (ed.), *Michel Foucault: Ethics, Subjectivity and Truth, The Essential Works of Michel Foucault 1954–1984, Vol 1* (London: The Penguin Press, 1997).

M. Foucault, *Fearless Speech* (New York: Semiotexte, 2001).

P. French, 'What is the evidence on evidence-based nursing? an epistemological concern', *Journal of Advanced Nursing,* 37.3 (2002) 250–257.

D. Freshwater and G. Rolfe, *Deconstructing Evidence-based Practice* (London: Routledge, 2004).

H.-G. Gadamer, *Truth and Method* (New York: Continuum, 1976).

H.-G. Gadamer, *The Enigma of Health: The Art of Healing in a Scientific Age,* trans. Jason Gaiger and Nicholas Walker (Stanford: Stanford University Press, 1996).

S. Gadow, Existential advocacy: philosophical foundation of nursing. In: S.F. Spicker and S. Gadow (eds), *Nursing Images and Ideals: Opening Dialogue with the Humanities* (New York: Springer Publishing Company, 1986).

J. Gall, *The Systems Bible: The Beginner's Guide to Systems Large and Small* (Walker, MN: General Systemantics Press, 2002).

P. Gallagher, 'How the metaphor of a gap between theory and practice has influenced nursing education', *Nurse Education Today*, 24 (2004) 263–268.

T. Gallwey, *The Inner Game of Golf* (New York: Random House, 1981).

E.J. Gibson, *Principles of Perceptual Learning and Development* (New York: Appleton-Century-Crofts, 1969).

J.J. Gibson, *The Ecological Approach to Visual Perception* (Hillsdale, NJ: Lawrence Erlbaum Associates, 1986).

R.N. Giere, Scientific cognition as distributed cognition. In: P. Carruthers, S. Stitch and M. Siegal (eds), *Cognitive Bases of Science* (Cambridge, UK: Cambridge University Press, 2002).

M. J. Goldenberg, 'On evidence and evidence-based medicine: lessons from the philosophy of science', *Social Science & Medicine*, 62 (2006) 2621–2632.

P.M. Gollwitzer and J.A. Bargh (eds), *The Psychology of Action: Linking Cognition and Motivation to Behaviour* (New York: Guilford Press, 1996).

I. Gough, *The Political Economy of the Welfare State* (London: The MacMillan Press, 1979).

H. Graham, 'Women's smoking and family health', *Social Science & Medicine*, 25, 1(1987) 47–56.

J. Gray, *Mill on Liberty: A Defense*, 1st edn (London: Routledge & Kegan Paul, 1983).

T. Greenhalgh and B. Hurwitz, *Narrative Based Medicine: Dialogue and Discourse in Clinical Practice* (London: BMA Books, 1998).

T. Greenhalgh and B. Hurwitz, 'Narrative based medicine: why study narrative?' *British Medical Journal*, 318, 7175 (1999) 48–50.

M.H.F. Grypdonck, *Qualitative Evidence in Health Care*. Keynote address delivered at the 11th International Qualitative Health Research Conference (Utrecht, Netherlands, May 11, 2005).

M. Gueret, 'Neary's profound errors of judgement took place in silence', *Irish Times* (Dublin: Friday August 22nd, 2003).

J. Habermas, 'Modernity – an incomplete project', *New German Critique*, 22 (1981) 3–15.

P. Hadot, Reflections on the notion of the 'cultivation of the self'. In: T.J. Armstrong (ed.), *Michel Foucault Philosopher* (Hemel Hempstead: Harvester Wheatsheaf, 1992).

D.H. Hargreaves, *Teaching as a Research Based Profession* (London: Teacher Training Agency, 1996).

D. Hartley, *Re-schooling Society* (London: The Falmer Press, 1997).

D. Hartley, 'Shoring up the pillars of modernity: teacher education and the quest for certainty', *International Studies in Sociology of Education*, 10.2 (2000) 113–131.

M. Heidegger, *Being and Time*, trans. J. Macquarrie and E. Robinson (Oxford: Basil Blackwell, 1962)

T. Hendel and D. Kidron, 'Staff nurses' role in long-term care hospitals in Israel: nurses' perspectives', *International Journal of Nursing Practice*, 6 (2000) 324–332.

V. Henderson, *The Nature of Nursing: A Definition and its Implications for Practice, Research and Education*. (New York: Macmillan, 1966).

E. Herrigal, *Zen in the Art of Archery* (New York: Vintage Books, 1971).

A. Hewison and S. Wildman, 'The theory-practice gap in nursing: a new dimension', *Journal of Advanced Nursing*, 24 (1996) 754–761.

J. Higgs and A. Titchen (eds), *Practice Knowledge and Expertise in the Health Professions* (Oxford: Butterworth Heinemann, 2001).

P. Hirskyj, *An Application of Habermas's Work on Communication and Discourse Ethics to Advocacy*, Unpublished PhD Thesis (Swansea: University of Wales, 2004).

H. Hodgson, *Changing the Method of Photofrin Dose Calculation: An Innovative Approach*. Unpublished report, Department of Nursing and Midwifery (Stirling: University of Stirling, 2004).

J.D. Hollan, E. Hutchins and D. Kirsh, 'Distributed cognition: towards a new foundation for human-computer interaction research', *Transactions on Human-Computer Interaction*, 7.2 (2000) 174–196.

R.M. Holloway, C. Wilkinson, T.J. Peters, I. Russell, D. Cohen D, J. Hale J, C. Rogers and H. Lewis, 'Cluster-randomised trial of risk communication to enhance informed uptake of cervical screening', *British Journal of General Practice*, 53.493 (2003) 620–625.

S. Holm, *Ethical Problems in Clinical Practice* (Manchester: Manchester University Press, 1997).

J. Holt, The unexamined life is not worth living. In: S.D. Edwards (ed.) *Philosophical Issues in Nursing* (Basingstoke: Macmillan, 1998).

S. Horrocks, Heidegger and the nurse curriculum. In: S.D. Edwards (ed.) *Philosophical Issues in Nursing* (Basingstoke: Macmillan, 1998).

R.I. Hughes, 'Look out for those medication errors that are just waiting to happen', *The Pharmaceutical Journal*, 266.7149 (2001) 717.

G. Hunt, *Whistleblowing in the Health Service: Accountability, Law and Professional Practice* (London: Edward Arnold, 1995).

K. Hunt and C. Emslie, 'Commentary: the prevention paradox in lay epidemiology – Rose revisited', *International Journal of Epidemiology*, 30 (2001) 442–446.

S.L. Hurley, *Consciousness in Action* (Cambridge, MA: Harvard University Press, 1998).

D.J. Husband, 'Malignant spinal cord compression: prospective study of delays in referral and treatment', *British Medical Journal*, 317 (1998) 18–21.

E. Hutchins, *Cognition in the Wild* (Cambridge, MA: The MIT Press, 1995).

E. Hutchins and T. Klausen, Distributed cognition in an airline cockpit. In: Y. Engeström and D. Middleton (eds), *Cognition and Communication at Work* (Cambridge, UK: Cambridge University Press, 1996).

C. Hutchison, 'Delayed diagnosis of malignant spinal cord compression', Unpublished report, Department of Nursing and Midwifery (Stirling, University of Stirling, 2003).

B.M. Hutton, 'Nursing mathematics: the importance of application', *Nursing Standard*, 13.11 (1998) 35–38.

I. Illich, 'Why We Must Abolish Schooling', *New York Review of Books*, 15.1 (1970), at http://www.preservenet.com/theory/Illich.html (accessed 14/05/04).

I. Illich, *Medical Nemesis* (New York: Pantheon, 1976).

I. Illich, 'Brave new biocracy: health care from womb to tomb. Life, death and the boundaries of the person', *NPQ: New Perspectives Quarterly*, Winter, 11.1 (1994) at http://homepage.mac.com/tinapple/illich/1994_biocracy.html (accessed 14/05/04).

R. Jacques, 'Untheorized dimensions of caring work: caring as a structural practice and caring as a way of seeing', *Nursing Administration Quarterly*, 17.2 (1993) 1–10.

A. Jenkins, *Invitations to Responsibility: The Therapeutic Engagement of Men who are Violent and Abusive* (Adelaide: Dulwich Centre Publications, 1990).

A.M. Jinks and P. Hope, 'What do nurses do? An observational survey of the activities of nurses on acute surgical and rehabilitation wards', *Journal of Nursing Management*, 8 (2001) 273–279.

J.L. Johnson, 'A dialectical examination of nursing art', *Advances in Nursing Science*, 17.1 (1994) 1–14.

J.L. Johnson and P.A. Ratner, The nature of the knowledge used in nursing practice. In: S.E. Thorne and V.E. Hayes (eds), *Nursing Praxis: Knowledge and Action* (Thousand Oaks: Sage, 1997), pp. 3–22.

R.A. Johnston, 'The management of acute spinal cord compression', *Journal of Neurology, Neurosurgery and Psychiatry*, 56 (1993) 1046–1054.

J. Kellett, 'Taking the blame', *Nursing Standard*, 11.12 (1996) 21–22.

S.D. Kelly, Grasping at straws: motor intentionality and the cognitive science of skilled behaviour. In: M. Wrathall and J. Malpass (eds), *Heidegger, Coping, and Cognitive Science: Essays in Honour of Hubert L. Dreyfus, Volume 2* (Cambridge, MA: The MIT Press, 2000).

J.W. Kenney (ed.), *Philosophical and Theoretical Perspectives for Advanced Nursing Practice* (Boston: Jones & Bartlett, 1999).

L. Kerr, *The Administration of Oxycodone*, Unpublished report, Department of Nursing and Midwifery (Stirling: University of Stirling, 2004).

J.F. Kikuchi, Nursing questions that science cannot answer. In: P.G. Reed, N.C. Shearer and L.H. Nicoll (eds), *Perspectives on Nursing Theory*, 4th edn (Philadelphia: Lippincot, 2004) pp. 23–30.

J.F. Kikuchi and H. Simmons (eds), *Philosophic Inquiry in Nursing* (London: Sage, 1992).

M. Kingwell, 'The abandoned alphabet of freedom: D (Drapetomania, a Southern plantation slave's uncontrollable urge to run away from slavery)' *Queens Quarterly* 110 (2003) 515–523.

A. Kirlik, Everyday life environments. In: W. Bechtel and G. Graham (eds), *A Companion to Cognitive Science* (Oxford: Blackwell, 1998).

A. Kitson, 'Research utilization: current issues, questions, and debates', *Canadian Journal of Nursing Research*, 31.1 (1999) 13–22.

A. Kitson, 'Recognising relationships: reflections on evidence-based practice', *Nursing Inquiry*, 9.3 (2002) 179–186.

T. Kuhn, *The Structure of Scientific Revolutions* (Chicago: University of Chicago Press, 1966).

T. Kuhn, *The Essential Tension: Studies in Scientific Tradition and Change* (Chicago: University of Chicago University Press, 1977).

J. Latimer, *The Conduct of Care: Understanding Nursing Practice* (Oxford: Blackwell Science, 2000).

B. Latour, *The Pasteurization of France* (Cambridge MA: Harvard University Press, 1993).

B. Latour, *Politics of Nature: How to Bring the Sciences into Democarcy* (Cambridge MA, Harvard: Harvard University Press, 2004).

J. Launer, *Narrative Based Primary Care: A Practical Guide* (Oxford: Radcliffe Medical Press, 2002)

J. Launer, 'Narrative-based medicine: a passing fad or a giant leap for general practice?', *British Journal of General Practice*, 53, 487 (2003) 91–92.

J. Le Fanu, *The Rise and Fall of Modern Medicine* (London: Little Brown, 1999).

M. Leininger and J. Watson, *The Caring Imperative in Education* (New York: National League for Nursing, 1990).

M. Levine, 'Nursing ethics and the ethical nurse', *American Journal of Nursing* Special AJN feature (May 1977) pp. 847–849.

D.A. Loblaw and N.J. Laperriere, 'Emergency treatment of malignant extradural spinal cord compression: an evidence-based guideline', *Journal of Clinical Oncology*, 16.4 (1998) 1613–1624.

L. Lovlie, 'On the uses of example in moral education', *Journal of Philosophy of Education*, 31.3 (1997) 409–425.

R.V. Luepker, J.M. Raczynski, S. Osganian, R.J. Goldberg, J.R. Finnegan, J.R. Hedges, D.C. Goff, M.S. Eisenberg, J.G. Zapka, H.A. Feldman, D.R. Labarthe, P. G. McGovern, C.E. Cornell, M.A. Proschan, D.G. Simons-Morton and REACT Study Grp 'Effect of a community intervention on patient delay and emergency medical service use in acute coronary heart disease – The Rapid Early Action for Coronary Treatment (REACT) trial', *Jama-Journal of the American Medical Association*, 284 (2000) 60–67.

G.B. Lum, 'Where's the competence in competence-based education and training', *Journal of Philosophy of Education*, 33.3 (1999) 403–418.

G.B. Lum, 'Towards a richer conception of vocational preparation', *Journal of Philosophy of Education*, 37.1 (2003) 1–15.

G.B. Lum, 'On the non-discursive nature of competence', *Educational Philosophy and Theory*, 36.5 (2004) 485–496.

M. Luntley, 'Knowing how to manage: expertise and embedded knowledge', *Reason in Practice*, 2.3 (2002) 3–14.

M. Luntley, 'Nonconceptual content and the sound of music', *Mind & Language*, 18.4 (2003a) 402–426.

M. Luntley, 'Ethics in the face of uncertainty – judgement not rules' *Business Ethics: A European Review*, 12 (2003b) 325–333.

M. Luntley, 'Growing awareness', *Journal of Philosophy of Education*, 38.1 (2004) 1–20.

M. Luntley, 'The character of learning', *Educational Philosophy & Theory*, 37.5 (2005) 689–704.

S. Lyftingsmo, 'Let the UK be a forerunner in the user-testing of patient pack labels and leaflets – a European perspective', *The Pharmaceutical Journal*, 270.7251 (2003) 753.

J.-F. Lyotard, *The Postmodern Condition: A Report On Knowledge*, trans. G. Bennington and B. Massumi (Manchester: Manchester University Press, 1984).

J.-F. Lyotard, *The Differend: Phrases In Dispute*, trans. G. Van Den Abbeele (Minneapolis: University of Minnesota Press, 1988).

J.-F. Lyotard, *The Postmodern Explained To Children*, trans. J. Pefanis and M. Thomas (London: Turnaround, 1992).

J.-F. Lyotard and J.-L. Thébaud, *Just Gaming*, trans. W. Godzich (Minneapolis: University of Minnesota Press, 1985).

G. Macdonald and R. Bunton, Health promotion: discipline or disciplines? In: G. Macdonald and R. Bunton (eds), *Health Promotion: Disciplines and Diversity* (London: Routledge, 1992).

A. MacIntyre, *After Virtue: A Study in Moral Theory* (London: Duckworth, 1985).

A. MacIntyre and J. Dunne, Alasdair MacIntyre on Education: in Dialogue with Joseph Dunne. In: J. Dunne and P. Hogan (eds), *Education and Practice: Upholding the Integrity of Teaching and Learning* (Oxford: Blackwell, 2004).

D.G. Mackay, *The Organization of Perception and Action: A Theory for Language and Other Cognitive Skills* (New York: Springer-Verlag, 1987).

D. Mant, 'Can randomized trials inform clinical decisions about individual patients?' *Lancet*, 353 (1999) 743–746.

J.D. Marshall, *Michel Foucault: Personal Autonomy and Education* (London: Kluwer Academic Publishers, 1996).

J. Masschelein, 'The discourse of the learning society and the loss of childhood', *Journal of Philosophy of Education*, 35.1 (2001) 1–20.

J. McKay, *Referrals to Cardiac Rehabilitation*. Unpublished report, Department of Nursing and Midwifery (Stirling, UK: University of Stirling, 2003).

J. McLeod, 'The development of narrative-informed theory, research and practice in counselling and psychotherapy: European perspectives', *European Journal of Psychotherapy Counselling and Health*, 3.3 (2000) 331–333.

C. Megone, 'Potentiality and persons: an Aristotelian perspective' In: Kuczewski and R. Polansky (eds), *Bioethics* (London: MIT Press, 2000).

K. Melia, *Learning and Working: The Occupational Socialization of Nurses* (London: Tavistock Publications, 1987).

J. Mill, *On Liberty* (London: Dent, 1972).

A. Miller, 'The relationship between nursing theory and nursing practice', *Journal of Advanced Nursing*, 10 (1985) 417–424.

C.W. Mills, *The Sociological Imagination* (Harmondsworth: Penguin, 1970).

G.M. Mitchell, 'Evidence-based practice: critique and alternative view', *Nursing Science Quarterly*, 12.1 (1999) 30–35.

G. Monk, J. Winslade, K. Crocket and D. Epston (eds), *Narrative Therapy in Practice: The Archaeology of Hope* (San Francisco: Jossey-Bass, 1997).

M.A. Moon, 'Nurse counselling raises smoking cessation rates', *Family Practice News*, 32.17 (2002) 16.

K. Montgomery Hunter, 'Narrative, literature and the clinical exercise of practical reason, *Journal of Medicine and Philosophy*, 21 (1996) 303–320.

D. Moore, *Assuring Fitness for Practice: Policy Review Commissioned by the Nursing and Midwifery, Council* (London, NMC, 2005). Available at http://www.nmc-uk.org Accessed February, 2006.

D. Moran, 'The role of knowledge in competence-based measurement', *Educa*, 115 (1991) 8–9.

A. Morgan, *What is Narrative Therapy?* (Adelaide: Dulwich Centre Publications, 2000).

K.P. Morgan, Contested bodies, contested knowledges: women, health, and the politics of medicalization. In: S. Sherwin (ed.), *The Politics of Women's Health: Exploring Agency and Autonomy* (Philadelphia: Temple University Press, 2003), pp. 83–121.

P. Morrison and P. Burnard, *Caring and Communicating: The Interpersonal Relationship in Nursing* 2nd edn (London: Macmillan, 1997).

I. Murdoch, *Sovereignty of Good* (London: Routledge and Kegan Paul, 1970).

I. Murdoch, *Existentialists and Mystics*, P.J. Conradi (ed.) (London: Allen Lane, 1998).

M. Murray (ed.) *Heidegger and Modern Philosophy* (London: Yale University Press, 1978).

V. Navarro, 'The political economy of the welfare state in developing countries', *International Journal of Health Services*, 29.1 (1999) 1–50.

National Council for the Professional Development of Nursing and Midwifery, *Agenda for the Future Professional Development of Nursing and Midwifery* (Dublin: National Council for the Professional Development of Nursing and Midwifery, 2003).

F. Nietzsche, *On the Genealogy of Morals* (New York: Doubleday, 1956).

C.A. Niven and P.A. Scott, 'The need for accurate perception and informed judgement in determining the appropriate use of the nursing resource: hearing the patient's voice', *Nursing Philosophy*, 4.3 (2003) 201–210.

N. Noddings, *Caring, A Feminine Approach to Ethics & Moral Education* (Berkeley, CA: University of California Press, 1984).

D.A. Norman, *The Design of Everyday Things* (London: The MIT Press, 1998).

N. Northcott, 'The place of practice', *Senior Nurse*, 8.2 (1988) 9–10.

G. Nurse, *Counselling and the Nurse: An Introduction* 2nd edn (Aylesbury: HM+M, 1980).

Nursing and Midwifery Council, *The NMC Code of Professional Conduct: Standards for Conduct, Performance and Ethics* (London: NMC, 2002).

Nursing and Midwifery Council, *Code of Professional Conduct: Standards for Conduct, Performance and Ethics* (London: NMC, 2004a) (currently under review).

Nursing and Midwifery Council, *Standards of Proficiency for Pre-registration Nursing Education* (London: NMC, 2004b).

Nursing and Midwifery Council, *Standards for Maintenance and Renewal of Registration* (London: NMC, 2006a).

Nursing and Midwifery Council, *The PREP Handbook* (London: NMC, 2006b).

M. Oakeshott, Education: the engagement and its frustration. In: R.F. Dearden, P.H. Hirst and R.S. Peters (eds), *Education and the Development of Reason* (London: Routledge & Kegan Paul, 1972).

A. Oakley, *Essays on Women, Medicine and Health* (Edinburgh: Edinburgh University Press, 1993).

J. Oakley and D. Cocking, *Virtue Ethics and Professional Roles* (Cambridge: Cambridge University Press, 2001).

A.M. O'Connor, A. Rostom, V.J. Fiset, J. Tetroe, V. Entwistle and H.A. Llewellyn-Thomas, 'Decision aids for patients facing health treatment or screening decisions: systematic review', *British Medical Journal*, 319 (1999) 731–734.

S. Orbell, S. Hodgkins and P. Sheeran, 'Implementation intentions and the theory of planned behaviour', *Personality and Social Psychology Bulletin*, 23 (1997) 945–954.

B. Orser, 'Reducing medication errors', *Canadian Medical Association Journal*, 162.8 (2000) 1150.

E. O'Shea, 'Factors contributing to medication errors: a literature review', *Journal of Clinical Nursing*, 8 (1999) 496–504.

A.D. Oxman, M.A. Thompson, D.A. Davis and R.B. Haynes, 'No magic bullets: a systematic review of 102 trials of intervention to improve professional practice', *Canadian Medical Association Journal*, 153.10 (1995) 1423–1431.

J. Paley, 'How not to clarify concepts in nursing', *Journal of Advanced Nursing*, 24.3 (1996) 572–578.

J. Paley, 'Benner's remnants: culture, tradition and everyday understanding', *Journal of Advanced Nursing*, 38.6 (2002) 566–573.

J. Paley, 'Clinical cognition and embodiment', *International Journal of Nursing Studies*, 41.1 (2004) 1–13.

J. Paley, 'Evidence and expertise', *Nursing Inquiry*, 13.2 (2006) 82–93.

A. Parry and R. Doan, *Story Re-visions: Narrative Therapy in the Post-modern World* (New York: Guilford Press, 1994).

R.R. Parse, *Man-Living-Health: A Theory of Nursing* (New York: John Wiley, 1981).

M. Payne, *Narrative Therapy: An Introduction for Counsellors* (London: Sage, 2000).

R.D. Pea, Practices of distributed intelligence and designed for education. In: G. Saloman (ed.) *Distributed Cognitions: Psychological and Educational Considerations* (Cambridge, UK: Cambridge University Press, 1993).

E.D. Pellegrino, *Humanism and the Physician* (Knockville, Tennessee: University of Tennessee Press, 1979).

E.D. Pellegrino, 'Philosophy of Medicine: towards a definition', *Journal of Medicine and Philosophy*, 11 (1986) 9–16.

H. Peplau, 'Interpersonal constructs for nursing practice', *Nurse Education Today*, 7 (1987) 201–208.

M.A. Peters, *Poststructuralism, Politics and Education* (Westport, CT: Bergin and Garvey, 1996).

M.A. Peters, '(Posts-) Modernism and Structuralism: Affinities and Theoretical Innovations', *Sociological Research Online*, 3.4 (September 1999) at: http://www.socresonline.org.uk/4/3/peters.html Accessed March, 2006.

M.A. Peters, *Poststructuralism, Marxism, and Neoliberalism: Between Theory and Politics* (Lanham, MD: Rowman and Littlefield, 2001).

M.A. Peters and N.C. Burbules, *Poststructuralism and Educational Research* (Lanham, MD: Rowman & Littlefield, 2004).

R. Peto, S. Darby, H. Deo, P. Silcocks, E. Whitley and R. Doll, 'Smoking, smoking cessation, and lung cancer in the UK since 1950: combination of national statistics with two case-control studies', *British Medical Journal*, 321 (2000) 323–329.

M.E. Pieterse, E.R. Seydel, H. DeVries, A.N. Mudde and G.J. Kok, 'Effectiveness of a minimal contact smoking cessation program for Dutch general practitioners: A randomized controlled trial', *Preventive Medicine*, 32 (2001) 182–190.

G. Pink, *Truth From the Bedside* (London: Charter 88, 1992).

M. Polanyi, *Personal Knowledge: Towards a Post-Critical Philosophy* (New York: Harper and Row, 1964).

M. Polanyi, *The Tacit Dimension* (London: Routledge and Kegan Paul, 1967).

E.C. Polifroni and M. Welch (eds), *Perspectives on Philosophy of Science in Nursing: An Historial and Contemporary Anthology* (Philadelphia: Lippincott, 1999).

A.M. Pollock and D. Price, 'Rewriting the regulations: how the World Trade Organisation could accelerate privatisation in health care systems', *Lancet*, 356 (2000) 1995–2000.

S. Proctor and J. Reed, Teaching reflective practice: possibilities and constraints. In: J. Reed and S. Proctor (eds), *Nurse Education – A Reflective Approach* (London: Edward Arnold, 1993).

H. Putnam, *Meaning and the Moral Sciences* (London: Routledge and Kegan Paul, 1978).

Quality Assurance Agency for Higher Education. Available at: http://www.qaa.ac:uk (see benchmarking) (Gloucester, QAAHE, 2001) Accessed February, 2006.

Quality Assurance Agency for Higher Education, *Handbook for Institutional Audit* (Gloucester, UK: QAAHE, 2002).

Quality Assurance Agency for Higher Education, *Handbook for Enhancement-led Institutional Review: Scotland* (Gloucester: QAAHE, 2003).

Quality Assurance Agency for Higher Education, *Recognition Scheme for Subject Benchmark Statements* (Gloucester: QAAHE, 2004) Available at: http://www.qaa.ac.uk Accessed February, 2006.

S. Radhakrishna, 'Syringe labels in anaesthetic induction rooms', *Anaesthesia*, 54.10 (1999) 963–968.

B. Readings, *Introducing Lyotard* (London: Routledge, 1991).

B. Readings, *The University in Ruins* (Cambridge, MA: Harvard University Press, 1996).

J. Reed and I. Ground, *Philosophy for Nursing* (London: Edward Arnold, 1997).

L. Rew, 'Intuition: nursing knowledge and the spiritual dimension of persons', *Holistic Nursing Practice*, 3.3 (1989) 56–68.

D. Reynolds, 'School effectiveness: retrospect and prospect', *Scottish Educational Review*, 29.1 (1997) 97–113.

M. Richard, *Propositional Attitudes: An Essay on Thoughts and How We Ascribe Them* (Cambridge, UK: Cambridge University Press, 1990).

G.B. Risse, *Hospital Life in Enlightenment Scotland: Care and Teaching at the Royal Infirmary of Edinburgh* (Cambridge: Cambridge University Press, 1986).

G. Rolfe (ed.), *Research, Truth, Authority: Postmodern Perspectives on Nursing* (Basingstoke: Palgrave Macmillan, 2000).

D.M. Romyn, M.N. Allen, G. Boschma, S.M. Duncan, N. Edgecombe, L.A. Jensen, J.C. Ross-Kerr, P. Marck, M. Salsali, A.E. Tourangeau and F. Warnock, 'The notion of evidence in evidence-based practice by the Nursing Philosophy Working Group', *Journal of Professional Nursing*, 19.4 (2003) 184–188.

R. Rorty (ed.), *The Linguistic Turn: Recent Essays in Philosophical Method*, Ed. and introd. R. Rorty (Chicago: University of Chicago Press, 1967).

R. Rorty, *Philosophy and the Mirror of Nature* (Oxford: Blackwell, 1980).

R. Rorty, *Objectivity, Relativism, and Truth* (Cambridge: Cambridge University Press, 1991).

G. Rose, 'Sick individuals and sick populations', *International Journal of Epidemiology*, 14 (1) (1985) 32–38.

N. Rose, *Powers of Freedom: Reframing Political Thought* (Cambridge: Cambridge University Press, 1999).

C. Rowe, T. Koren and G. Koren, 'Errors by paediatric residents in calculating drug dosages', *Archives of Disease in Childhood*, 79 (1998) 56–58.

RTE Primetime Programme Monday (May 30th 2005), 9.30 p. m.

J. Rycroft-Malone, K. Seers, A. Titchen, G. Harvey, A. Kitson and B. McCormack, 'What counts as evidence in evidence-based practice?', *Journal of Advanced Nursing*, 47.1 (2004) 81–90.

G. Ryle, *The Concept of Mind* (London: Hutchinson, 1949).

M. Sabin, Competence in practice-based calculation: issues for nursing education. Learning and Teaching Support Network, Higher Education Academy, York, UK (2004). On line at: http://www.health.heacademy.ac.uk/publications/occasionalpaper/occasionalpaper03.pdf. Accessed 31/10/05.

D.L. Sackett, W.M.C. Rosenberg, J.A. Muir Gray, R.B. Haynes and W.S. Richardson, 'Evidence-based medicine: what it is and what it isn't: it's about integrating individual clinical expertise and the best external evidence', *British Medical Journal*, 312 (1996) 71–72.

D.L. Sackett, S.E. Straus, W.S. Richardson, W. Rosenberg and R.B. Haynes, *Evidence-Based Medicine: How to Practice and Teach EBM*, 2nd edn (Edinburgh: Churchill Livingstone, 2000).

G.P. Salkeld, P. Phongsavan, M. Oldenburg, P. Johannesson, P. Convery, G. Clarke, S. Walker and J. Shaw, 'The cost-effectiveness of a cardiovascular risk reduction program in general practice', *Health Policy*, 41 (1997) 105–119.

N. Salmon and S. Soames (eds), *Propositions and Attitudes* (Oxford: Oxford University Press, 1989).

G. Salomon (ed.) *Distributed Cognitions: Psychological and Educational Considerations* (Cambridge, UK: Cambridge University Press, 1993).

D. Sanders, *The Struggle for Health.* (Hampshire, UK: Macmillan Education, 1985).

D. Sanders, 'The Medicalization of Health Care and the Challenge of Health for All' (n.d.) at http://phmovement.org/about/background3.html (accessed 14/05/04).

G. Scambler (ed.), *Habermas, Critical Theory and Health* (London: Routledge, 2001).

G. Scambler, *Health and Social Change: A Critical Theory* (Buckingham: Open University Press, 2002).

G. Scambler and P. Higgs (eds), *Modernity, Medicine and Health* (London: Routledge, 1998).

H.R. Schaffer (ed.), *Studies in Infant Mother Interaction* (New York: Academic Press, 1977) 4–17.

L. Schiff, 'Study links nurse counseling with lower hysterectomy rate', *RN*, 66.2 (2003) 16.

P.A. Scott, *Virtue, Moral Imagination and the Health Care Practitioner*, Unpublished PhD Thesis (Glasgow: University of Glasgow, 1993).

P.A. Scott, 'Care, attention and imaginative identification in nursing practice', *Journal of Advanced Nursing*, 21 (1995) 1196–1200.

P.A. Scott, 'Ethics, education and nursing practice', *Nursing Ethics*, 3.1 (1996) 53–63.

P.A. Scott, 'Imagination in practice', *Journal of Medical Ethics*, 23.1 (1997) 45–50.

P.A. Scott, 'Emotion, moral perception and nursing practice', *Nursing Philosophy*, 1.2 (2000) 123–133.

P.A. Scott, A. Matthews and M. Corbally, *Nurses' and Midwives' Understanding and Experiences of Empowerment in Ireland: Research Report for the Department of Health and Children* (Dublin: Department of Health and Children, 2003)

P.A. Scott, M. Hanrahan, M.p. Treacy, P, MacNeela, A. Hyde and K. Irving, *An Investigation into How Mental Health Nurses Document their Contribution to Care.* (Dublin: Dublin City University, 2004).

P.A. Scott, M. Corbally, M.P. Treacy, P. MacNeela, A. Hyde, M. Butler and K. Irving, *Mental Health Nurses' Contribution to Patient Care: Report of a Qualitative Study Using Focus Group Method* (Dublin: Dublin City University, 2005).

Scottish Executive, Towards the knowledge economy: various at http://www. scotland.gov.org(Edinburgh: Scottish Executive, 2001) Accessed 30th January, 2006.

Scottish Executive, *Learning Together: A Strategy for Education, Training and Lifelong Learning for all Staff in the National Health Service in Scotland* (Edinburgh, Health Department, Management Executive, 1999).

Scottish Commission for the Regulation of Care (Dundee: The Care Commission, 2006), available at: http://www.carecommission.com

Scottish Office, *Opportunity Scotland: A Paper on Lifelong Learning* (Edinburgh: Scottish Office, 1998).

D. Seedhouse, *Health Promotion: Philosophy, Prejudice and Practice* (Chichester: Wiley, 1997).

D. Seedhouse, *Values-based Decision-making for the Caring Professions* (Chichester: Wiley, 2005).

P. Sheeran and S. Orbell, 'Using implementation intentions to increase attendance for cervical cancer screening', *Health Psychology*, 19 (2000) 283–289.

Scientific Committee on Tobacco and Health (SCOTH) *Secondhand Smoke: Review of Evidence Since 1998* (London: Department of Health, 2004).

P. Simons, 'Education through research at European universities', *Journal of Philosophy of Education*, 40.1 (2006) 31–50.

P. Skrabanek, 'Why is preventive medicine exempted from ethical constraints', *Journal of Medical Ethics* 16 (1990) 187–190.

C. Smith and D. Nylund, *Narrative Therapies with Children and Adolescents* (New York: Guilford Press, 1997).

R. Smith and P. Standish, P. (2001) 'It lifted my sights': Revaluing higher education in an age of new technology. In: M. Fielding (ed.), *Taking Education Really Seriously: Three Years Hard Labour* (London: Routledge Falmer) 119–129.

L.K. Smith, C. Pope and J.L. Botha, 'Patients' help-seeking experiences and delay in cancer presentation: a qualitative synthesis', *Lancet*, 366 (2005) 825–831.

J. Speedy, 'The "storied" helper', *European Journal of Psychotherapy Counselling and Health*, 3.3 (2000) 361–374.

P. Standish, 'Why we should not speak of an educational science', *Studies in Philosophy and Education*, 14.2–3 (1995) 267–281.

P. Standish, 'Heidegger and the technology of further education', *Journal of Philosophy of Education*, 31.3 (1997) 439–460.

P. Standish, 'Centre without substance: Cultural capital and the university in ruins', *Jahrbuch Fur Bildungs – Und Erziehungsphilosophie*, 2 (1999) 83–103.

P. Standish, 'Data Return: the sense of the given in educational research', *Journal of Philosophy of Education*, 35.3 (2001) 497–518.

P. Standish, 'Euphoria, Dystopia, and practice today', in symposium on H. Dreyfus, *On the Internet*, London and New York: Routledge, 2001, *Educational Philosophy and Theory*, 34.4 (2002) 407–412.

P. Standish, Equal recognition: Identity politics and the idea of a Social Science. In: M. Depaape and P. Smeyers (eds), *Philosophy and History of Education*, Leuven: KU Leuven, 2003).

P. Standish, John Wilson's confused 'Perspectives on the Philosophy of Education', *Oxford Review of Education*, 32.2 (2006) 265–279.

S. Starkings, 'Drug calculation and the mathematics required for nursing', *MSOR Connections*, 3.4 (2003) 46–49.

N. Stehr, *Knowledge Societies* (London: Sage, 1994).

J. Stevens, 'An observational study of skilled memory in a waitress', *Applied Cognitive Psychology*, 7 (1993) 205–217.

J. Stiglitz, *Public Policy for a Knowledge Economy*, paper presented at the Department of Trade and Industry and Centre for Economic Policy Research, UK (London: DTI, January 27, 1999).

L. Suchman, *Plans and Situated Actions: The Problem of Human-Machine Communication* (Cambridge, UK: Cambridge University Press, 1987).

J. Sutton, *Philosophy and Memory Traces: Descartes to Connectionism* (Cambridge, UK: Cambridge University Press, 1998).

A. Tannahill, 'What is health promotion?', *Health Education Journal* 44 (1985) 167–168.

A. Tannahill, 'Health education and health promotion: Planning for the 1990s', *Health Education Journal*, 49 (1990) 194–198.

C. Taylor, *Sources of the Self: The Making of the Modern Identity* (Cambridge, MA: Harvard University Press, 1992).

G. Teeple, *Globalization and the Decline of Social Reform* (Toronto: Garamond Press, 1995).

T.O. Tengs, N.D. Osgood and L.L. Chen, 'The cost-effectiveness of intensive national school-based anti-tobacco education: Results from the Tobacco Policy Model', *Preventive Medicine*, 33 (2001) 558–570.

S. Tennant and R. Field, 'Continuing professional development: Does it make a difference?', *Nursing in Critical Care*, 9.4 (2004) 167–172.

C. Thompson, 'Clinical experience as evidence in evidence-based practice', *Journal of Advanced Nursing*, 43.3 (2003) 230–237.

S.E. Thorne, *Negotiating Health Care: The Social Context of Chronic Illness* (London: Sage, 1993).

S. Timmermans and M. Berg, *The Gold Standard: The Challenge of Evidence-Based Medicine and Standardization in Health Care* (Philadelphia: Temple University Press, 2003).

S. Todes, *Body and World*, with introductions by Hubert L. Dreyfus and Piotr Hoffman (Cambridge, Mass, and London: MIT Press, 2001).

M.R. Tonelli, 'The limits of evidence-based medicine', *Respiratory Care*, 46.12 (2001) 1435–1440.

B. Tones, 'Education for health promotion: new directions', *Journal of the Institute for Health Education*, 21 (1983) 121–131.

M. Traynor, 'The oil crisis, risk and evidence-based practice', *Nursing Inquiry*, 9.3 (2002) 162–169.

M.P. Treacy, K. Irving, P.A. Scott, A.Hyde, P.MacNeela and M. Butler, *An Investigation into How General Nurses Document their Contribution to Care* (Dublin: University College Dublin, 2004).

M.P. Treacy, K. Irving, P.A. Scott, A. Hyde, P. MacNeela, M. Butler and M. Corbally, *General Nurses' Contribution to Patient Care: Report of a Qualitative Study Using Focus Group Method* (Dubin: University College Dublin, 2005).

C. Trevarthen (ed.), *Brain Circuits and Functions of the Mind: Essays in Honour of Roger W Sperry* (Cambridge, UK: Cambridge University Press, 1990).

V. Tschudin, *Counselling Skills for Nurse*. 4th edn (London: Baillière Tindall, 1995).

UK Clinical PDT Study Group, *Clinical Guidelines for Performing Photodynamic Therapy (PDT) on Patients with Bronchopulmonary or Oesophageal Cancer* (Barnham, W Sussex, UK: Eurocommunica Publications, 2002).

United Kingdom Central Council for Nursing, Midwifery and Health Visiting, Commission for Nursing and Midwifery Education, *Fitness for Practice* (London: UKCC, 1999).

United Kingdom Central Council for Nursing, Midwifery and Health Visiting The UKCC and PREP: The Continuing Professional Development Standard, *Register*, No. 28, Summer (London: UKCC, 1999).

United Kingdom Central Council for Nursing, Midwifery and Health Visiting, *Requirements for Pre-registration Nursing Programmes* (London: UKCC, 2001).

R.E.G. Upshur, 'If not evidence, then what? Or does medicine really need a base?', *Journal of Evaluation in Clinical Practice*, 8.2 (2002) 113–119.

V. Velanovich, 'Does the philosophy of Medicine exist? a commentary on Caplan', *Theoretical Medicine*, 15 (1994) 77–81.

P. Wainright, P. (2000) 'Towards an aesthetics of nursing', *Journal of Advanced Nursing*, 32.3 (2000) 750–756.

K. Walker, 'Why evidence-based practice now?' *Nursing Inquiry*, 10 (2003) 145–155.

J. Watson, *Postmodern Nursing and Beyond* (New York: Elsevier Science, 1999).

S. Weil, *Waiting on God* (Glasgow: Collins, 1978).

M. White, *Narrative of Therapists' Lives* (Adelaide: Dulwich Centre Publications, 1997).

M. White and D. Epston, *Narrative Means to Therapeutic Ends* (New York: W.W. Norton, 1990).

J. White, W. Carr, T. McLaughlin, R. Smith and P. Standish, 'Five critical stances against Liberalism', *Journal of Philosophy of Education*, 37.1 (2003) 169–173.

I. Willaing and S. Ladelund, 'Nurse counseling of patients with an overconsumption of alcohol', *Journal of Nursing Scholarship*, 37.1 (2005) 30.

J. Williams, *Understanding Poststructuralism* (Chesham, Bucks: Acumen, 2005).

J. Wilson, 'Perspectives on the philosophy of education', *Oxford Review of Education*, 29.2 (2003) 279–293.

R.A. Wilson, *Boundaries of the Mind: The Individual in the Fragile Sciences: Cognition* (Cambridge, UK: Cambridge University Press, 2004).

P. Winch, *The Idea of a Social Science: And its Relation to Philosophy* (London: Routledge, 1958; 1990).

S. Winch, D. Creedy and W. Chaboyer, 'Governing nursing conduct: the rise of evidence-based practice', *Nursing Inquiry*, 9.3 (2002) 156–161.

T. Winograd and F. Flores, *Understanding Computers and Cognition: A New Foundation for Design* (Norwood, NJ: Ablex, 1986).

J. Winslade and G. Monk, *Narrative Counselling in Schools: Powerful and Brief* (Thousand Oaks, CA: Corwin Press, 1999).

J. Winslade and G. Monk, 'Nurse counselling key to fewer smear tests?', *Practice Nurse*, 26.3 (2003) 13.

L. Wittgenstein, *Philosophical Investigations*, trans. G.E.M. Anscombe (Oxford: Basil Blackwell, 1958).

A. Wolf, Can competence and knowledge mix? In: J. Burke (ed.), *Competency Based Education and Training* (London: Falmer Press, 1989).

World Bank, *World Development Report 1998/1999: Knowledge for Development* (Washington DC: World Bank Publications, 1998).

C.M. Yu, C.P. Lau, J. Chan, S. McGhee, S.L. Kong, B.M.Y. Cheung and L.S.W. Li, 'A short course of cardiac rehabilitation program is highly cost effective in improving long-term quality of life in patients with recent myocardial infarction or percutaneous coronary intervention', *Archives of Physical Medicine and Rehabilitation*, 85 (2004) 1915–1922.

Index